Dementia with Lewy Bodies
and Parkinson's Disease
Dementia

Dementia with Lewy Bodies
and Parkinson's Disease Dementia

Edited by

John O'Brien BM BCh MA FRCPsych DM
Professor of Old-Age Psychiatry
Wolfson Research Centre
Institute for Ageing and Health
Newcastle General Hospital
Newcastle-upon-Tyne, UK

Ian McKeith MD FRCPsych F Med Sci
Professor of Old Age Psychiatry
Wolfson Research Centre
Institute for Ageing and Health
Newcastle General Hospital
Newcastle-upon-Tyne, UK

David Ames BA MD FRCPsych FRANZCP
Professor of Psychiatry of Old Age
University of Melbourne,
Academic Unit for Psychiatry of Old Age
St. George's Hospital, Kew
Australia

Edmond Chiu AM MBBS DPM, FRANZCP
Professorial Fellow in Psychiatry of Old Age
University of Melbourne
Academic Unit for Psychiatry of Old Age
St. George's Hospital, Kew
Australia

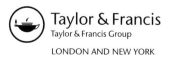

Taylor & Francis
Taylor & Francis Group

LONDON AND NEW YORK

First published in the United Kingdom in 2006
by Taylor & Francis, an imprint of the Taylor & Francis Group, 2 Park Square, Milton Park, Abingdon, Oxon OX14 4RN

Tel: +44 (0) 20 7017 6000
Fax: +44 (0) 20 7017 6699
E-mail: info.medicine@tandf.co.uk
Website: http://www.tandf.co.uk/medicine

A CIP record for this book is available from the British Library.

Library of Congress Cataloging-in-Publication Data

Data available on application

ISBN 1 84184 395 4
ISBN 9781 84184 395 7

Distributed in North and South America by
Taylor & Francis
2000 NW Corporate Blvd
Boca Raton, FL 33431, USA

Within Continental USA
Tel: 800 272 7737; Fax: 800 374 3401

Outside Continental USA
Tel: 561 994 0555; Fax: 561 361 6018
E-mail: orders@crcpress.com

Distributed in the rest of the world by
Thomson Publishing Services
Cheriton House
North Way
Andover, Hampshire SP10 5BE, UK
Tel: +44 (0) 1264 332424
E-mail: salesorder.tandf@thomsonpublishingservices.co.uk

Composition by J&L Composition, Filey, North Yorkshire, UK

Printed and bound in the UK by CPI Bath

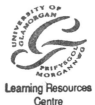

Contents

Contributors

Dag Aarsland
Professor of Geriatric Psychiatry
Centre for Clinical Neuroscience
Research
Stavanger University Hospital and
School of Medicine
University of Bergen
Norway

Louise M Allan
Institute for Ageing and Health and
MRC Development Centre for
Clinical Brain Ageing
Falls and Syncope Service
Victoria Wing
Royal Victoria Infirmary
Newcastle upon Tyne, UK

David Ames
Professor of Psychiatry of Old Age
University of Melbourne
Academic Unit for Psychiatry of
Old Age
St. George's Hospital
Kew, Australia

Liana G Apostolova
Reed Neurological Research
Center
University of California
Los Angeles
USA

Thomas H. Bak
MRC Cognition and Brain Sciences
Unit
Cambridge, UK
and
Department of Neurology
Addenbrooke's Hospital
Cambridge, UK

Carol Brayne
Professor of Public Health
Medicine /
Honorary Consultant in Public
Health Medicine
Department of Public Health and
Primary Care
University of Cambridge
Cambridge, UK

David J Burn
Consultant Neurologist & Reader in
Movement Disorder Neurology
Regional Neuroscience Centre
Newcastle General Hospital and
Institute of Ageing and Health
University of Newcastle upon Tyne
Newcastle upon Tyne, UK

Jaume Campdelacreu
Movement Disorders Unit
Neurology Service
Institut Clinic de Neurosciencies
Hospital Clinic i Universitari
Barcelona, Spain

Edmond Chiu
Professorial Fellow in Psychiatry of
Old Age
Academic Unit for Psychiatry of
Old Age
St. George's Hospital
Kew, Australia

Jiska Cohen-Mansfield
Director, Research Institute on
Aging
Hebrew Home of Greater
Washington
Rockville, USA

Sean Colloby
Research Associate
Institute for Ageing and Health
Wolfson Research Centre
Newcastle General Hospital
Newcastle upon Tyne, UK

Jeffrey L Cummings
Reed Neurological Research
Center
University of California,
Los Angeles, USA

Dennis Dickson
Professor of Pathology
(Neuropathology) and
Neuroscience
Department of Pathology &
Neuroscience
Mayo Clinic College of Medicine
Jacksonville, USA

John E Duda
Co-Director, Parkinson's Disease
Research, Education and Clinical
Center
Philadelphia VA Medical Center
Philadelphia, USA

Tom Foltynie
Neurology Registrar
Cambridge Centre for Brain Repair
University of Cambridge Forvie Site
Cambridge, UK

Paul T Francis
Reader in Neurochemistry
King's College London
Wolfson Centre for Age-Related
Diseases
London, UK

Serge Gauthier
Director
Alzheimer Disease and Related
Disorders Unit
McGill Center for Studies in Aging
Montreal, Canada

John Hardy
Chief, Laboratory of Neurogenetics,
National Institute on Aging,
National Institutes of Health,
Bethesda, USA
and
Visiting Professor
Reta Lila Weston Institute of
Neurological Studies
University College London
London, UK

Joanne M Hamilton
Assistant Project Scientist
Department of Neurosciences
University of California, San Diego
La Jolla, USA

Rose Anne Kenny
Institute for Ageing and Health and
MRC Development Centre for
Clinical Brain Ageing
Falls and Syncope Service
Victoria Wing
Royal Victoria Infirmary
Newcastle upon Tyne, UK

Graham L Lennox
Department of Neurology
Addenbrooke's Hospital
Cambridge, UK

Maria J Marti
Movement Disorders Unit
Neurology Service
Institut Clinic de Neurosciencies
Hospital Clinic i Universitari
Barcelona, Spain

Cherie McCracken
Lecturer in Statistics
University Department of
Psychiatry
Royal Liverpool University
Hospital
Liverpool, UK

Ian G McKeith
Professor of Old Age Psychiatry
Institute for Ageing and Health
Wolfson Research Centre
Newcastle General Hospital
Newcastle upon Tyne, UK

John O'Brien
Professor of Old Age Psychiatry
Wolfson Research Centre
Institute for Ageing and Health
Newcastle General Hospital
Newcastle upon Tyne, UK

Elaine K Perry
Professor of Neurochemical
Pathology
IAH Research Laboratories
Brain Ageing and Dementia
Group
Institute for Ageing and Health
Newcastle General Hospital
Newcastle upon Tyne, UK
and
King's College London
Wolfson Centre for Age-Related
Diseases
London, UK

Margaret A Piggott
IAH Research Laboratories
Brain Ageing and Dementia Group
Institute for Ageing and Health
Newcastle General Hospital
Newcastle upon Tyne, UK

Niall P Quinn
Professor of Clinical Neurology
Sobell Department of Motor
Neuroscience and Movement
Disorders
Institute of Neurology
University College London
and
Honorary Consultant Neurologist
National Hospital for Neurology
and Neurosurgery
London, UK

David P Salmon
Professor in Residence
Department of Neurosciences
University of California, San Diego
La Jolla, USA

Eduardo Tolosa
Hospital Clinic
Neurology Service
Villarroel
Barcelona, Spain

Zuzana Walker
Senior Lecturer in Psychiatry of the
Elderly
Department of Mental Health
Sciences
Royal Free & University College
Medical School
University College London; and
St. Margaret's Hospital
Epping, UK

Meg Wilkes
Private address:
The Mount
St. John's Hill
Ellesmere, Shropshire

Julia Zaccai
Department of Public Health and
Primary Care
University of Cambridge
Cambridge, UK

Acknowledgments

David Ames and Edmond Chiu would like to thank their personal assistants Marilyn Kemp and Roz Seath for their dedication to the task of compiling this book and for their cheerful efficiency in ensuring its completion.

Dr Salmon and Dr Hamilton wish to acknowledge that preparation of their chapter was supported by funds from NIA grants AG-05131 and AG-12963 to the University of California, San Diego. Professor Dickson wishes to acknowledge the support of NIH Grants P50–NS42056, P01–AG14449, P01–AG03949 and P50–AG16574 and the Mayo Foundation.

Preface

Although the history of dementia with Lewy bodies (DLB) is considerably shorter than that of Alzheimer's or Parkinson's disease, a comprehensive text about the disorder is already long overdue. The only other book published about DLB (Perry E, McKeith I, Perry R, Dementia with Lewy Bodies. Cambridge University Press: New York, 1996) chronicled the debates that led up to the formulation of International Consensus Criteria for clinical and pathological diagnosis of the disorder. This was a landmark publication, but it was very technical and therefore not easily accessible to the wide range of potential readers interested in learning about DLB. In the following decade, a great deal of new information about DLB and experience of its diagnosis and management have been accumulated. This is what we have tried to capture in this volume.

Writing about DLB, shortly after the Consensus Criteria had been published, one of us referred to it as 'an unwelcome newcomer'. There were several reasons for this. Most importantly, DLB appeared as a new 'type' of dementia at a time when clinicians and researchers had finally become comfortable with the idea that Alzheimer's disease (AD) and multi-infarct dementia (MID), as it was then called, were the two common causes of dementia and that all other types were rare. It was bad enough to rock the boat by suggesting that a third common cause of dementia existed, but even worse was the implication that this carried with it. The fact that relatively large numbers of people with DLB were apparently being (mis)diagnosed as having AD or MID, and that our classification systems were happy to accommodate that, suggested that our understanding of those two disorders was also imperfect.

Secondly, there were problems over nomenclature. A variety of terms were being used in the early 1990s to describe what were essentially the same group of patients. Diagnostic labels such as Lewy body dementia, Lewy body variant of AD (LBV), senile dementia of Lewy body type (SDLT), and diffuse Lewy body disease (DLBD) were all in use at the same time, and each had its proponents. The existence of this multiple terminology inevitably led many clinicians to reject the disorder as something too uncertain and imprecise for routine use.

Thirdly, there was the issue of the relationship between DLB and Parkinson's disease (PD). Lewy bodies are seen in the brain in both disorders, and, on the basis of neuropathological examination alone, it is impossible to say whether a person has had DLB or PD during life. Partly because of this, movement disorder specialists in particular considered that DLB was simply a variant, or an end-stage, of PD. It is certainly true that the dementia that commonly occurs late in the course of PD is often clinically similar to DLB.

An academic debate about the nosological status of LBV, SDLT, DLBD and PD with dementia might still be in progress were it not for two things. Firstly, the dementia field was beginning to move along very quickly in the early 1990s. New discoveries in molecular genetics were revolutionizing our understanding of AD, and the early cholinesterase inhibitor treatment trials were in progress. This was a climate in which new ideas were more likely to be accepted. Secondly, there was the suggestion that diagnosing DLB (whatever name it was given) might be justified on the grounds that many patients could than avoid suffering severe neuroleptic sensitivity reactions that carried increased morbidity and mortality.

Recognizing a need to act, the interested parties resolved their differences over nomenclature at a Consensus Meeting in Newcastle upon Tyne, UK in October 1995. The term DLB was picked for good reasons. It described exactly what had been observed up to that time – namely, a particular clinical syndrome of dementia with fluctuating cognition, visual hallucinations and parkinsonism that seemed to occur almost exclusively in patients with Lewy bodies (LBs) at autopsy. So, dementia with LB it was. The term was deliberately chosen to be agnostic about the role of LBs in causing the dementia, because that was (and still is) an unknown. Opinion is currently in favor of LBs being 'good guys' that scavenge and sequester toxic α-synuclein protofibrils into less toxic aggregates within the cell body. The term DLB also had the advantage of being a new one, belonging to no particular individual researcher or group. Despite being a little unwieldy and containing the word 'dementia', which is disliked by many, it has been adopted globally and in its abbreviated format seems useable by clinicians, carers and patients alike. This action to coalesce the various terms under the

DLB umbrella was probably the single most important step in progressing its acceptance as a clinical diagnosis. Now DLB is widely diagnosed across the globe and over the last decade we have witnessed a 30-fold expansion in the published literature. It has, for example, made it possible to use standard criteria to recruit DLB patients into clinical and neuroimaging trials and other investigative studies. The problem over the boundary between DLB and PD dementia was resolved by an arbitary time cutoff, which stated that DLB should be diagnosed if the dementia features occur within 12 months or less of the onset of parkinsonism.

Each of these decisions and compromises that have been made remain open for discussion and deeper understanding in the light of new research, and all are addressed in this book. The role of Alzheimer-type pathology, for example, is now better understood. Whereas the debate was originally about whether DLB was simply a variant of AD (LBV) or a separate entity, it now seems clear that both Alzheimer and LB pathologies frequently coexist in the brains of elderly people with dementia. The clinical profile that emerges depends to some extent on the relative load and distribution of each pathology – neocortical neurofibrillary tangles in particular altering the clinical profile to look more like AD with prominent amnestic symptoms and reducing the probability of fluctuation, visual hallucinations and parkinsonism. The implication of this is that some DLB cases will lack these core features and be extremely difficult to recognize clinically. This explains at least in part why clinicians have so much trouble diagnosing DLB. It is not they who are lacking in their powers of observation, nor are the clinical diagnostic criteria incorrect. It is simply that not all DLB cases present with the typical picture. To detect these patients, additional pieces of clinical evidence are required, for example a history of REM sleep behavior disorder (RBD) or of severe neuroleptic sensitivity. The other approach to improving diagnostic sensitivity for DLB is to use biological tests, the most promising of which so far are neuroimaging methods, particularly those labeling the dopamine transporter site in the basal ganglia.

Modifications to pathological and clinical criteria for DLB were discussed at the 3rd International DLB Workshop in September 2003 and are currently under review for publication. Most of the information and opinion that contributed to that process is reflected in the chapters that follow, many of which were written by members of the consensus process.

For families dealing with DLB, the recognition that the clinical picture and burden of care is different for them compared with people affected with AD is a major step forward. But it carries with it many frustrations, not least that they often are more aware of DLB than their professional carers. The Alzheimer's and Parkinson's Associations and Societies, nationally and internationally, provide rapid access via the internet to a growing range of fact-sheets and other sources of information about DLB. More recently a carer-based organization specifically for DLB has been established offering on-line communication with other families and providing more detailed and up-to-date information. The range of topics about which people who have DLB and their carers need to know is extensive. In addition to the fluctuating cognitive impairments, which predominantly affect attention and visuoperceptual abilities, there may also be psychiatric and behavioral abnormalities, motor deficits, autonomic dysfunction and sleep disorders. How to impart such a diverse range of facts without instilling pessimistic anticipation of the worst is truly a challenge. The reality is that many of these symptoms of DLB are amenable to treatment – often, but not always, pharmacological. As treatment guidelines for DLB emerge, clinicians should become more confident about not only prescribing single therapies but also combining them to target all symptoms identified by patient and carer as troublesome enough to warrant intervention.

If so much progress has been made in the last decade, what can be hoped for in the next? The ideal would be a drug that significantly interrupted the pathological processing of α-synuclein and other proteins, arresting the neurodegenerative process. A useful clinical objective would be for our clinical diagnostic methods to have improved to such a point that patients with DLB were reliably identifiable in the earliest stages of disease when application of such a treatment would be of most benefit. If one makes analogy with the current status of amnestic mild cognitive impairment (MCI) as a predictor for AD, it is clear that defining the MCI equivalent of LB disease is likely to be a difficult task. Research effort needs to be directed towards early detection of LB disease, likely using biological markers such as dopamine transporter imaging in patients showing evidence of possible early symptoms. For those with established DLB, we need better symptomatic treatments. This may involve new drug discovery, but there is huge scope for improvement in the management of individual patients using tailored regimes of currently available medications. Specialist clinics for DLB patients may be one way to deliver these, and they could be embedded within existing provisions for people with dementia or movement disorders.

The chapters that follow trace the historical development of DLB, pathological and clinical issues, pharmacological and nonpharmacological treatments, pathophysiology and a personal perspective of this disorder, which has moved over a short space of time from unawareness, through reluctant acceptance, to now being the subject of intense activity. We hope that out of these pages will come further acceleration of the process of understanding DLB and its boundaries.

John O'Brien
Ian McKeith
David Ames
Edmond Chiu
August 2005

chapter 1

Historical background

Thomas H Bak and Graham G Lennox

The development of the concept of dementia with Lewy bodies (DLB) mirrors the history of neuroscience in general over the last 200 years. The first contributions, in the 19th century, were entirely based on observation at a time when the examination of the nervous system had not yet been systematized. By the early 20th century, these clinical observations began to be supplemented by pathological data of gradually increasing sophistication. Progress accelerated when immunohistochemical techniques provided a way of identifying cortical Lewy bodies easily, and allowed clinicians to go back and improve the descriptions of the clinical correlates and their epidemiology. Most recently we have moved into an era where molecular genetic studies are starting to contribute to our understanding of the condition. This whole process has seen a move from the geographically-defined schools of thought (which provided, for example, predominantly French and German early clinical and pathological reports and a period of almost exclusively Japanese clinicopathological progress) to the present international approach.

The first detailed description of a Lewy body disorder was probably James Parkinson's Essay on the Shaking Palsy (1817). He outlined many of the motor symptoms of what we now call Parkinson's disease, then termed paralysis agitans. Perhaps as a consequence of limited opportunity to follow the progress of his six patients, he made no mention of the cognitive aspects of Parkinson's disease and believed that the intellect was 'uninjured'. He appealed to morbid anatomists to clarify the anatomical and pathological cause. The late 19th century brought recognition that dementia may complicate the course of Parkinson's disease. In 1861–62, whilst still a junior member of the Salpetriere faculty, Charcot with Vulpian baldly stated that 'in general, psychic faculties are definitely impaired'. He later added that 'the mind becomes clouded and the memory is lost', an assertion amplified by his pupil Ball (1882) in a detailed description of seven cases. The positions taken by Parkinson and Charcot respectively, had a long lasting influence on the predominant views in their countries: while French authors regularly reported dementia, depression, hallucinations and bradyphrenia in their parkinsonian patients, Anglo-Saxon authors usually stressed normal behavior and cognition.

It was not until 1912 that Friedrich Heinrich Lewy began to answer Parkinson's call for pathological clarification. In a chapter on the pathological anatomy of paralysis agitans, Lewy observed intracytoplasmic inclusion bodies in the basal forebrain (substantia innominata) and dorsal motor nucleus of the vagus nerve in brains of patients with Parkinson's disease. With the limited staining techniques of the time, he classified them as similar to the amyloid inclusions described previously in myoclonus epilepsy by Lafora (1911). Lafora replicated Lewy's results the following year and demonstrated that the inclusions described by Lewy form a separate category, which he called 'cuerpos hialinos' (Lafora, 1913). The term 'Lewy Body' ('corps de Lewy') was introduced by Tretiakoff (1919), who was also the first to detect them in the substantia nigra and stress the importance of this location for the pathogenesis of Parkinson's disease. Lewy himself (1923) went on to describe the occurrence of Lewy bodies in different parts of the brain, including the cerebral cortex, in a group of 56 patients, 64% of whom had marked mental alteration. The existence of cortical Lewy bodies was widely confirmed (Hallervorden, 1933; Helfland, 1939; von Braunmühl, 1949).

The first study linking dementia directly to the cortical Lewy bodies was presented at the Annual Meeting of the American Association of Neuropathologists in 1958 and published three years later (Okazaki et al, 1961). The authors described two cases with progressive dementia, disorientation, hallucinations and profound motor disability which they regarded as 'terminal quadriparesis in flexion' rather than parkinsonism. The pathological examination revealed the presence of Lewy bodies, 'morphologically and histochemically indistinguishable from those initially described by Lewy in Parkinson's Disease', but 'widely disseminated in all lobes and all cortical layers except Layer I'. Although the authors did not propose any specific name for the new putative syndrome, they stressed that the 'morphologic singularity and close clinical resemblance' of their two cases suggested the possibility that 'this complex represents a defined entity'. The study of Okazaki et al (1961) contained not only many clinical and pathological features which today would be considered as characteristic of DLB, but also discussed its differential diagnosis. The clinical picture of dementia in the absence of parkinsonism and the strikingly different distribution of Lewy bodies set the cases clearly apart from idiopathic Parkinson's disease. The absence of senile plaques or neurofibrillary tangles distinguished them from Alzheimer's disease. Indeed, the authors went as far as to claim that Lewy body and Alzheimer pathology are 'to a large measure, mutually exclusive', a statement which, as we will see, has been called into question by subsequent studies.

After a hiatus lasting more than 10 years, a series of detailed case reports of dementia associated with cortical Lewy bodies began to emerge from Japan (Kosaka et al, 1976; Ogasawara et al, 1978; Kosaka and Mehraein 1979, Ikeda et al, 1980). In terms of the clinical picture the cases were often referred to as 'unclassifiable' or 'atypical', but a comparison of their main features reveals a remarkable similarity. The majority of cases showed a combination of dementia and parkinsonism, although the latter was often mild; only very few studies reported cases of dementia without parkinsonism (Ikeda et al, 1980) or parkinsonism without dementia (Ikeda et al, 1975). The most prominent and frequent cognitive symptoms were disorientation, confusion, forgetfulness and restlessness (Kosaka et al, 1976; Ogasawara et al, 1978; Kosaka and Mehraein, 1979; Ikeda et al, 1980). Psychotic features such as hallucinations and paranoid delusions were also reported (Kosaka and Mehraein, 1979). In terms of pathology the cases were characterized by widespread cortical Lewy bodies but, in contrast to the study of Okazaki et al (1961), the majority of the brains showed additional signs of a variable degree of Alzheimer-type pathology (Kosaka et al, 1976; Kosaka, 1978; Kosaka and Mehraein, 1979; Ogasawara et al, 1978; Ikeda et al, 1980).

In 1984, Kosaka, Yoshimura, Ikeda and Budka reviewed the existing literature and proposed that these cases should be regarded as a new disease entity, which they termed 'diffuse Lewy body disease'. Shortly thereafter the disease became increasingly recognized also in Britain and North America. Gibb et al (1987) described four of their own cases and discussed 23 of previously published ones, all with remarkably similar clinical and pathological findings. The next few years saw the publication of further series including some that were reasonably large and from relatively unselected sources (Eggerton and Sima, 1986; Ditter and Mirra, 1987; Joachim et al, 1988; Burkhard et al, 1988; Byrne et al, 1989; Hansen et al, 1990; Perry et al, 1990). The triad of dementia, parkinsonism and psychotic symptoms was established as the core syndrome of the new disease. In addition, new symptoms, now considered to be key features of DLB, were first recognized in that period: fluctuating level of consciousness with episodic confusion (Gibb et al, 1987; Byrne et al; 1989), frequent unexplained falls (Byrne et al, 1989; McKeith et al, 1992), excessive sensitivity to side effects of neuroleptic medication (McKeith et al, 1992) and syncope with transient loss of consciousness (McKeith et al, 1992). The profile of the dementia was elaborated upon, highlighting deficits in attention (Sahgal et al, 1992), visuospatial abilities (Sahgal et al, 1995) and executive function (Salmon and Galasko, 1996).

While the clinical description of DLB became more precise and specific, the underlying pathology, in particular the relative significance of Lewy bodies and Alzheimer-type changes, remained controversial. This uncertainty was reflected in the terms used to describe the emerging diagnosis. Some authors stressed the importance of the Alzheimer-type pathology, proposing names such as 'Alzheimer disease with Parkinson's disease changes' (Ditter & Mirra, 1978), 'Alzheimer's disease with incidental Lewy bodies' (Joachim et al, 1988) or 'Lewy body variant of Alzheimer's disease' (Hansen et al, 1990). Others focused on the importance of cortical Lewy bodies, preferring terms such as 'diffuse Lewy body disease' (Kosaka et al, 1984), 'dementia with cerebral Lewy bodies' (Eggerton & Sima, 1986), 'diffuse cortical Lewy body disease' (Gibb et al, 1987) or 'senile dementia of Lewy body type' (Perry et al, 1990). The consensus conference in Newcastle upon Tyne in October 1995 recognized the crucial importance of cortical Lewy bodies in the pathogenesis of the disease and recommended the designation 'Dementia with Lewy bodies' – DLB (McKeith et al, 1996).

The recognition of DLB as an entity created a need for operational, clinically applicable diagnostic criteria. The first attempt to formulate such criteria, based on the largest case series of its time (Byrne et al, 1989), came from the Nottingham group (Byrne et al, 1991). The criteria included parkinsonism, dementia and psychiatric features as well as fluctuations in cognition. In the following year, a comparison of 57 autopsy-confirmed AD patients with 41 'senile dementia of Lewy body type' cases led McKeith et al (1992) to formulate new criteria, emphasizing cognitive dysfunction and neuropsychiatric features and adding excessive sensitivity to neuroleptic medication to the list of clinical characteristics of the disease; in contrast to the Nottingham criteria, the presence of parkinsonian features was not considered mandatory. The Newcastle criteria formed the basis of the consensus criteria (McKeith et al, 1996), which soon became adopted worldwide. Fluctuations, visual hallucinations and spontaneous motor features of parkinsonism (not provoked by a neuroleptic medication) were classified as the key features of the disease. The presence of any two indicated a probable, the presence of one a possible DLB. Supportive features included falls, syncope, transient loss of consciousness, neuroleptic sensitivity, systematized delusions and nonvisual hallucinations. Several retrospective and prospective studies have examined the accuracy of the consensus criteria (McKeith et al, 2000; Litvan et al, 2003) and the Second (July 1998) and Third (September 2003) International DLB Workshop recommended the continuation of their use (McKeith et al, 1999; Cummings, 2004).

The last 10 years have witnessed an enormous progress in the methodology applied in DLB research, such as neuropathological staining techniques, molecular biology and neuroimaging. However, the fundamental question troubling researchers since the first descriptions of the disease, the relation between DLB and its two principal differential diagnoses, Parkinson's disease (PD) and Alzheimer's (AD), remains an issue of lively debate, made more topical by recent scientific discoveries. By the time of the first descriptions of DLB in the 1960s and 1970s PD was generally considered, at least in the Anglo-Saxon literature, to be almost exclusively a motor disorder. The difference between the 'demented' DLB and the 'cognitively intact' PD patients seemed, therefore, clear and unequivocal. In the last 30 years, however, cognitive impairment has been increasingly recognized as a frequent and often pronounced feature of PD. The estimated prevalence of dementia in PD patients has increased dramatically from 3% (Mjones, 1949) to 78% (Aarsland et al, 2003). The term Parkinson disease dementia (PDD) came into use to refer to PD with prominent cognitive deficits. DLB and PDD can be indistinguishable on neuropsychological testing (Noe et al, 2004; Mosiman et al, 2004), differing only in the sequence of the symptoms: a patient presenting with dementia followed by parkinsonism is diagnosed as DLB, a patient presenting with parkinsonism followed by dementia as PDD (Cummings, 2004). In this context DLB could be considered a part of a spectrum.

Also in the field of pathology, the boundary between DLB and PD is not always clear-cut. Both diseases are associated with Lewy bodies, which, as noted by Okazaki et al (1961) and Kosaka et al (1976), show only minor differences in morphology between the brainstem and cortex. The main difference observed by Kosaka and Mehraein (1979) was their distribution: in the brainstem they were distributed in accordance with the monoamine nerve terminals; this was not the case in cortex, suggesting that both types of Lewy body might affect different transmitter systems, later identified as cholinergic and dopaminergic. The efficacy of cholinesterase inhibitors in DLB (McKeith et al, 2000) provided an additional confirmation of the importance of the cholinergic pathways in this disease. However, none of these features is

DLB-specific: cholinergic deficits have been implicated in the cognitive dysfunction of PD (Dubois et al, 1990) and positive effects of cholinesterase inhibitors have also been reported in PD patients (Aarsland et al, 2004). More importantly, not only have cortical Lewy bodies been detected in PD patients, their density has also been related to cognitive symptoms (Kövari et al, 2003). Moreover, the identification of alpha-synuclein as the main component of Lewy bodies in DLB and PD (Spillantini, 1997) placed both diseases, together with multiple system atrophy (MSA), in the emerging class of alpha-synucleinopathies (Goedert, 2001). Indeed, an interaction between alpha-synuclein and beta-amyloid (a protein implicated in the pathogenesis of AD) may explain the frequently reported co-occurrence of Lewy body and Alzheimer-type pathology and contribute significantly to the clinical overlap between DLB and AD (Masliah et al, 2001).

Looking back over 50 years of DLB research we see a remarkable evolution: beginning with single cases of a rare condition, reported as a curiosity at neuropathological meetings, DLB has come to be recognized as the second commonest form of dementia, accounting for around 15–20% of all cases (Perry et al, 1990; Kosaka & Iseki, 1996). Initially regarded as an atypical mixture of PD and AD, it has evolved into a distinct entity with operationalized diagnostic criteria (McKeith et al, 1996). From a disease with rapid progression and bleak prognosis it has transformed into one of the few forms of dementia in which significant benefits can be derived from pharmacotherapy (McKeith et al, 2000). With its wide range of psychiatric, neuropsychological and neurological symptoms DLB continues to stimulate interdisciplinary research and consequently, an improved understanding of brain function.

References

Aarsland D, Andersen K, Larsen JP, Lolk A et al, Prevalence and characteristics of dementia in Parkinson disease: an 8-year prospective study. Arch Neurol (2003) 60:387–92.

Aarsland D, Mosimann UP, McKeith IG, Role of cholinesterase inhibitors in Parkinson's disease and dementia with Lewy bodies. J Geriatr Psychiatry Neurol (2004) 17:164–71.

Ball B, De l'insanite dans la paralysie agitante. Encephale J Mal Ment Nerv (1882) 2:22–32.

Burkhardt CR, Filley CM, Kleinschmidt-DeMasters BK, Diffuse Lewy body disease and progressive dementia. Neurology (1988) 38:1520–8.

Byrne EJ, Lennox G, Lowe J, Godwin-Austen RB, Diffuse Lewy body disease; clinical features in 15 cases. J Neurol Neurosurg Psychiatry (1989) 52:709–17.

Byrne EJ, Lennox G, Godwin-Austen RB, Dementia associated with cortical Lewy bodies. Proposed diagnostic criteria. Dementia (1991) 2:283–4.

Charcot JM, Vulpian A, De la paralysie agitante. Gaz Hebdomadaire Med Chir (1861–62) 8:765–7; 9:54–9.

Cummings JL, Reconsidering diagnostic criteria for dementia with Lewy bodies. Meeting review. Reviews in Neurological Diseases (2004) 1:31–34.

Ditter SM, Mirra SS, Neuropathologic and clinical features of Parkinson's disease in Alzheimer's patients. Neurology (1987) 37:754–60.

Dubois B, Pilon B, Lhermitte F, Agid Y, Cholinergic deficiency and frontal dysfunction in Parkinson's disease. Ann Neurol (1990) 28:117–21.

Eggerton DE, Sima AAF, Dementia with cerebral Lewy bodies. Arch Neurol (1986) 43:524–7.

Gibb WRG, Esiri MM, Lees AJ, Clinical and pathological features of diffuse cortical Lewy body disease (Lewy body dementia). Brain (1987) 110:1131–53.

Goedert M, Alpha-synuclein and neurodegenerative diseases. Nature Reviews Neuroscience (2001) 2:492–501.

Hallervorden J, Zur Pathogenese des postencephalitischen Parkinsonismus. Klin Wochenschrift (1933) 12:692–5.

Hansen L, Salmon D, Galasko D, The Lewy body variant of Alzheimer's disease: a clinical and pathological entity. Neurology (1990) 40:1–8.

Helfand M, Status pigmentosus. Its pathology and its relation to Hallervorden–Spatz disease. J Nerv Ment Dis (1939) 81:662.

Ikeda K, Yoshimura T, Kato H, A case of idiopathic Parkinsonism with many Lewy bodies in the cerebral cortex. No to Shinkei [Brain and Nerve] (1975) 27:733–42.

Ikeda K, Hori A, Bode G, Progressive dementia with 'diffuse Lewy-type inclusions' in cerebral cortex. Arch Psychiatrie und Nervenkr (1980) 228, 243–8.

Joachim CL, Morris JH, Selkoe DJ, Clinically diagnosed Alzheimer's disease: autopsy results in 150 cases. Ann Neur (1988) 24; 50–6.

Kosaka K, Oyanagi S, Matsushita M, Hori A, Presenile dementia with Alzheimer-, Pick- and Lewy-body changes. Acta Neuropathologica (1976) 36:221–33.

Kosaka K, Lewy bodies in cerebral cortex. Report of three cases. Acta Neuropathologica (1978) 42:127–34.

Kosaka K, Mehraein P, Dementia-Parkinsonism syndrome with numerous Lewy bodies and senile plaques in cerebral cortex. Arch Psychiatr Nervenkr (1979) 226:241–50.

Kosaka K, Yoshimura M, Ikeda K, Budka H, Diffuse type of Lewy body disease. Progressive dementia with abundant cortical Lewy bodies and senile changes of varying degree: a new disease? Clin Neuropathol (1984) 3:185–92.

Kosaka K, Iseki E, Diffuse Lewy Body disease within the spectrum of Lewy Body disease. In Perry R, McKeith I, Perry E (eds) (1996) Dementia with Lewy Bodies. Cambridge, Cambridge University Press; 238–47.

Kövari E, Gold G, Herrmann F et al, Lewy body densities in the entorhinal and anterior cingulate cortex predict cognitive deficits in Parkinson's disease. Acta Neuropathologica (2003) 106:83–8.

Lafora GR, Ueber das Vorkommen amyloider Körperchen im Innern der Ganglienzellen; zugleich ein Beitrag zum Studium der amyloiden Substanz im Nervensystem. Virchows Arch (1911) 4:356.

Lafora GR, Nuevas investigaciones sobre los cuerpos amilaceos del interior de las células nerviosas. Trab Lab Invest biol Univ Madrid (1913) 11:29.

Lewy FH, Paralysis agitans:pathologische Anatomie. In: Lewandowsky M, ed, Handbuch der Neurologie (Springer: Berlin, 1912) Vol 3:920–33.

Lewy FH, Die Lehre vom Tonus und der Bewegung. (Springer: Berlin, 1923)

Litvan I, Bhatia KP, Burn DJ, Task force appraisal of clinical diagnostic criteria for parkinsonian disorders. Movt Dis (2003) 18:467–86.

McKeith IG, Perry RH, Fairbairn AF, Operational criteria for senile dementia of Lewy body type. Psychol Med (1992) 22:911–22.

McKeith IG, Galasko D, Kosaka K, Consensus guidelines for the clinical and pathologic diagnosis of dementia with Lewy bodies. Neurology (1996) 47:1113–24.

McKeith IG, Perry EK, Perry RH, Report of the second dementia with Lewy bodies international workshop. Neurology (1999) 53:902–5.

McKeith IG, Ballard CG, Perry RH, Prospective validation of consensus criteria for the diagnosis of dementia with Lewy bodies. Neurology (2000) 54:1050–8.

McKeith I, Del Ser T, Spano P et al, Efficacy of rivastigmine in dementia with Lewy bodies: a randomised, double-blind, placebo-controlled international study. Lancet (2000) 356:2031–6.

Masliah E, Rockenstein E, Veinbergs I et al, Beta-amyloid peptides enhance alpha-synuclein accumulation and neuronal deficits in a transgenic mouse model linking Alzheimer's disease and Parkinson's disease. Proc Natl Acad Sci USA (2001) 98:12245–50.

Mjones H, Paralysis agitans. Acta Psychiatr Neurolog (1949) 54:1–195.

Mosimann UP, Mather G, Wesnes KA et al, Visual perception in Parkinson disease and dementia with Lewy bodies. Neurology (2004) 63:2091–6.

Noe E, Marder K, Bell KL et al, Comparison of dementia with Lewy bodies to Alzheimer's disease and Parkinson's disease with dementia. Movt Disord (2004) 19:60–7.

Ogasawara N, Takamatsu K, Monma Y, Itoh T, Presenile Demenz mit senilen Veränderungen, argentophilen Kugeln and Levy Körperchen. J Neuropath Exp Neurol (1978) 37:667.

Okazaki H, Lipkin LE, Aronson SM, Diffuse intracytoplasmic ganglionic inclusions (Lewy type) associated with progressive dementia and quadriparesis in flexion. J Neuropath Exp Neurol (1961) 20:237–44.

Parkinson J, An Essay on the Shaking Palsy. (Sherwood, Neely and Jones: London, 1817).

Perry RH, Irving D, Blessed G, Senile dementia of Lewy body type. A clinically and neuropathologically distinct type of Lewy body dementia in the elderly. J Neurol Sci (1990) 95:119–39.

Sahgal A, Galloway PH, McKeith IG, A comparative study of attentional deficits in senile dementias of Alzheimer and Lewy body types. Dementia (1992) 3:350–4.

Sahgal A, McKeith IG, Galloway PH, Do differences in visuospatial ability between senile dementias of Alzheimer and Lewy body types reflect differences solely in mnemonic function. J Clin Expl Neuropsychol (1995) 17:35–43.

Salmon D, Galasko D, Neuropsychological aspects of Lewy body dementia. In: Perry R, McKeith I, Perry E, eds, Dementia with Lewy Bodies. (Cambridge University Press: New York, 1996) 99–114.

Spillantini MG, Alpha-synuclein in Lewy bodies. Nature (1997) 388:839–40.

Tretiakoff C, Contribution à l'étude de l'anatomie pathologique du locus niger de Soemmering. Thèse de Paris, 1919.

von Braunmühl, Encephalitis epidemica und Synäresislehre. Grundsätzliches zur Anatomie und Pathogenese des postencephalitischen Parkinsonismus. Archiv Psychiatrie (1949) 181:543–76.

chapter 2

Clinical spectrum of Lewy body disease

Maria J Martí, Jaume Campdelacreu and Eduardo Tolosa

Lewy bodies (LB) are rounded, eosinophilic, intracytoplasmatic neuronal inclusions named after FH Lewy who first described them in 1912 (Lewy, 1912). LB are chiefly composed of altered neurofilaments and contain α-synuclein and proteolytic stress proteins such as ubiquitin and sometimes β-crystalline (Wakabayashi et al, 2002). LB are classically associated with Parkinson's disease (PD) where they are found in selected brainstem nuclei (substantia nigra, locus ceruleus, dorsal vagal nucleus), the nucleus basalis of Meynert, hypothalamus and sympathetic ganglia. Small numbers of LB are also found in the cortex. Cortical LB are less eosinophilic and often surrounded by a pale halo and are therefore more difficult to recognize with traditional staining methods. The most specific method of detecting LBs and Lewy neurites is synuclein immunocytochemistry (Lowe and Leigh, 2002).

LB are also typically associated with another disorder initially called diffuse LB disease (DLBD) and more recently dementia with Lewy bodies (DLB). The first cases with DLBD were described by Okazaki et al (1961) and the term DLBD was first used by Yoshimura (1983). Patients with this form of LB disorder have a progressive dementia syndrome associated with parkinsonism and prominent involvement of the cortex by LB pathology.

Kosaka et al (1980) originally proposed a classification for the pathological spectrum of Lewy body disease (LBD): diffuse LBD (type A) with numerous LBs in the brainstem and diencephalon, limbic structures and cortex; transitional form of LBD (type B), with numerous LBs in brainstem and diencephalon but less frequent LB in limbic structures and fewer in the cortex; and brainstem LB disease (type C) with numerous LBs in the brainstem and diencephalon but few or none in limbic structures and cortex, which corresponds to our notion of classical PD. Later, Kosaka also separated the common forms from the pure forms of LBD depending on the concomitant presence (common form) or absence (pure form) of senile plaques and/or neurofibrillary tangles on pathological examination (Kosaka, 1990).

The studies by Kosaka and others strongly support the concept that there is a spectrum of disorders characterized neuropathologically by the presence of LBs with the clinical manifestation in part reflecting the topography of the neuropathological lesions. To the disorders mentioned above one could add to the spectrum of LBD the disorder called pure autonomic failure (PAF) characterized by prominent dysautonomia clinically and central and peripheral nervous system LBs and those clinically normal individuals with 'incidental' LBs found on autopsy ('incidental' LBD) (Gibb and Lees, 1988).

The concept of a spectrum of LB disorders ranging from incidental to diffuse LBD is attractive and would presume that these disorders would have somewhat similar pathophysiology and possibly similar etiology. It is a concept that can be backed on the bases of clinical, neuropathological and current molecular genetic findings. There is, for example, remarkable clinical overlap between PD and dementia with Lewy bodies (DLB) and there is frequently no distinction between advanced PD and DLB on neuropathological examination. Like PD, DLB has been shown to be related to mutations of α-synuclein (Zarranz et al, 2004). However, the spectrum concept has its detractors who highlight the differences rather than the commonalities among these disorders and who point out that LB occur in many unrelated disorders of variable etiology such as Alzheimer's disease, traumatic brain lesions or Hallervorden–Spatz disease. Despite intensive research it remains to be proven if the various disorders discussed above indeed reflect a spectrum of disorders determined by similar etiological and pathophysiological factors or are actually distinct clinicopathological entities.

Clinical features of Lewy body disorders

Many signs and symptoms are common to the various disorders associated with prominent LB pathology in the central nervous system. Common to all these disorders is the occurrence of neuropsychiatric alterations, parkinsonism and dysautonomia. In PD, parkinsonism predominates, in DLB dementia and in PAF dysautonomia. In the text that follows we attempt to describe these clinical manifestations as well as some other, less common clinical features associated with LB diseases (see Table 2.1).

Table 2.1 Clinical features of Lewy body diseases

Main clinical features	*Other clinical features*
Motor	**Motor**
Tremor	Speech disorders
Rigidity	Motor blocks (freezing)
Bradykinesia	Myoclonus
Postural instability	
	Psychiatric
Cognitive	Anxiety
Cognitive impairment	Apathy
Executive dysfunction	Agitation
Attention deficit	Delirium
Visuospatial dysfunction	Behavioral disorders
Reduced verbal fluency	Nonvisual hallucinations
Cognitive fluctuations	
	Dysautonomic
Psychiatric	Diarrhea
Visual hallucinations	Decreased sweating
Delusions	Heat intolerance
Depression	Facial flushing
	Oral dryness
Dysautonomic	
Orthostatic hypotension	**Sleep disorders**
Syncope	REM sleep behavior disorder
Urinary dysfunction	Insomnia
Constipation	Excessive daytime sleepiness
Sexual dysfunction	Restless legs
	Periodic limb movements
	Sleep apnea
	Fragmented sleep architecture
	Nightmares
	Others
	Olfactory deficits
	Akathisia
	Pain
	Cramps
	Fatigue

Parkinsonism

Parkinsonism is the cardinal and defining clinical feature of PD, manifesting with the classical motor syndrome of bradykinesia, rigidity, rest tremor, and gait and postural reflex abnormalities.

On the basis of clinicopathological studies (Hughes et al, 1992a), diagnosis of PD is highly probable when a patient presents progressive slowness of movements, pill-rolling tremor or rigidity, and excellent and sustained response to levodopa. Asymmetry at onset and absence of atypical features strongly support the diagnosis. Two different clinical phenotypes of PD have been proposed (Jankovic et al, 1990): one characterized by postural instability and gait disorder (PIGD) and another where tremor is dominant. The tremor subtype is associated with preserved mental status, earlier age at onset and a slower progression than the PIGD subtype. Likewise, patients with young onset have a slower rate of progression and present levodopa-induced dyskinesias earlier than those with older onset (Jankovic and Kapadia, 2001).

Familial PD, caused by specific mutations, usually presents with an earlier onset. The phenotype is variable even among patients with the same mutation. Up to now, 11 types of familial PD (loci Park 1–Park 11) have been identified in which seven causative genes have been found (Huang et al, 2004; Valente et al, 2004; Healy et al, 2004). The discovery of α-synuclein mutations allowed the identification of this protein as the main component of LBs. α-synuclein mutations cause autosomal dominant PD. The Ala53Thr mutation has been reported in 13 families of Greek and Italian descent. Clinical features include an initially good response to levodopa, younger age at onset than PD (mean 45 years), more rapid progression and frequent dementia (Mori et al, 2003). Other reported symptoms are central hypoventilation, postural hypotension, myoclonus, and urinary incontinence (Spira et al, 2001). The Ala30Pro mutation has been reported in only one family (Krüger et al, 1998), and recently the E46K mutation has been found in a family with DLB (Zarranz et al, 2003). α-synuclein locus duplication has also been recently reported as a cause of familial young onset Parkinson's disease (Ibanez et al, 2004; Chartier-Harlin et al, 2004), and triplication has been described in a family leading to a variable phenotype ranging from PD to DLB (Singleton et al, 2003). Interestingly, Lewy bodies are not found in brains of patients with *parkin* gene mutations, which is the most common known cause of familial PD, causing autosomal recessive juvenile parkinsonism (Lücking et al, 2000). The other types of familial PD are rare and restricted to a few families (Sethi, 2002; Healy et al, 2004) and hardly any information is available on their pathological substrate.

Dementia with Lewy bodies (DLB) is characterized by progressive dementia, parkinsonism, fluctuating cognitive impairment and persistent visual hallucinations. Parkinsonism is a prominent feature of DLB and will appear in up to 75% of patients, usually presenting with a symmetric akinetic-rigid syndrome or 'PIGD' phenotype (Burn et al, 2003), and is sometimes associated with action tremor and myoclonus (Aarsland et al, 2001a; Louis et al,1997). Axial symptoms, like gait abnormalities and postural instability are prominent, probably reflecting involvement of nondopaminergic structures. However, some patients may have unilateral rest tremor and are clinically indistinguishable from idiopathic PD (Louis et al, 1995). The efficacy of levodopa on DLB parkinsonism is unclear since it has not been systematically evaluated. Although a 'good' response has been reported in some retrospective clinical (Rojo et al, 2002) or pathological series (Louis et al, 1995) the range of responder patients is probably lower than in patients fulfilling PD clinical diagnostic criteria (Bonelli et al, 2004). Neuroleptic sensitivity with marked motor worsening and mental status changes has also been claimed as a distinctive feature of DLB (McKeith et al, 1992) but differences in tolerability of neuroleptic treatment between patients with PD dementia and DLB have never been established.

Dementia and neuropsychiatric symptoms

Cognitive impairment is the most frequent presenting feature of DLB. It is characterized by a prominent frontosubcortical and visuospatial dysfunction, with attention deficits and memory loss (Salmon and Galasko, 1996). Prominent or persistent memory impairment must not necessarily occur in early stages but it becomes eventually evident. A rapidly progressive dementia, accompanied by aphasia, dyspraxia and spatial disorientation suggestive of temporoparietal dysfunction can be seen as the disease progresses. When comparing with Alzheimer's disease (AD), patients with DLB have more neuropsychiatric features and more intense attention fluctuations (Ballard et al, 1999; Walker et al, 2000a). Fluctuations in cognition have been observed in up to 90% of patients with DLB (Byrne et al, 1989). They are difficult to assess because of the lack of agreement on their definition and a wide range of presentations. They have been described as day-to-day changes of more than 50% on performing the Mini-Mental State Examination (MMSE), or as variations in alertness, the same patient sometimes ranging from stupor to alertness (Gibb et al, 1987). The use of semi-structured scales can be useful to clinically identify cognitive fluctuations (Walker et al, 2000a). Recently, standardized assessment methods (Walker et al, 2000b) have found that they are more common and severe in DLB than in other major dementias, such as AD and vascular dementia.

Specific cognitive domains such as visuospatial or executive function are frequently affected in patients with PD, with or without dementia. Patients perform poorly on visuospatial and perceptual tasks, but language function is spared. Dementia is difficult to examine in PD due to interference of the motor syndrome in the assessment of certain domains and activities of daily living, as well as the effect of drugs. The prevalence of dementia in PD is variable in different studies, and has been estimated as 20–40%. Recently, long-term follow-up studies showed that 60–80% of PD patients will develop dementia 10–15 years after motor symptoms appear (Aarsland et al, 2003). Several features have been associated with an increased risk of developing dementia: older age, older age at onset, greater motor disability, akinetic parkinsonism, depression, reduced verbal fluency, executive dysfunction, slow EEG, previous hallucinations and excessive daytime sleepiness (Emre, 2003). When present, dementia is more frequent in the PIGD subtype than in tremoric PD (Burn et al, 2003).

The dementia of PD has been characterized as subcortical in type, but in advanced stages cognitive deficits are generalized and can be indistinguishable from AD. The main features of PD dementia, as in DLB, are the dysexecutive syndrome, attention deficits and visuospatial and constructional dysfunction (Pillon et al, 1986, 1991; Litvan et al, 1991). Memory recall is impaired, with benefit from external cues, while learning of new information is less affected, and recognition is more preserved, suggesting a deficit in the generation of coding and retrieval strategies with relatively preserved information storage. Language and praxis are preserved, except for a marked impairment of verbal fluency that could be due to a deficit in search strategies rather than in language itself. Cognitive fluctuations seem to be related to fluctuations of attention and are similar to those found in patients with DLB (Ballard et al, 2002). Although the neuropathological basis of dementia in PD is heterogeneous, recent reports suggest that diffuse cortical LBs are the main pathological substrate in the majority of cases (Hurtig et al, 2000; Calopa et al, 2002; Apaydin et al, 2002).

As for neuropsychiatric symptoms, patients with DLB can present early in the course of the disease with visual and auditory hallucinations and delusions (Ballard et al, 1999). Similar to the visual hallucinations induced by dopaminergic drugs in PD patients, hallucinations in DLB have complex forms and are rich in details and colour, involving human figures and animals. Other psychiatric manifestations include apathy, depression or anxiety.

Psychotic symptoms, including hallucinations, delusions, paranoid beliefs, agitation and delirium, constitute a relatively frequent but nevertheless serious complication of PD. Visual hallucinations and paranoid delusions often are the most prominent manifestation, the prevalence of visual hallucinations being similar in both DLB and PD with dementia (Harding et al, 2002), generally with a more preserved insight in PD. They are common in patients with PD with dementia but are also observed as a drug-induced complication in patients without apparent cognitive deficit. Age, disease duration and severity, cognitive impairment, depression and sleep disorders have been identified as risk factors for developing psychosis (Poewe, 2003). Depression is also frequent in PD, and often begins several years before the motor symptoms (Santamaria et al, 1986; Shiba et al, 2000). Cross-sectional surveys have reported depression rates of 20–50% in patients with PD (Mayeux et al, 1981; Schrag et al, 2001; Starkstein et al, 1990). Although minor depressive symptoms are frequent, major depression is uncommon, affecting 3–8% of patients, with higher rates in patients with associated dementia (Hantz et al, 1994; Tandberg et al, 1996) Other factors associated with depression in PD are disease severity, advanced age and lower cognitive scores (Cubo et al, 2000; Giladi et al, 2000; Schrag et al, 2001). Other frequent neuropsychiatric symptoms are anxiety, apathy, behavior disorders and agitation (Aarsland et al, 1999).

Dysautonomia

The paradigm of autonomic dysfunction within the LB disorders is pure autonomic failure (PAF). It is an uncommon progressive, adult-onset, sporadic disorder characterized by orthostatic hypotension as the cardinal symptom, usually with evidence of more widespread autonomic failure (Consensus, 1996). Postural related symptoms as dizziness, syncope, visual disturbances and suboccipital/paracervical 'coat-hanger' neck pain are common in these patients (Mathias et al, 1999). Patients may also present with decreased sweating and heat intolerance, urinary dysfunction (frequency, urgency and incontinence), constipation or diarrhoea and erectile dysfunction (Hague et al, 1997; Arai et al, 2000). No other neurological symptoms are present. However, some patients who initially present with features of PAF develop years later symptomatology that prompt reclassification of the diagnosis within the Lewy body disorders spectrum (Larner et al, 2000; Kaufmann et al, 2004).

Sympathetic autonomic system is also affected in PD. Nearly all PD patients experience some degree of autonomic disturbances throughout the course of the illness. The most common are constipation, sexual dysfunction due to loss of libido and impotence, and urinary symptoms. Constipation is frequent in patients with PD, probably related to LB pathology in the myenteric plexus (Edwards et al, 1992; Wakabayashi and Takahashi, 1997), and infrequent bowel movements have been associated with an elevated risk of future PD (Abbott et al, 2001). Orthostatic hypotension, symptomatic or asymptomatic, is present in 20–47% of patients (Senard et al, 1997; Allcock et al, 2004), even in early stages (Bonucelli et al, 2003), and the prevalence may be higher, according to a retrospective study on patients with neuropathologically confirmed PD (Wenning et al, 1999). Impaired vascular response can manifest with non-specific symptoms such as giddiness, nausea, transitory defect of vision, and rarely loss of consciousness. Dysautonomic symptoms may also appear as nonmotor fluctuations manifesting as drenching sweats, facial flushing, oral dryness, dyspnea, dysphagia, and constipation (Witjas et al, 2002).

In DLB patients, features like repeated falls, syncope, and transient loss of consciousness can be attributed in part to autonomic nervous system abnormalities. Orthostasis, either asymptomatic or associated with syncope, can be present in these patients, although prevalence of symptomatic orthostatic hypotension has been found in a lesser frequency (15%) than in other types of parkinsonism such as multiple system atrophy (Wenning et al, 1999; Thaisetthawatkul et al, 2004). Recently, in a retrospective study for autonomic symptoms, urinary incontinence and constipation were respectively found in 97% and 83% of 29 cases with neuropathologically confirmed DLB. Severe autonomic failure was present in 62% of patients (Horimoto et al, 2003). Quantification of postganglionic sympathetic cardiac innervation by means of [123I]MIBG scintigraphy might detect early disturbances in DLB, and help to separate this dementia from AD (Yoshita et al, 2001). This technique is also useful to discriminate between PD and multiple system atrophy (Braune et al, 1999).

Other symptoms encountered in the LB disorders

Rapid eye movement (REM) sleep behavior disorder (RBD) is a parasomnia characterized by loss of normal skeletal muscle atonia during REM sleep with prominent motor activity and dreaming. This disorder is frequently associated with the synucleinopathies (DLB, PD and multiple system atrophy) but rarely occurs in neurodegenerative disorders associated with amyloid or tau protein deposition. RBD can precede the onset of dementia or parkinsonism by many years (Boeve et al, 2001). The majority of autopsied cases have the neuropathological diagnosis of Lewy body disease (Boeve et al, 2003). While RBD is common in PD and DLB, it seems to be absent throughout the course of PAF (Plazzi et al, 1998). Dysfunction of the pedunculo-pontine nucleus or other key brainstem structures associated with REM sleep is hypothesized to underlie the pathophysiology of this disorder.

In PD, excessive daytime sleepiness is common and correlates with advanced disease and the use of dopamine agonists. Other sleep disorders reported in PD are restless legs syndrome, periodic limb movements, insomnia, sleep apnea, fragmented sleep architecture and reduced slow wave and REM sleep (Ondo et al, 2001; Henderson et al, 2003). Impairment of different brainstem and subcortical structures, and several motor and neuropsychiatric disturbances associated with PD, as well as the effect of treatments, contribute to sleep disruption in PD (Chaudhuri, 2003). In DLB, excessive daytime sleepiness, insomnia, nightmares, and confusion on waking are also common (Grace et al, 2000).

Olfactory deficits are frequent in PD and occur early in the course of the disease. Severity ranges from subtle deficits to anosmia, which are unresponsive to levodopa (Henderson et al, 2003). Recent studies have shown that hyposmia may be an early 'preclinical' manifestation of PD. It can occur among asymptomatic relatives of parkinsonian patients and be associated with reduced striatal dopamine transporter (DAT) binding (Ponsen et al, 2004). Increased tyrosine hydroxylase-positive neurons and dopamine in the glomerular layer of the olfactory bulb could underlie these deficits (Huisman et al, 2004). Anosmia has also been reported in patients with DLB (McShane et al, 2001).

Patients with PD can also experience fluctuating sensory symptoms such as akathisia or tightening and tingling sensations (Witjas, et al, 2002). Painful episodes, especially musculoskeletal cramps, usually occur in 'off state'. Fatigue is reported by almost half of the patients with PD, even without depression. Its cause is unknown and it seems to be an independent symptom of the disease not related to other motor or nonmotor symptoms (Herlofson and Larsen, 2002).

Diagnostic criteria of Lewy body disorders

The diagnostic criteria for PD developed by the UK Parkinson's Disease Society Brain Bank (Hughes et al, 1992b) are the most frequently accepted.

They allow a diagnostic accuracy of up to 90% if strictly applied (Hughes et al, 2001). Gelb et al (1999) based on an extensive review of the literature, have proposed another clinical diagnostic classification. Three levels of certainty can be differentiated: probable and possible PD, based on clinical criteria, and definite PD, which requires neuropathologic confirmation. The accuracy of the diagnosis improves when atypical features such as symmetry at onset, early marked dysautonomia or dementia, corticospinal tract dysfunction or supranuclear gaze palsy are absent and possible causes for secondary parkinsonism have been ruled out.

Table 2.2 Clinical diagnostic criteria of Parkinson's disease (Hughes et al, 1992), dementia with Lewy bodies (McKeith et al, 1996) and pure autonomic failure (Consensus, 1996)

Parkinson's disease (PD)

Bradykinesia and at least 1 of:
    Rigidity
    Rest tremor at 4–6 Hz
    Postural instability not caused by
    visual, vestibular, cerebellar or
    proprioceptive dysfunction

Features that support diagnosis (3 or more required for diagnosis of clinically definite PD):
    Unilateral onset
    Rest tremor present
    Progressive disorder
    Persistent asymmetry affecting the side of onset most
    Excellent (70–100%) response to levodopa
    Severe levodopa-induced chorea
    Levodopa response for $\geq$ 5 years
    Clinical course of $\geq$ 10 years

Exclusion criteria:
    History of repeated strokes with stepwise progression of parkinsonian features
    History of repeated head injury
    History of definite encephalitis
    Neuroleptic treatment at onset of symptoms
    >1 affected relatives
    Sustained remission
    Strictly unilateral features after 3 years
    Supranuclear gaze palsy
    Cerebellar signs
    Early severe autonomic involvement
    Early severe dementia with disturbances of memory, language and praxis
    Babinski's sign
    Presence of a cerebral tumor or communicating hydrocephalus on CT scan
    Negative response to large doses of levodopa (if malabsorption excluded)
    Methylphenyltetrahydropyridine (MPTP) exposure

Dementia with Lewy bodies (DLB)

Progressive cognitive decline of sufficient magnitude to interfere with normal social or occupational function, and:

Two (probable DLB) or one (possible DLB) of the following:

Fluctuating cognition with pronounced variations in attention and alertness

Recurrent visual hallucinations which are typically well-formed and detailed

Spontaneous motor features of parkinsonism

Features supportive of the diagnosis are:
Repeated falls
Syncope or transient loss of consciousness
Neuroleptic sensitivity
Systematized delusions
Hallucinations in other modalities

Diagnosis is less likely in the presence of:
Stroke disease, evident as focal neurological signs or on brain imaging
Evidence on physical examination and investigation of any physical illness or other brain disorder sufficient to account for the clinical picture

Pure autonomic failure (PAF)
Idiopathic sporadic disorder
Orthostatic hypotension, usually with evidence of more widespread autonomic failure
No other neurological features are present

CT, computed tomographic

Clinical criteria for DLB, established by consensus during the 1996 International Workshop on DLB (McKeith et al, 1996) and updated in 1999 (McKeith et al, 1999), are based on the presence of progressive dementia plus one (possible DLB) or two (probable DLB) of three major criteria: fluctuations on cognition, recurrent visual hallucinations and spontaneous parkinsonism. The presence of repeated falls, syncope, transient loss of consciousness, hypersensitivity to neuroleptics, systematized delusions and other modalities of hallucinations help to support the diagnosis. Specificity of the clinical diagnosis with these criteria is very high when validated by autopsy but sensitivity is low and variable. However, a recent prospective study reported a sensitivity and specificity of 0.83 and 0.95, respectively (McKeith et al, 2000). PAF was defined in a Consensus Conference in 1995. Clinical diagnostic criteria of these disorders is shown in Table 2.2.

Conclusions

A number of neurological disorders are characterized by the presence of LB in the nervous system. LB are composed mostly of α-synuclein and its presence is frequently associated with other synuclein pathology such as Lewy neuritis. It has been suggested that a spectrum of LB disorders occurs ranging from incidental Lewy body disease (asymptomatic individuals with few, mostly brainstem, Lewy bodies) to diffuse Lewy body disease (characterized predominantly by parkinsonism and dementia clinically and pathologically by abundant brainstem, limbic and cortical LBs). Included in the so-called Lewy body spectrum besides incidental LB disease and DLB are conditions such as PD and pure autonomic failure. The prominent clinical and pathological overlap that exists among these disorders support the spectrum concept. Studies in molecular genetics have furthermore shown that mutations in the α-synuclein gene and in other genes as well, can cause synucleinopathies presenting in a given family member as PD or as DLB.

The main clinical features shared by the LB disorders outlined above consist of parkinsonism, dysexecutive dementia and dysautonomia. Other clinical abnormalities frequently encountered in these disorders include RBD, hyposmia and excessive daytime sleepiness. Some nonmotor manifestations of PD such as RBD, depression or constipation may pre-date the development of the typical motor syndrome of PD. Consequently isolated RBD, hyposmia, depression or constipation, could in some individuals represent manifestation of an underlying LB disorder.

The concept of a spectrum of LB disorders is indeed appealing but several issues need to be clarified until we can embrace it. Although we know LB pathology has many causes, both genetic and environmental, we still do not know through which mechanism synuclein is deposited in the brain and how cell death occurs in these disorders. And we are unclear about how LB are formed and what they represent, whether an adaptive response or actually a pathogenic process. Until we clarify these and other relevant issues we suggest that clinicians should consider the various LB disorders as separate entities. After all each of them has its own clinical peculiarities and requires a differential clinical management.

References

Aarsland D, Larsen JP, Lim NG et al, Range of neuropsychiatric disturbances in patients with Parkinson's disease. J Neurol Neurosurg Psychiatry (1999) 67:492–6.

Aarsland D, Ballard C, McKeith I et al, Comparison of extrapyramidal signs in dementia with Lewy bodies and Parkinson's disease. J Neuropsychiatry Clin Neurosci (2001a) 13:374–9.

Aarsland D, Andersen K, Larsen JP et al, Risk of dementia in Parkinson's disease: a community-based, prospective study. Neurology (2001b) 56:730–6.

Aarsland D, Andersen K, Larsen JP et al, Prevalence and characteristics of dementia in Parkinson disease: an 8-year prospective study. Arch Neurol (2003) 60:387–92.

Abbott RD, Petrovitch H, White LR et al, Frequency of bowel movements and the future risk of Parkinson's disease. Neurology (2001) 57:456–62.

Allcock LM, Ullyart K, Kenny RA, Burn DJ, Frequency of orthostatic hypotension in a community based cohort of patients with Parkinson's disease. J Neurol Neurosurg Psychiatry (2004) 75:1470–1

Apaydin H, Ahlskog JE, Parisi JE et al, Parkinson disease neuropathology: later-developing dementia and loss of the levodopa response. Arch Neurol (2002) 59:102–12.

Arai K, Kato N, Kashiwado K, Hattori T, Pure autonomic failure in association with human α-synucleinopathy. Neurosci Lett (2000) 296:171–3.

Ballard C, Holmes C, Neill D et al, Psychiatric morbidity in dementia with Lewy bodies: A prospective clinical and neuropathological comparative study with Alzheimer's disease. Am J Psychiatry (1999) 156:1039–45.

Ballard CG, Aarsland D, McKeith I et al, Fluctuations in attention: PD dementia vs DLB with parkinsonism. Neurology (2002) 59:1714–20.

Boeve BF, Silber MH, Ferman TJ et al, Association of REM sleep behaviour disorder and neurodegenerative disease may reflect any underlying synucleinopathy. Mov Disord (2001) 16:622–30.

Boeve BF, Silber MH, Parisi JE et al, Synucleinopathy and REM sleep behaviour disorder plus dementia or parkinsonism. Neurology (2003) 61:40–5.

Bonelli SB, Ransmayr G, Steffelbauer M et al, L-Dopa responsiveness in dementia with Lewy bodies, Parkinson disease with and without dementia. Neurology (2004) 63:376–8.

Bonucelli U, Lucetti C, Del Dotto P et al, Orthostatic hypotension in de novo Parkinson disease. Arch Neurol (2003) 60:1400–4.

Braune S, Reinhardt M, Schnitzer R et al, Cardiac uptake of [123I]MIBG separates Parkinson's disease from multiple system atrophy. Neurology (1999) 53:1020–5.

Burn DJ, Rowan EN, Minnet T et al, Extrapyramidal features in Parkinson's disease with and without dementia and dementia with Lewy bodies: A cross-sectional comparative study. Mov Disord (2003) 18:884–9

Byrne EJ, Lennox G, Lowe J, Godwin-Austen RB, Diffuse Lewy body disease: clinical-features in 15 cases. J Neurol Neurosurg Psychiatry (1989) 52:709–17.

Calopa M, Tolosa E, Ferrer I et al, Cortical Lewy bodies in Parkinson's disease with dementia. In: Tolosa E, Schulz JB, McKeith IG, Ferrer I, eds, Neurodegenerative Disorders Associated with Alpha-Synuclein Pathology (Medicina stm editores: Barcelona, 2002) 127–34.

Chartier-Harlin MC, Kachergus J, Roumier C et al, Alpha-synuclein locus duplication as a cause of familial Parkinson's disease. Lancet (2004)364:1167–9

Chaudhuri KR, Nocturnal symptom complex in PD and its management. Neurology (2003) 61:S17–S23.

Consensus Committee of the American Autonomic Society and the American Academy of Neurology. Consensus statement of the definition of orthostatic hypotension, pure autonomic failure and multiple system atrophy. Neurology (1996) 46:1460.

Cubo E, Bernard B, Leurgans S, Ramam R, Cognitive and motor function in patients with Parkinson's disease with and without depression. Clin Neuropharmacol (2000) 23:331–4.

Edwards L, Quigley EMM, Pfeiffer RF, Gastrointestinal dysfunction in Parkinson's disease. Frequency and pathophysiology. Neurology (1992) 42:726–32.

Emre M, Dementia associated with Parkinson's disease. Lancet Neurol (2003) 2:229–37.

Gelb DJ, Oliver E, Gilman S, Diagnostic criteria for Parkinson disease. Arch Neurol (1999) 56:33–9.

Gibb WRG, Esiri MM, Lees AJ, Clinical and pathological features of diffuse Lewy body disease (Lewy body dementia). Brain (1987) 110:1131–57.

Gibb WR, Lees AJ, The relevance of the Lewy body to the pathogenesis of idiopathic Parkinson's disease. J Neurol Neurosurg Psychiatry (1988) 51:745–52

Giladi N, Treves TA, Paleacu D et al, Risk factors dementia, depression and psychosis in long-standing Parkinson's disease. J Neural Transm (2000) 107:59–71.

Grace JB, Walker MP, Mckeith IG, A comparison of sleep profiles in patients with dementia with Lewy bodies and Alzheimer disease. Int J Geriatr Psychiatry (2000) 15:1028–33.

Hague K, Lento P, Morgello S et al, The distribution of Lewy bodies in pure autonomic failure: autopsy findings and review of the literature. Acta Neuropathol (1997) 94:192–6.

Hantz P, Caradoc-Davies G, Caradoc-Davies T et al, Depression in Parkinson's disease Am J Psychiatry (1994) 151:1010–14.

Harding AJ, Broe GA, Halliday GM, Visual hallucinations in Lewy body disease relate to Lewy bodies in the temporal lobe. Brain (2002) 125:391–403.

Healy DG, Abou-Sleiman MA, Wood NW, PINK, PANK, or PARK? A clinician's guide to familial parkinsonism. Lancet Neurol (2004) 3:652–62.

Henderson JM, Lu Y, Wang S et al, Olfactory deficits and sleep disturbances in Parkinson's disease: a case-control survey. J Neurol Neurosurg Psychiatry (2003) 74:956–8.

Herlofson K, Larsen JP, Measuring fatigue in patients with Parkinson's disease – the Fatigue Severity Scale. Eur J Neurol (2002) 9:595–600.

Horimoto Y, Matsumoto M, Akatsu H et al, Autonomic dysfunction in dementia with Lewy bodies. J Neurol (2003) 250:530–3.

Huang Y, Cheung L, Rowe D, Halliday G, Genetic contributions to Parkinson's disease. Brain Res Brain Res Rev (2004) 46:44–70.

Hughes AJ, Ben-Shlomo Y, Daniel SE, Lees AJ, What features improve the accuracy of clinical diagnosis in Parkinson's disease: a clinicopathologic study. Neurology (1992a) 42:1142–6.

Hughes AJ, Daniel SE, Kilford L, Lees AJ, Accuracy of clinical diagnosis of idiopathic Parkinson's disease: a clinico-pathological study of 100 cases. J Neurol Neurosurg Psychiatry (1992b) 55:181–4.

Huisman E, Uylings HBM, Hoogland PV, A 100% increase of dopaminergic cells in the olfactory bulb may explain hyposmia in Parkinson's disease. Mov Disord (2004) 19:687–92.

Hurtig HI, Trojanowski JQ, Galvin J et al, Alpha-synuclein cortical Lewy bodies correlate with dementia in Parkinson's disease. Neurology (2000) 54:1916–21.

Ibanez P, Bonnet AM, Debarges B et al, Causal relation between alpha-synuclein gene duplication and familial Parkinson's disease. Lancet (2004) 364 (9440):1169–71

Jankovic J, Kapadia AS, Functional decline in Parkinson disease. Arch Neurol (2001) 58:1611–15.

Jankovic J, McDermott M, Carter J et al, Variable expression of Parkinson's disease: a base-line analysis of the DATATOP cohort. The Parkinson Study Group. Neurology (1990) 40:1529–34

Kaufmann H, Nahm K, Purohit D, Wolfe D, Autonomic failure as the initial presentation of Parkinson disease and dementia with Lewy bodies. Neurology (2004) 63:1093–5

Kosaka, Matsushita M, Oyanagi S, Mehraein P, A clinicopathological study of the 'Lewy body disease'. Seishin Shinkeugaku Zasshi (1980) 82:292–311

Kosaka K, Diffuse Lewy body disease in Japan. J Neurol (1990) 237:197–204.

Kruger R, Kuhn W, Muller T et al, Ala30Pro mutation in the gene encoding alpha-synuclein in Parkinson's disease. Nat Genet (1998) 18:106–8.

Larner AJ, Mathias CJ, Rossor MN, Autonomic failure preceding dementia with Lewy bodies. J Neurol (2000) 247:229–31.

Lewy FH, Paralysis agitans 1 pathologische anatomie. In: Handbuch der Neurologie. (Springer: Berlin 1912) Vol III: 920–3.

Litvan I, Mohr E, Williams J, Differential memory and executive functions in demented patients with Parkinson's and Alzheimer's disease. J Neurol Neurosurg Psychiatry (1988) 54:25–9.

Louis Ed, Goldman JE, Powers JM, Fahn S, Parkinsonian features of eight pathologically diagnosed cases of difuse Lewy body disease. Mov Disord (1995) 10:188–94.

Louis ED, Klatka LA, Liu Y, Fahn S, Comparison of extrapyramidal features in 31 pathologically confirmed cases of diffuse Lewy body disease and 34 pathologically confirmed cases of Parkinson's disease. Neurology (1997) 48:376–80.

Lowe J, Leigh PN, Disorders of movement and system degeneration. In: Graham D, Lantos PL, eds. Greenfield's Neuropathology (7th edn). Arnold: London (2002) 325–430.

Lücking CB, Durr A, Bonifati V et al, Association between early-onset Parkinson's disease and mutations in the parkin gene. French Parkinson's Disease Genetics Study Group. N Engl J Med (2000) 342:1560–7.

McKeith I, Fairbairn A, Perry R et al, Neuroleptic sensitivity in patients with senile dementia of Lewy body type. BMJ (1992) 19:673–8.

McKeith IG, Galasko D, Kosaka K et al, Consensus guidelines for the clinical and pathological diagnosis of dementia with Lewy bodies (DLB): report of the consortium on DLB international workshop. Neurology (1996) 47:1113–24.

McKeith IG, Perry EK, Perry RH, Report of the dementia with Lewy body international workshop. Neurology (1999) 53:902–5.

McKeith IG, Ballart CG, Perry RH et al, Prospective validation of consensus criteria for the diagnosis of dementia with Lewy bodies. Neurology (2000) 54:1050–8.

McShane RH, Nagy Z, Esiri MM et al, Anosmia in dementia is associated with Lewy bodies rather than Alzheimer's pathology. J Neurol Neurosurg Psychiatry (2001) 70:739–43.

Mathias CJ, Mallipeddi R, Bleasdalc-Barr K, Symptoms associated with orthostatic hypotension in pure autonomic failure. J Neurol (1999) 246:893–8

Mayeux R, Stern Y, Rosen J, Leventhal J, Depression, intellectual impairment and Parkinson's disease. Neurology (1981) 31:645–50.

Mori H, Hattori N, Mizuno Y, Genotype–phenotype correlation: familial Parkinson disease. Neuropathology (2003) 23:90–4.

Okazaki H, Lipkin LE, Aronson SM, Diffuse intracytoplasmatic ganglionic inclusions (Lewy type) associated with progressive dementia and quadriparesis in flexion. J Neuropathol Exp Neurol (1961) 20:237–44

Ondo WG, Dat Vuong K, Khan H et al, Daytime sleepiness and other sleep disorders in Parkinson's disease. Neurology (2001) 57:1392–6.

Pillon B, Dubois B, Lhermite F, Agyd Y, Heterogeneity of cognitive impairment in progressive supranuclear palsy, Parkinson's disease and Alzheimer's disease. Neurology (1986) 36:1179–85.

Pillon Ddubois B, Ploska A, Agyd Y, Severity and specifity of cognitive impairment in Alzheimer's, Huntington's and Parkinson's diseases and progressive supranuclear palsy. Neurology (1991) 41:634–43.

Plazzi G, Cortelli P, Montagna P et al, REM sleep behaviour disorder differentiates pure autonomic failure from multiple system atrophy with autonomic failure. J Neurol Neurosurg Psychiatry (1998) 64:683–5.

Poewe W. Psychosis in Parkinson's disease. Mov Disord (2003) 18:S80–S87

Ponsen MM, Stoffers D, Booij J et al, Idiopathic hyposmia as a preclinical sign of Parkinson's disease. Ann Neurol (2004) 56:173–81.

Rojo AA, Aguilar MM, Navas II, Quintana SS, Parkinsonism and the response to treatment in dementia with Lewy bodies (DLB). Mov Disord (2002) 17:S257–S258.

Salmon D, Galasko D, Neuropsychological aspects of Lewy body dementia. In: Perry R, McKeith I, Perry E, eds, Dementia with Lewy bodies. (Cambridge University Press: New York, 1996) 99–114.

Santamaria J, Tolosa E, Valles A, Parkinson's disease with depression: a possible subgroup of idiopathic parkinsonism. Neurology (1986) 36:1130–3.

Senard JM, Rai S, Lapeyre-Mestre M et al, Prevalence of orthostatic hypotension in Parkinson's disease. J Neurol Neurosurg Psychiatry (1997) 63:584–9.

Sethi KD, Clinical aspects of Parkinson disease. Curr Opin Neurol (2002) 15:457–60.

Schrag A, Jahanshahi M, Quinn NP, What contribute to depression in Parkinson's disease. Psychol Med (2001) 31:65–73.

Shiba M, Bower JH, Maraganore DM et al, Anxiety disorders and depressive disorders preceding Parkinson's disease: a case-control study. Mov Disord (2000) 15:667–669.

Starkstein SE, Preziosi TJ, Bolduc PL, Robinson RG, Depression in Parkinson's disease. J Nerv Ment Dis (1990) 178:27–31.

Singleton AB, Farrer M, Johnson J et al, Alpha-Synuclein locus triplication causes Parkinson's disease. Science (2003) 302(5646):841

Spira PJ, Sharpe DM, Halliday G et al, Clinical and pathological features of a Parkinsonian syndrome in a family with an Ala53Thr alpha-synuclein mutation. Ann Neurol (2001) 49:313–19.

Tandberg E, Larsen JP, Aarslan D, Cummings JL, The occurrence of depression in Parkinson's disease. A community-based study. Arch Neurol (1996) 53:175–9.

Thaisetthawatkul P, Boeve BF, Benarroch EE et al, Autonomic dysfunction in dementia with Lewy bodies. Neurology (2004) 62:1804–9.

Valente EM, Abou-Sleiman PM, Caputo V et al, Hereditary early-onset Parkinson's disease caused by mutations in PINK1. Science (2004) 304:1158–60.

Wakabayashi K, Takahashi H, Neuropathology of autonomic nervous system in Parkinson's disease. Eur Neurol (1997) 38(Suppl 2):2–7.

Wakabayashi K, Engelender S, Tanaka Y et al, Immunocytochemical localization of synphilin-1, an alpha-synuclein-associated protein, in neurodegenerative disorders. Acta Neuropathol (2002)103:209–14.

Walker MP, Ayre GA, Cummings JL et al, The clinical assessment of fluctuation and the one day fluctuation assessment scale. Two methods to assess fluctuating confusion in dementia. Br J Psychiatry (2000a) 177:252–6.

Walker MP, Ayre GA, Cummings JL et al, Quantifying fluctuation in dementia with Lewy bodies, Alzheimer's disease and vascular dementia. Neurology (2000b) 54:1616–24.

Wenning GK, Scherfler C, Granata R et al, Time course of symptomatic orthostatic hypotension and urinary incontinence in patients with postmortem confirmed parkinsonian syndromes: a clinicopathological study. J Neurol Neurosurg Psychiatry (1999) 67:620–3.

Witjas T, Kaphan E, Azulay JP et al, Nonmotor fluctuations in Parkinson's disease: frequent and disabling. Neurology (2002) 59:408–13.

Yoshimura M, Cortical changes in the parkinsonian brain: a contribution to the delineation of 'diffuse Lewy body disease'. J Neurol (1983) 329:17–32

Yoshita M, Taki J, Yamada M, A clinical role for ((123)I(MIBG myocardial scintigraphy in the distinction between dementia of the Alzheimer's type and dementia with Lewy bodies. J Neurol Neurosurg Psychiatry (2001) 71:574–5.

Zarranz JJ, Alegre J, Gomez-Esteban JC et al, The new mutation, E46K, of alpha-synuclein causes Parkinson and Lewy body dementia. Ann Neurol (2004) 55:164–73.

chapter 3

Classification and diagnostic criteria for dementia with Lewy bodies

Serge Gauthier and Ian G McKeith

The diagnosis of dementia with Lewy bodies (DLB) has been facilitated by the availability of diagnostic criteria based on expert consensus opinions followed by a number of validation studies. These diagnostic criteria are being re-examined periodically through international conferences, taking into account all available evidence, such as the International Psychogeriatric Association Expert Meeting on DLB, McKeith et al (2004). Despite all this work, there are still challenges in defining clearly what is DLB for the average practicing clinician. This chapter presents published diagnostic criteria for DLB along-side those currently accepted for Alzheimer's disease (AD), vascular dementia (VaD) and Parkinson's disease dementia (PDD), which often overlap clinically and pathologically with DLB.

Diagnostic criteria for DLB

The currently accepted diagnostic criteria for DLB were published in 1996 by the Consortium on Dementia with Lewy bodies (McKeith et al, 1996), and included central features, core features and supportive features (Table 3.1).

DLB can be recognized by clinicians on the basis of a progressive, disabling and fluctuating cognitive impairment with problem solving and visuospatial difficulties rather than memory and language impairment as seen in AD. Visual hallucinations are present in most patients early in the course of DLB, and less frequently parkinsonian-type rigidity. A number of validation studies

Table 3.1 Consensus criteria for the clinical diagnosis of probable DLB (McKeith et al, 1996)

Central features:
Progressive cognitive decline of sufficient magnitude to interfere with normal social or occupational function. Prominent or persistent memory impairment may not necessarily occur in the early stages but is usually evident with progression. Deficits on tests of attention and of fronto-subcortical skills and visuospatial ability may be especially prominent.

Core features, two of:
Fluctuating cognition with pronounced variations in attention and alertness
Recurrent visual hallucinations typically well formed and detailed
Spontaneous motor features of parkinsonism

Supportive features include:
Repeated falls
Syncope
Transient loss of consciousness
Neuroleptic sensitivity
Systematized delusions
Hallucinations in other modalities

have been published since the original publication of the Consortium on Dementia with Lewy bodies which suggest that these diagnostic criteria offer high specificity but relatively low sensitivity, which would improve if a biological marker for DLB was available. New recommendations and revised clinical criteria for diagnosing DLB have been proposed by the DLB Consortium and are due for publication (McKeith et al, 2005). The core features remain unchanged but greater diagnostic weighting has been given to severe neuroleptic sensitivity reactions and rapid eye movement (REM) sleep behavior disorder. Abnormal (low) activity of the dopamine uptake site in the basal ganglia, visualized by PET or SPECT neuro-imaging, is also recommended as suggestive of DLB compared with other dementia subtypes. The list of features supportive of a DLB diagnosis has also been extended to include severe autonomic dysfunction e.g. orthostatic hypotension, urinary incontinence, relative preservation of medial temporal lobe structures on CT/MRI scan, generalized low uptake on SPECT/PET perfusion scan with reduced occipital activity, abnormal (low uptake) on MIBG myocardial scintigraphy and prominent slow wave activity on EEG with temporal lobe transient sharp waves.

Diagnostic criteria for other causes of dementia

AD being the most common cause of dementia, there is no surprise in finding an overlap between AD and DLB on clinical and pathological grounds. Diagnostic criteria for probable, possible and definite AD have been proposed by the NINDS-ADRDA Work Group (McKhann et al, 1984) and are widely used since in epidemiological as well as therapeutic research (Table 3.2).

Criteria for VaD are still under debate, but the most widely used set of criteria (Table 3.3) have been proposed by the NINCDS-AIREN Work Group (Román et al, 1993).

There are no research criteria for PDD beyond the nonspecific DSM-IV definition of 'dementia due to other medical condition' (American Psychiatric Association, 1994). Fortunately, a number of clinical features (Table 3.4) have been identified (Emre, 2003) and will facilitate the work of a new Task Force on PDD of the Movement Disorders Society towards publishing research diagnostic criteria.

Conclusions

Today, clinicians with interest and experience in the diagnosis and management of dementia can differentiate DLB from AD, VaD and PDD. Research diagnostic criteria for these conditions are at different stages of maturity in terms of consensus opinion based on autopsy confirmation. Special efforts should be made on consensus opinions for biological and pathological criteria, and there must be recognition of the clinical and pathological overlap

Table 3.2 Criteria for the clinical diagnosis of probable AD (McKhann et al, 1984

Criteria for the diagnosis of probable Alzheimer's disease include:
- Dementia established by clinical examination and documented by MMSE, Blessed Dementia Scale or some similar examination, and confirmed by neuropsychological tests
- Deficits in two or more areas of cognition
- Progressive worsening of memory and other cognitive functions
- No disturbance of consciousness
- Onset between ages 40 and 90, most often after age 65
- Absence of systemic disorders or other brain diseases that in and of themselves could account for the progressive deficits in memory and cognition

Table 3.3 Criteria for the clinical diagnosis of probable VaD (Román et al, 1993)

Criteria for the clinical diagnosis of probable VaD include all of the following:

- Dementia defined by cognitive decline from a higher level of functioning and manifested by impairment of memory and of two or more cognitive domains, preferably established by clinical examination and documented by neuropsychological testing; deficits should be severe enough to interfere with activities of daily living not due to physical effects of stroke alone
- Cerebrovascular disease (CVD), defined by the presence of focal signs on neurologic examination consistent with stroke (with or without a history of stroke), and evidence of CVD by brain imaging
- A relationship between dementia and CVD, manifested or inferred by onset of dementia within 3 months following a recognized stroke and/or abrupt deterioration in cognitive functions, or fluctuating, stepwise progression of cognitive deficits

Table 3.4 Clinical features of dementia associated with PD (Emre et al, 2003)

Impaired attention with fluctuations

Impaired executive functions

Concept formation
Problem solving
Set elaboration, shifting, and maintenance
Internally cued behavior; benefit from external cues

Impaired memory

Impaired free recall; benefit from external cues
Well preserved recognition

Impaired visuospatial functions

Language largely preserved, except for verbal fluency

Praxis largely preserved

Personality changes

Multiple behavioral symptoms

between these conditions. Etiological research requires as homogeneous a disease as possible, but clinical and therapeutic research should take into account the fact that mixed dementias may predominate over pure cases of DLB, AD, VaD and PDD.

References

American Psychiatric Association. Diagnostic and Statistical Manual of Mental Disorders (4th edn). (APA: Washington DC, 1994).

Emre M, Dementia associated with Parkinson's disease. Lancet Neurol (2003) 3:229–37.

McKhann G, Drachman D, Folstein M et al, Clinical diagnosis of Alzheimer's disease: report of the NINCDS-ADRDA Work Group under the auspices of Department of Health and Human Services Task Force on Alzheimer's Disease. Neurology (1984) 34:939–44.

McKeith IG, Galasko D, Kosaka K et al, Consensus guidelines for the clinical and pathologic diagnosis of dementia with Lewy bodies (DLB): report of the consortium on DLB international workshop. Neurology (1996) 47:1113–24.

McKeith I, Mintzer J, Aarsland D, et al, Dementia with Lewy bodies. Lancet Neurol (2004) 3:19–28.

McKeith IG, Dickson DW, Lowe J, et al, for the Consortium on DLB. Dementia with Lewy Bodies: Diagnosis and Management: Third Report of the DLB Consortium. Neurology 2005; (in press).

Román GC, Tatemichi TK, Erkinjuntti T et al, Vascular dementia : diagnostic criteria for research studies. Report of the NINDS-AIREN International Workshop. Neurology (1993) 43:250–60.

chapter 4

Epidemiology of dementia with Lewy bodies

Carol Brayne, Julia Zaccai and Cherie McCracken

Introduction

Epidemiology underpins good clinical research, as it anchors it to population relevance. It aims to study the distribution and determinants of disease frequency, drawing on techniques and methodologies from biostatistics, social sciences and clinical medicine, as well as from the range of biological sciences such as genetics, toxicology and pathology. Descriptive epidemiology is concerned with the variation in patterns of disease in persons, place and time; and analytical epidemiology is concerned with testing specific hypotheses, usually regarding etiology. Through pattern variation and specific testing, potential determinants of, or risk factors for, disease can be elucidated. Such information is crucial to planning interventions and allocating resources. In the first instance, management of the disease requires knowledge of its prevalence and incidence. Prevalence is the cases existing at a given time in a given population, usually expressed as a percentage. Incidence is the rate of the numbers of new cases accruing over a given period in a given population, expressed either as a percentage or per person-years of risk. Two main factors are important when considering epidemiological studies because of their impact on estimates of the prevalence and incidence of any disorder: the definition of the disorder, or case criteria, and the population (sample) in which it is studied.

Case criteria

Dementia with Lewy bodies (DLB), once thought to be a syndrome described in isolated case reports, has been claimed to be the second most common type of degenerative dementia in older people. Depending on the case criteria used and the nature of the population studied, estimates from community-based clinical studies have been as high as one-quarter of all demented cases over the age of 65 (Shergill et al, 1994), similar to estimates from autopsy series which have ranged between 15% and 25% (Perry et al, 1990; Heidebrink, 2002).

The term DLB arose from the 1996 Proceedings of the First International Workshop of the Consortium on Dementia with Lewy Bodies (McKeith et al, 1996). Before this, there were several terms to describe the appearance of Lewy bodies in dementia. Among these were diffuse Lewy body disease, Lewy body variant of Alzheimer's disease, and dementia in Parkinson's disease (PDD). It was recognized that they have overlapping clinical and pathological features, and debate continues as to whether these represent the same disease approached from different perspectives. The neurologist and movement disorder specialists might diagnose PDD and the psychiatrist DLB. Estimates of prevalence and incidence may vary according to the discipline generating the definition and the range and sensitivity of diagnostic procedures used. If case criteria are not sufficiently precise and reproducible, conclusions from neuropsychological testing, imaging studies and neuropathology may result in various case classifications even when dealing with one disease entity. DLB undoubtedly has been included in other dementia subtypes in the past, and its importance can only be assessed if case criteria can be developed to allow clear separation of the disorder from other types of dementia. This is emphasized by the clinical implications of medication with neuroleptics versus cholinesterase inhibitors in DLB patients.

The World Health Organization's International Classification of Disease (ICD) and the American Psychiatric Association's Diagnostic and Statistical Manual (DSM) have not incorporated diagnostic criteria for DLB, which has hampered any attempt to identify it in many population-based epidemiological studies of dementia subtypes. For example, no separate category of cortical Lewy body disease was made in the Honolulu Asia Aging Study because White et al (1996) felt it was too difficult to make a valid diagnosis without the benefit of autopsy findings. The advent of diagnostic guidelines, such as the 1996 Consensus criteria (McKeith et al, 1996) (Table 4.1) has allowed its inclusion in more recently initiated epidemiological surveys with assessment by clinicians. These criteria derive from the Nottingham (Byrne et al, 1991) and Newcastle (McKeith et al, 1992) clinical criteria (Tables 4.2 and 4.3). There is a large degree of overlap between the two, with the main differences being that the Nottingham criteria do not allow acute confusion brought

Table 4.1 Newcastle criteria (adapted from McKeith et al, 1996)

1. The central feature required for a diagnosis of DLB is progressive cognitive decline of sufficient magnitude to interfere with normal social or occupational function. Prominent or persistent memory impairment may not necessarily occur in the early stages, but is usually evident with progression. Deficits on tests of attention and of frontal–subcortical skills and visuospatial ability may be especially prominent.

2. Two of the following core features are essential for a diagnosis of probable DLB, and one is essential for possible DLB:
   (a) Fluctuating cognition with pronounced variations in attention and alertness
   (b) Recurrent visual hallucinations that are typically well formed and detailed
   (c) Spontaneous motor features of parkinsonism

3. Features supportive of the diagnosis are:
   (a) Repeated falls
   (b) Syncope
   (c) Transient loss of consciousness
   (d) Neuroleptic sensitivity
   (e) Systematized delusions
   (f) Hallucinations in other modalities

4. A diagnosis of DLB is less in the presence of
   (a) Stroke disease, evident as focal neurological signs or on brain imaging
   (b) Evidence on physical examination and investigation of any physical illness or other brain disorder sufficient to account for the clinical picture

about by medication and have no requirement for visual hallucinations. The development of the criteria may have been influenced by the discipline of the groups responsible for them, namely, predominantly old-age psychiatry for the Newcastle criteria, and neurology, old-age medicine and old-age psychiatry for the Nottingham criteria (Shergill et al, 1994).

Fitting DLB into an epidemiological context

Prevalence and incidence can only be estimated from cases derived from defined populations. Within this defined population, there are two main methods for case-finding. The first is by relying on referrals from various healthcare services and patient groups that serve this known population. The second is by direct examination of the whole population sample. The latter is particularly valuable for direct generalization of findings, because participants are from all relevant subgroups of a population and not solely those already

Table 4.2 Nottingham criteria (adapted from Byrne et al, 1991)

- Diagnostic criteria for dementia associated with cortical Lewy bodies – A, B, C and D should be present to make a diagnosis of *probable* dementia associated with cortical Lewy bodies:

    A. Either (1), (2) or (3):

    (1) Gradual onset of dementia syndrome (which fulfils DSM-IIIR criteria) with prominent attentional deficits *or* the appearance early in the course of apparent acute confusional states for which no underlying toxic metabolic infective or other cause is identified, *or*

    (2) 'classical' Parkinson's disease (defined as levodopa-responsive parkinsonism) at onset with the later emergence of dementia syndrome (as described in 1), *or*

    (3) the simultaneous occurrence at onset of dementia (as described in 1) and parkinsonism.

    B. Both (1) and (2) should be fulfilled: (1) The absence of any unequivocal history of stroke; (2) no focal signs other than parkinsonism (note that the Hatchinski score is not reliable in this respect).

    C. Three or more of the following should be present: (1) tremor, (2) rigidity; (3) postural change; (4) bradykinesia; (5) gait abnormality. These symptoms may be mild and may develop late in the course of the illness, and abnormal involuntary movements resulting from levodopa treatment are unusual in parkinsonism with cortical Lewy bodies.

    D. Other causes of dementia syndrome or parkinsonism have been excluded (e.g. boxer's encephalopathy, chronic phenothiazine poisoning) after thorough clinical and laboratory investigation.

- A, B, C and D should be present to make a diagnosis of *possible* dementia associated with cortical Lewy bodies:

    A. Either (1) or (2):

    (1) Dementia (as described above) with acute onset and rapid course, sometimes associated with plateaux (periods where the symptoms do not progress) and frequently associated with psychiatric symptoms (depression or delusional states), *or*

    (2) dementia (as described above) with late presentation or parkinsonian symptoms will fulfil B.

    B. One or two of the following: (1) tremor; (2) rigidity; (3) bradykinesia; (4) postural change; (5) gait abnormality.

    C. (1) The absence of any unequivocal history of stroke; (2) no focal signs other than parkinsonism. Both should be fulfilled (note that the Hatchinski score is not reliable in this respect)

    D. Other causes of dementia syndrome and parkinsonism have been excluded, after clinical and laboratory investigation.

Table 4.3 Proposed operational criteria for senile dementia of Lewy body type (SDLT) (adapted from McKeith et al 1992)

A. Fluctuating cognitive impairment affecting both memory and higher cortical functions (such as language, visuospatial ability, praxis or reasoning skills). The fluctuation is marked with the occurrence of both episodic confusion and lucid intervals, as in delirium, and is evident either on repeated tests of cognitive function or by variable performance in daily living skills.

B. At least one of the following:
   (1) visual and/or auditory hallucinations which are usually accompanied by secondary paranoid delusions;
   (2) mild spontaneaous extrapyramidal features or neuroleptic sensitivity syndrome, i.e. exaggerated adverse responses to standard doses of neuroleptic medication;
   (3) repeated unexplained falls and/or transient clouding or loss of consciousness.

C. Despite the fluctuating pattern the clinical features persist over a long period of time (weeks or months) unlike delirium which rarely persists as long.

D. Exclusion of any underlying physical illness adequate to account for fluctuating cognitive state, by appropriate examination and investigation.

E. Exclusion of past history of confirmed stroke and/or evidence of cerebral ischaemic damage on structural brain imaging.

in contact with the healthcare system. Selection bias caused by the referral of patients from primary to secondary or tertiary care centers can affect the results of clinical or epidemiological studies (Sackett et al, 1979). Referral may differ according to the burden of symptoms, access to care, the 'popularity' of the disorder and institutions. In many cultures, dementia has been regarded as a normal part of aging, and patients are brought for help only when their behavior becomes troublesome (McKeith et al, 2004). The diversity between the general population and achieved research respondents is shown in Figure 4.1. It illustrates the problem of not knowing whether the findings on the research group are generalizable to the whole population.

The total dementia 'burden' in most populations is not identified. A case study conducted for the Organization for Economic Cooperation and Development (OECD) revealed that there generally has been no organized population-based or primary care effort directed at the early detection of dementia in the USA (to be published). In the English 'Forget-Me-Not' report by the Audit Commission (2002), fewer than half of the General Practitioners, who are the gatekeepers for specialized care, felt that they had sufficient basic and

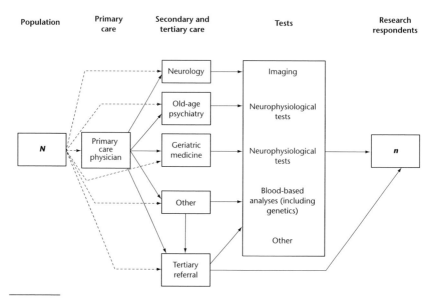

Figure 4.1 *Pathways through which individuals are filtered before becoming potential research participants. **N** = true population; **n** = study sample. Note: In systems such as in the UK, referral from secondary and tertiary services is almost always through primary care. This is not the case in all health care systems.*

postqualifying training for dementia. Thus, although dementia and its subtypes are becoming more recognized, one can fairly assume that many dementia cases go unnoticed by the healthcare system if one does not specifically screen the population. It is not known whether the prevalence of DLB would be higher in the general population than in a referred group, as these are groups with different denominators. The effect of the referral bias on the prevalence of DLB amongst the dementia group is also not straightforward to predict (see Figure 4.1).

A selected sample of papers reporting the prevalence and incidence of DLB has been chosen for this review as they illustrate the various methods used to date in DLB epidemiological research. These papers can be divided into two groups based on their choice of target population. The first group includes papers that base their results on participants who were recruited via secondary or tertiary referral centers. The data were either sourced from case notes or collected especially for the study. The second group includes papers that base their results on older participants recruited from within a defined geographical area. Details on the main characteristics and findings of each selected paper can be found in Tables 4.4 and 4.5.

Table 4.4 Main characteristics of a selected sample of studies reporting the incidence or prevalence of dementia with Lewy bodies (DLB)

Study	Population	Sample	Age (years)	Diagnosis	Dementia criteria	DLB criteria	DLB/ population	DLB/10000 population	DLB/ dementia	%
Case referrals										
Shergill et al (1994)	Dementia patient series, London	Case series	≥65	Psychiatrist	ICD-10	McKeith et al (1992) Byrne et al (1991)			30 of 114 27 of 114	26.3 23.7
Chan et al (2002)	Psychogeriatric inpatients, Hong Kong	Case series	≥65	Psychiatrist	DSM-IV, ADRDA, AIREN	McKeith et al (1992) Byrne et al (1991)			3 of 102	3.0
Harvey et al (2003)	In contact with medical, social and voluntary services	Reported cases	<65	Psychiatrist	ICD-10, DSM-IV, ADRDA, AIREN	McKeith et al (1996)			12 of 185	6.5
Population-based: prevalance										
Yamada et al (2001)	Rural town, Japan	Community census	≥65	Neurologist	DSM-IIIR, ADRDA, AIREN	McKeith et al (1996)	4 of 3715 (1.08/1000)	10 (3–30)	4 of 142	2.8
Herrera et al (2002)	Urban, Catanoluva, Brazil	Community random	≥65	Neurologist	DSM-IV, ADRDA, AIREN	McKeith et al (1996)	2 of 1656 (1.21/1000)	10 (2–40)	2 of 118	1.7
Stevens et al (2002)	Urban, North London	Community random	≥65	Psychiatrist	ICD-10, DSM-IV, ADRDA, AIREN	McKeith et al (1995)	22 of 1085 (20.27/1000)	200 (130–310)	22 of 72	30.5

Table 4.4 Main characteristics of a selected sample of studies reporting the incidence or prevalence of dementia with Lewy bodies (DLB) *cont.*

Study	Population	Sample	Age (years)	Diagnosis	Dementia criteria	DLB criteria	DLB/ population	DLB/10000 population	DLB/ dementia	%
Yamada et al (2002)	Urban, Japanese—Brazilian	Community census	≥70	Neurologist	DSM-IIIR, ADRA, AIREN	McKeith et al (1996)	0 of 157 (0/1000)	0	0 of 19	0.0
de Silva et al 2003	Urban, Ragama, Sri Lanka	Community random	≥65	Not known	DSM-IV, ADRDA, Hachinski	McKeith et al (1996)	1 of 703 (1.42/1000)	10 (1–80)	1 of 28	3.6
Haan et al (2003)	City, California, Latino only	Community census	≥60	Neurologist	None specified		1 of 1789 (0.56/1000)	10 (1–30)	1 of 138	0.7
Rahkonen et al (2003)	Urban, Kuopio, Finland	Community random	≥75	Neurogeriatric	DSM-IIIR, DSM-IV	McKeith et al (1996)	30 of 601 (49.92/1000)	500 (340–710)	30 of 137	22.0

aConfidence interval in parentheses.

Table 4.5 Study population characteristics from a selected sample of studies reporting the prevalence of dementia with Lewy bodies (DLB)

Study	Total no. included	Source	Urban	Method of recruitment	Criteria used
Case referrals					
Shergill et al (1994)	114	Consecutive referrals to old-age psychiatry services (case notes), UK	NA	NA	McKeith et al (1992) Byrne et al (1991)
Chan et al (2002)	102	Inpatient psychogeriatric population, Hong Kong	–	All dementia patients admitted in 1999–2000	Combined Byrne et al (1991) and McKeith et al (1992)
Harvey et al (2003)	227	Residents of selected London boroughs – referrals for further investigation	Yes	Asked for referrals	McKeith et al (1992)
Population-based					
Yamada et al (2001)	3715	Residents in Amino-cho rural town, Japan	Rural town	Door-to-door two-phase design	McKeith et al (1996)
Herrera et al (2002)	1656	Area of Catanduva (institutionalized included), Brazil	Yes	Selected every fourth address from census list plus all nursing home residents	McKeith et al (1996)
Stevens et al (2002)	1085	Geographical catchment area, 5% lived in care (residential or nursing care facilities), UK	Yes	Random enumeration districts in Islington, London	Altered McKeith et al (1995)
Yamada et al (2002)	157	Japanese–Brazilian residents of Campo Grande, members of 'Okinawa Kenjinnkai' association, Brazil	Yes	Random sample contacted by mail	McKeith et al (1996)
De Silva et al (2003)	703	Ragama town	Semi-urban	Randomly selected from four public health midwife areas	McKeith et al (1996)
Haan et al (2003)	1789	Self-designated Latino residents of the Sacramento Metropolitan Statistical Area and surrounding counties in California, USA	Urban and rural	Contacted all eligible candidates	?
Rahkonen et al (2003)	601	Kuopio City, including institutions	Yes	Random sample, all those > 75	McKeith et al (1996)

NA, Not applicable.

DLB prevalence estimates from case series and referral groups

Three papers are shown in Table 4.4 that fit into this first category. The Harvey et al (2003) study was a review of reported cases of DLB in contact with medical social and voluntary services, but as it is the only study that examines people under the age of 65 years, there is no basis for comparison of estimates. The next two studies used both the McKeith et al (1992) and the Byrne et al (1991) criteria, either separately or separately and in combination to review the case notes of patients who had been referred to a psychogeriatric service. The Shergill et al (1994) study, an analysis for subtype of all patients referred to a district general hospital in one year, shows wide variation in estimates, depending on which criteria were used. Thirty patients were found using the McKeith et al criteria (26%) and 27 patients (probable and possible combined) the Byrne criteria (24%), with some overlap of individuals between diagnostic criteria. Overall 82% of the cases according to Byrne et al fulfilled the McKeith et al criteria. Conversely, only 47% (14 of 30) of the cases according to McKeith et al fulfilled the Byrne et al criteria. The authors concluded that these differences probably reflected the different populations from which the diagnostic criteria were themselves developed (see above). The Chan et al (2002) study reported all dementia cases referred for inpatient care over a 2-year period to a unit serving a catchment area of 100 000 Hong Kong Chinese aged 65 or over. Individuals were considered a case if they fulfilled either or both of the criteria. Of the 102 people admitted with dementia, only 3 were diagnosed as having DLB. The three cases were reported as having cognitive fluctuation and visual hallucinations, but no standardized assessment of these symptoms was reported. To explain this low prevalence (3%), the authors suggested a low diagnostic sensitivity, especially in cases with mixed Alzheimer's disease (AD) and DLB symptomatology combined with low rates of postmortem examination and a higher preponderance of vascular dementia in Asian populations.

Despite the fact that the case criteria used by both Chan et al (2002) and Shergill et al (1994) were the same, there was substantial variation between the estimates. Because there are few data on the provenance of the samples, it is not possible to assess whether this may be due to a true difference in population rates. Although one advantage of studying disease occurrence in referral groups is that more in-depth investigation into the diagnosis can be done, this can be outweighed by referral bias.

Referral bias might result in identification of cases with different socio-demographic characteristics and suggest spurious associations. Specialized research samples derived from referrals have typically employed stringent selection criteria where, for example, DLB patients may be selected to have fewer comorbid conditions. It is known that the older population is charac-terized by the multiplicity and coexistence of more than one disease or syn-drome. This has rarely been systematically investigated. An illustration of this potential bias is shown in one study that does provide the sociodemo-graphic characteristics of three groups of patients with AD, the groups being population-based patients, patients referred from a near distance or patients referred from a far distance (Kokmen et al, 1993). This possible bias in sociodemographic variables has important implications for research, because some of these variables have been implicated as risk factors for AD. For exam-ple, the age at onset of symptoms is a marker of the severity, the genetic nature and the clinical course of AD. Kokmen et al (1993) also found differ-ences across population-based and referral AD groups for education, living arrangement, marital status and household composition. If one continues research solely in referred samples, DLB cases may be 'tagged' wrongly with a typical age of onset, associated with unfounded risk factors. A comparison between nonresponders, participants and noncompleters can help clarify possible impacts of sociodemographic differences between groups, but this has not been done systematically in all the studies reporting DLB prevalence.

DLB incidence and prevalence estimates from population-based studies

Which population group?

In comparison with case series and referral groups, population-based studies are not prone, by definition, to referral bias. Several studies on the epidemi-ology of DLB are population-based and participants have been recruited from all relevant subgroups of a population. This is considered to be the gold stan-dard for assessing the prevalence and incidence of a condition. There are particular difficulties in assessing a complex disorder such as DLB in older population groups. There is naturally a high mortality in this population seg-ment and eligible persons are often fragile, functionally dependent or even moribund (Riedel-Heller et al, 2000). If there are long delays between the ini-tial recruitment and the assessment, and if the participants are protected by their relatives from possible stress related to the examination, researchers may lose key participants from their study.

Recruitment from all relevant subgroups is not easily achieved in all populations, and different approaches are necessary, such as household enumeration, general practice lists and residential lists, ensuring the inclusion of, for example, institutions. Participants in the Cache County Study (Miech et al, 2002) were chosen solely on the basis that they were permanent residents of Cache County, Utah and were aged 65 years or older on 1 January 1995. The maintenance of the population representativeness of the study was investigated throughout, and those who dropped out from second-wave screening were compared with participants in terms of differences in gender, mean education and *APOE* ε4 alleles recorded at baseline. Researchers found that dropouts were significantly older and less educated, while those who completed screening but refused diagnosis were significantly more likely to be women.

The requirement to include institutionalized persons in a representative community sample in dementia studies has been subject to scrutiny. Based on a meta-analysis covering prevalence studies from 1945 to 1985 Jorm et al (1987) found no effect on the overall prevalence rates. They argued that institutionalized individuals represent only a small proportion of the elderly population and thus effects are marginal. In LEILA75+ (Riedel-Heller et al, 2000), which included institutionalized individuals, it was found that these were older, more often single and less often married, and seven times more likely to be demented than community-dwelling individuals. Two studies specifically mention screening for DLB in institutions (Herrera et al, 2002; Stevens et al, 2002). Herrera et al (2002) reported the prevalence of DLB in an elderly Brazilian population in Catanduva by sampling all elderly subjects living in 25% of the domiciles, at the subjects' homes and in all nursing homes in the community. Since DLB has unknown prevalence and features that could increase institutionalization, not screening for DLB in institutions could lead to biased prevalence estimates. It is difficult at this point in time, however, when different criteria or types of source population are used, to record the impact of including those institutionalized in studies assessing the prevalence and incidence of DLB.

Comparing population-based estimates of prevalence and incidence using different case criteria for DLB

Of the seven studies of community prevalence of DLB reported here, rates vary from 0% to 5% and as a percentage of all dementias from 0% to 30.5%.

Five studies used the McKeith et al (1996) criteria, one study used McKeith et al (1995) and the other (Haan et al, 2003) did not explicitly state the use of any criteria. This last study aimed to estimate dementia prevalence in older Mexican–Americans and to determine the distribution of dementia by etiology. Dementia diagnosis was made through a three-stage screening including cognitive testing (diagnosis requiring impairment in two or more cognitive domains), a clinical adjudication by a team of neurologists and a neuropsychologist, followed by magnetic resonance imaging (MRI) scanning and laboratory tests. While this procedure is very clearly explained, there is no account of the methods for differential diagnosis and it is difficult to know how the results (0.1% in population and 0.7% of dementias) can be compared. The Stevens et al (2002) study used rigorous methodology and diagnostic criteria (see Tables 4.4 and 4.5) based on McKeith et al (1995), and explored the relationships between the application of those criteria on the 107 people they found to be demented, 22 of whom with a diagnosis of DLB (21%) (7 probable and 15 possible). Application of DSM-IV to the 7 probable cases resulted in a diagnosis of 4 people with AD, 1 with vascular dementia, 1 with PDD and 1 unspecified. A similar pattern was found with the application of ICD-10. This suggests that in studies using only the main psychiatric diagnostic criteria that do not include DLB, cases will be forced into an AD diagnosis.

Comparison of the five studies using the McKeith et al (1996) criteria still shows a variation in level of DLB as a percentage of all dementias, from 0% to 22%. The Finnish study (Rahkonen et al, 2003), undertaken in the city of Kuopio, found the same high level of DLB (22%) as the Stevens et al (2002) study (21%). Again, this study was specifically designed to estimate the prevalence of DLB according to the consensus criteria in a general population – although of older people (75 years and older rather than 65). The authors comment that the major source of diagnostic difficulty for them was the reliable identification of fluctuating cognition – despite a long clinical examination and information from proxies. This may lead to underdiagnosis, especially in people living alone. The authors also note that the individuals they diagnosed with DLB were at a less severe stage of dementia and that the greater the severity, the more that AD and DLB become similar. The remaining four community studies of an urban Japanese–Brazilian population (Yamada et al, 2002), a city in Brazil (Herrera et al, 2002), an urban area in Sri Lanka (de Silva et al, 2003) and a rural town in Japan (Yamada et al, 2001) all had similar low levels of DLB as a percentage of all dementias (0–4%). Most study diagnosticians were neurologists. The main difference between these and the former studies is their emphasis on the prevalence of dementia per se rather than focusing on subtypes.

Two community studies that have reported the incidence of dementia subtypes have included DLB. Copeland et al (1999) cite 3 out of 263 cases of dementia (1.14%) and Miech et al (2002) 6 out of 185 cases (3.24%). As the latter study makes no reference to the diagnostic criteria and the former states that diagnosis was on the basis of clinical judgment (two psychiatrists and a neurologist), comparison of rates is difficult. However, Copeland et al report that there were a further 17 cases of dementia associated with delirium, Parkinson's disease, Pick's disease or mental retardation. If only 6 of these 17 cases were misdiagnosed and the DLB clinical diagnosis was similar, as were the methods, then it is possible to claim similar incidence rates.

Conclusions

Although the literature on the prevalence and incidence of DLB is limited, it is still clear that Lewy bodies must be considered in the range of neuro-degenerative conditions in the elderly. Considering all 12 studies reported in this chapter, it is difficult to assess whether the differences in source populations or the use of different case criteria had more effect on the estimates of the incidence and prevalence of DLB. It is clear, however, from the population-based studies that the use of different criteria leads to different estimates of rates of disease. Of the seven studies of community prevalence of DLB reported here, rates vary from 0% to 5%, and as a percentage of all dementias from 0% to 30.5%. Were all seven population-based prevalence studies to have been identical in methodology, their varying prevalence rates would give vital clues to etiology, especially given their wide geographical and potentially genetic spread. The combination of a study in Japan, another in Brazil and a third in Japanese–Brazilian immigrants would be even more powerful in the search for risk and in disentangling genetic and environmental factors. The move towards the more widespread use of consensus criteria is welcome. Their application in a more routine way towards rigorously defined and selected study populations will lead to more informative studies in the future.

References

Audit Commission, Forget Me Not 2002 – Developing Mental Health Services for Older People in England, Update. (Audit Commission: London, 2002) 49.

Byrne EJ, Lennox GG, Godwin-Austen RB et al, Dementia associated with cortical Lewy Bodies: proposed clinical diagnostic criteria. Dementia (1991) 2:283–4.

Chan SS, Chiu HF, Lam LC, Leung VP, Prevalence of dementia with Lewy bodies in an inpatient psychogeriatric population in Hong Kong Chinese. Int J Geriatr Psychiatry (2002) 17:847–50.

Copeland JR, McCracken CF, Dewey ME et al, Undifferentiated dementia, Alzheimer's disease and vascular dementia: age- and gender-related incidence in Liverpool. The MRC–ALPHA Study. Br J Psychiatry (1999) 175:433–8.

de Silva HA, Gunatilake SN, Smith AD, Prevalence of dementia in a semi-urban population in Sri Lanka: report from a regional survey. Int J Geriatr Psychiatry (2003) 18:711–15.

Haan MN, Mungas DM, Gonzalez HM et al, Prevalence of dementia in older latinos: the influence of type 2 diabetes mellitus, stroke and genetic factors. J Am Geriatr Soc (2003) 51:169–77.

Harvey RJ, Skelton-Robinson M, Rossor MN, The prevalence and causes of dementia in people under the age of 65 years. J Neurol Neurosurg Psychiatry (2003) 74:1206–9.

Heidebrink JL, Is dementia with Lewy bodies the second most common cause of dementia? J Geriatr Psychiatry Neurol (2002) 15:182–7.

Herrera E, Jr, Caramelli P, Silveira AS, Nitrini R, Epidemiologic survey of dementia in a community-dwelling Brazilian population. Alzheimer Dis Assoc Disord (2002) 16:103–8.

Jorm AF, Korten AE, Henderson AS, The prevalence of dementia: a quantitative integration of the literature. Acta Psychiatr Scand (1987) 76:465–79.

Kokmen E, Beard CM, O'Brieu PC, Offord KP, Kurland LT, Is the incidence of dementing illness changing? A 25-year time trend study in Rochester, Minnesota (1960–1984). Neurology (1993) 43:1887–92.

McKeith IG, Perry RH, Fairbairn AF, Jabeen S, Perry EK, Operational criteria for senile dementia of Lewy body type (SDLT). Psychol Med (1992) 22:911–22.

McKeith IG, Galasko D, Wilcock G, Bryne JE, Lewy body dementia – diagnosis and treatment. Br J Psychiatry (1995) 167:709–17.

McKeith IG, Galasko D, Kosaka K et al, Consensus guidelines for the clinical and pathologic diagnosis of dementia with Lewy bodies (DLB): report of the consortium on DLB international workshop. Neurology (1996) 47:1113–24.

McKeith I, Mintzer J, Aarsland D et al, Dementia with Lewy bodies. Lancet Neurol (2004) 3:19–28.

Miech RA, Breitner JCS, Zandi PP et al, Incidence of AD may decline in the early 90s for men, later for women: The Cache County study. Neurology (2002) 58:209–18.

Perry RH, Irving D, Blessed G, Fairbairn A, Perry EK, Senile dementia of Lewy body type. A clinically and neuropathologically distinct form of Lewy body dementia in the elderly. J Neurol Sci (1990) 95:119–39.

Rahkonen T, Eloniemi-Sulkava U, Rissanen S et al, Dementia with Lewy bodies according to the consensus criteria in a general population aged 75 years or older. J Neurol Neurosurg Psychiatry (2003) 74:720–4.

Riedel-Heller SG, Schork A, Matschinger H, Angermeyer MC, Recruitment procedures and their impact on the prevalence of dementia. Results from the Leipzig Longitudinal Study of the Aged (LEILA75+). Neuroepidemiology (2000) 19:130–40.

Sackett DL, Bias in analytic research. J Chronic Dis (1979) 32:51–63.

Shergill S, Mullen E, D'Ath P, Katona C, What is the clinical prevalence of Lewy body dementia? Int J Geriatric Psychiatry (1994) 9:907–12.

Stevens T, Livingston G, Kitchen G et al, Islington study of dementia subtypes in the community. Br J Psychiatry (2002) 180:270–6.

White L, Petrovitch H, Ross GW et al, Prevalence of dementia in older Japanese-American men in Hawaii: The Honolulu-Asia Aging Study. JAMA (1996) 276:955–60.

Yamada T, Hattori H, Miura A, Tanabe M, Yamori Y, Prevalence of Alzheimer's disease, vascular dementia and dementia with Lewy bodies in a Japanese population. Psychiatry Clin Neurosci (2001) 55:21–5.

Yamada T, Kadekaru H, Matsumoto S et al, Prevalence of dementia in the older Japanese-Brazilian population. Psychiatry Clin Neurosci (2002) 56:71–5.

chapter 5

Neuropsychological features of dementia with Lewy bodies

David P Salmon and Joanne M Hamilton

Since the discovery of the clinicopathological condition known as dementia with Lewy bodies (DLB) in the 1980s (Kosaka et al, 1984; Gibb et al, 1985, 1989; Dickson et al, 1987; Lennox et al, 1989; Hansen et al, 1990; Kosaka, 1990; Perry et al, 1990a,b), there has been considerable effort to identify neuropsychological features that uniquely characterize the disorder and distinguish it from Alzheimer's disease (AD). These efforts have been informed by neuropathological studies that have identified the typical distribution of brain abnormalities that occur in DLB. Patients with DLB have been shown to have subcortical pathology similar to that of Parkinson's disease (PD), but with fewer Lewy bodies and a milder degree of cell loss in the substantia nigra and in other pigmented brainstem nuclei (e.g. locus ceruleus and dorsal vagal nucleus; for reviews, see Perry et al, 1990a,b; Hansen and Galasko, 1992; Ince et al, 1998). They also have diffusely distributed cortical Lewy body pathology that primarily occurs in the cingulate, insula, amygdala, hippocampus, entorhinal cortex and transentorhinal cortex, and in the neocortex of the temporal, parietal and frontal lobes (Double et al, 1996; Kosaka and Iseki, 1996; Ince et al, 1998; Gómez-Tortosa et al, 1999, 2000; Harding et al, 2002). Abnormalities have also been noted in the occipital cortex of patients with DLB (Kosaka and Iseki, 1996; Pellise et al, 1996; Rezaie et al, 1996; Gómez-Tortosa et al, 1999; Higuchi et al, 2000; Harding et al, 2002), but these usually take the form of white matter spongiform change with coexisting gliosis (Higuchi et al, 2000).

The search for neuropsychological features that might distinguish DLB from AD is complicated by the fact that the majority of patients with DLB have concomitant AD pathology (i.e. neuritic plaques, neurofibrillary tangles) that is sufficient to meet standard criteria for AD (e.g. Khachaturian, 1985; Mirra et al, 1993). This AD pathology occurs in the same general distribution throughout the brain as in 'pure' AD (Armstrong et al, 1998; Gómez-Tortosa et al, 2000) and affects many of the same cortical areas as the Lewy body pathology. Both patients with DLB and those with pure AD also have widespread depletion of cortical choline acetyltransferase (ChAT), although the depletion is greater in DLB and also affects the striatum (Reid et al, 2000; Tiraboschi et al, 2000, 2002). Unlike AD, DLB is further characterized by a disruption of dopaminergic input to the striatum due to the loss of pigmented substantia nigra neurons (Perry et al, 1990a,b; for review, see Ince et al, 1998).

Given the similarities in the nature and distribution of neuropathologic changes in DLB and AD, it is not surprising that the two disorders result in similar dementia syndromes. Both disorders are initially characterized by the insidious onset of cognitive decline with no other prominent neurological abnormalities (Hansen et al, 1990; McKeith et al, 1996). Memory impairment is often the earliest feature of both disorders and with time cognitive deficits become widespread and patients inexorably progress to severe dementia. Indeed, the clinical manifestations are so similar that patients with DLB are often clinically diagnosed as having probable or possible AD during life (e.g. Hansen et al, 1990; Merdes et al, 2003). There are, however, several clinical features that occur with a higher prevalence in patients with DLB than in those with pure AD. These features include mild spontaneous motor features of parkinsonism (e.g. bradykinesia, rigidity, masked facies; but without a resting tremor), recurrent and well-formed visual hallucinations and fluctuating cognition with pronounced variations in attention or alertness (Hansen et al, 1990; McKeith et al, 1992, 1996; Beck, 1995; McShane et al, 1995; Galasko et al, 1996; Hely et al, 1996; Weiner et al, 1996; Ala et al, 1997; Graham et al, 1997; Verghese et al, 1999; Ballard et al, 2001; Harding et al, 2002; Merdes et al, 2003; for reviews, see Perry et al, 1996; Cercy and Bylsma, 1997). These clinical distinctions form the basis for consensus criteria adopted by the International Consortium on DLB (McKeith et al, 1996) to clinically diagnose DLB and distinguish it from AD.

The general similarities in the dementia syndromes engendered by DLB and AD raises the question of whether or not Lewy body pathology contributes importantly to the syndrome above and beyond the contribution of AD pathology. To address this issue, Samuel and colleagues (1996) compared quantitative measures of pathology and dementia severity in 14 patients with autopsy-verified DLB and 12 patients with autopsy-verified pure AD. Despite being matched for disease duration and having similar scores on mental status tests (i.e. the Mini-Mental State Exam (MMSE) and the Blessed Information–Memory–Concentration Test) when last evaluated prior to death, the DLB patients had fewer neurofibrillary tangles and total plaques than the AD patients, and the number of neurofibrillary tangles was correlated with severity of dementia in the AD patients but not in the DLB patients. Importantly, the number of Lewy bodies was correlated with severity of dementia in the DLB patients. This latter finding was replicated in a second study with a larger number of DLB patients ($n=17$; Samuel et al, 1997), but in this study the number of neocortical neuritic plaques and the severity of ChAT activity loss also correlated with the severity of dementia in the DLB patients (but see Sabbagh et al, 1999).

The findings of Samuel and colleagues (1996, 1997) indicate that the Lewy body pathology in patients with DLB contributes importantly to the severity of their dementia above and beyond the impact of AD pathology. This also suggests that Lewy body pathology, alone or in combination with AD pathology, may 'flavor' the particular pattern of cognitive deficits exhibited by patients with DLB and allow the pattern to be distinguished from that of patients with pure AD. Studies that have attempted to identify distinct patterns of cognitive deficits in patients with DLB and AD are discussed below.

Patterns of cognitive deficits in DLB

A number of studies have examined the pattern of neuropsychological deficits exhibited by patients with DLB across tests of various cognitive domains, and many have compared the pattern to that shown by patients with AD. Several early studies clearly demonstrated that patients with DLB have global cognitive dysfunction that includes deficits in memory, attention, executive functions, constructional praxis, and language (Gibb et al, 1985; Byrne et al, 1989). While these studies did not directly compare DLB and AD patients, the observed pattern of deficits was consistent with previous reports of the pattern exhibited by patients with AD. This initial impression was confirmed by a study that found similar degrees of language, praxis and memory impairment on the cognitive portion of the Cambridge Mental Disorders of the Elderly Examination (CAMCOG) in eight autopsy-confirmed DLB patients and eight patients with AD (Förstl et al, 1993).

One of the first studies to demonstrate distinct profiles of cognitive deficits in patients with DLB and AD was reported by Hansen and colleagues (1990). These investigators retrospectively examined the performance of nine patients with autopsy-proven DLB and nine patients with pure AD on a comprehensive neuropsychological test battery that included measures of memory, language, executive functions, attention and visuospatial abilities. All of these DLB patients had concomitant AD pathology and were identified as patients with the Lewy body variant (LBV) of AD. The DLB and AD patients were matched one-to-one on the basis of age, education, overall level of global dementia as assessed by the Blessed Information–Memory–Concentration Test, and the interval between cognitive testing and death. The results of this study showed that the DLB and AD patients were equally impaired (relative to elderly normal control subjects) on tests of episodic memory, confrontation naming (e.g. the Boston Naming Test) and arithmetic (i.e. the WAIS-R Arithmetic subtest), but the patients with DLB performed significantly worse than those with AD on a test of attention (i.e. the WAIS-R Digit Span subtest) and on tests of visuospatial and constructional ability (i.e. the WISC-R Block Design subtest and the Copy-a-Cross test). In addition, the DLB patients scored significantly lower than the AD group on the phonemically-based letter fluency task (i.e. generating words that begin with a particular letter) but the two groups performed similarly on the semantically based category fluency task (i.e. producing words that belong to a particular category such as 'animals').

Subsequent studies have generally replicated these findings in much larger cohorts of autopsy-confirmed or clinically-diagnosed DLB and AD patients (Yeatman et al, 1994; Gnanalingham et al, 1996; Wagner and Bachman, 1996; Connor et al, 1998; Galasko et al, 1998; Noe et al, 2003; Hamilton et al, 2004). In one such study, Galasko and colleagues (1998) found that 50 patients with autopsy-verified DLB (all with LBV) performed significantly worse than 95 patients with autopsy-verified AD on tests of visuospatial ability, verbal fluency, psychomotor speed and abstract reasoning. The groups did not differ, however, on tests of global cognitive functioning (i.e. the MMSE) or on specific tests of confrontation naming, general semantic knowledge, attention or episodic memory. A logistic regression model designed to distinguish between DLB and AD patients on the basis of scores achieved on tests of verbal fluency (i.e. the Phonemic Fluency Test), visuospatial ability (i.e. the WISC-R Block Design Test, the Clock Drawing Test), psychomotor speed (i.e. Part A of the Trail-Making Test) and general semantic knowledge (i.e. the

Number Information Test) was highly significant and correctly classified approximately 60% of patients with DLB and 88% of patients with AD.

The distinct patterns of neuropsychological deficits exhibited by DLB and AD patients on large batteries of rigorous cognitive tests are robust enough to be detected on relatively brief, standardized tests of mental status (McKeith et al, 1992; Connor et al, 1998; Ala et al, 2002; Aarsland et al, 2003). Connor and colleagues (1998), for example found that 23 patients with autopsy-verified DLB (all with LBV) performed significantly worse than 23 patients with autopsy-verified AD on the Mattis Dementia Rating Scale (DRS) Initiation/Perseveration subscale, a subscale that is heavily weighted towards verbal fluency and other executive functions. In contrast, the AD patients performed significantly worse than those with DLB on the Memory subscale of the DRS. When Connor et al (1998) limited their analyses to mildly demented patients, the DLB patients also performed significantly worse than the AD patients on the Construction subtest, a subtest that engages visuospatial and visuoconstructive abilities. This pattern of results was recently replicated in a larger sample of 60 autopsy-verified patients with DLB whose performance was compared to 29 clinically diagnosed patients with AD (Aarsland et al, 2003). Despite comparable dementia severity at the time of testing, Aarsland and colleagues (2003) found that the DLB patients had higher Memory subscale scores than patients with AD, but lower scores on the Initiation/Perseveration and Construction subscales. Interestingly, the subscale score profiles of patients with DLB were identical to those of patients with Parkinson's disease (PD) with dementia (i.e. patients who initially presented with idiopathic PD and then subsequently developed dementia).

Consistent with the discrepant patterns of performance on memory and visuospatial aspects of the mental status examinations, Hamilton and colleagues (2004) recently found that 24 patients with autopsy-confirmed DLB (all with LBV) performed significantly worse than 24 patients with autopsy-confirmed AD on several rigorous tests of visuospatial ability (i.e. the WISC-R Block Design Test, copying figures from the Visual Reproduction Test) but significantly better than the AD patients on rigorous tests of verbal episodic memory (i.e. the California Verbal Learning Test; CVLT, the WMS-R Logical Memory Test). These group differences were apparent despite similar levels of impairment on tests of language production (i.e. the Boston Naming Test) or global dementia (i.e. the MMSE). Similarly, Shimomura and colleagues (Shimomura et al, 1998) found that patients with clinically diagnosed probable DLB scored significantly worse than those with probable AD on tests of executive functions and visuospatial ability (i.e. the Raven Colored Progressive Matrices Test, the WAIS-R Picture Arrangement, Block Design, Object Assembly and Digit Symbol Substitution subtests), but significantly better on tests of orientation and word recall. A discriminant function analysis showed that the two groups could be most effectively differentiated by their scores on a word recall measure and the WAIS-R Block Design subtest. A similar finding was reported by Walker and colleagues (1997).

The discrepancy in the pattern of visuospatial and memory deficits exhibited by patients with DLB and AD was verified in autopsy-confirmed groups in a recent study reported by Salmon and colleagues (2002). Comparison of the neuropsychological test profiles of 66 patients with autopsy-verified DLB and 132 patients with autopsy-verified AD (samples overlapping those of Galasko et al, 1998) showed that patients with DLB were significantly more impaired (relative to normal control subjects) on tests of visuoconstructive ability (i.e. the WISC-R Block Design Test) than on tests of memory (i.e. the DRS Memory Subtest), whereas the opposite pattern was true for patients with AD. A derived measure of the difference between memory test and visuoconstructive test standardized scores (i.e. z-scores) revealed that these dissociable patterns of performance were apparent in both mild and moderate stages of dementia (see Figure 5.1).

The persistence of the dissociable patterns of neuropsychological performance exhibited by DLB and AD patients across mild and moderate stages of dementia in the cross-sectional study by Salmon and colleagues (2002) suggests that there are distinct patterns of cognitive decline in the two disorders. To address this possibility, Salmon and colleagues (1998) examined patterns of decline in a 1-year longitudinal study of 20 patients with autopsy-confirmed DLB (all with LBV) and 20 patients with autopsy-confirmed AD. The results of this study showed that the two groups exhibited similar rates of decline on measures of confrontation naming (i.e. the Boston Naming Test), general semantic knowledge (i.e. the Number Information Test) and episodic memory (i.e. the DRS Memory subtest), but the DLB patients declined more rapidly than those with AD on measures of verbal fluency (also see Ballard et al, 1996) and visuospatial abilities (i.e. the WISC-R Block Design Test). A similar difference in patterns of decline was observed in a study (Soininen et al, 1992) of clinically diagnosed AD patients with and without extrapyramidal motor signs (EPS). The AD patients with EPS (and a higher likelihood of clinical DLB) declined more rapidly over one year than those without EPS on tests of reasoning and abstraction, visuospatial abilities, praxis, verbal fluency and

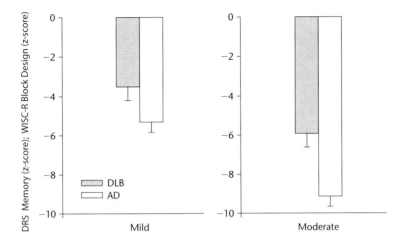

Figure 5.1 *The average discrepancy between Dementia Rating Scale (DRS) Memory and WISC-R Block Design standard scores (i.e. z-scores) for patients with Alzheimer's disease (AD; n=132) and patients with dementia with Lewy bodies (DLB; all with the Lewy body variant of AD; n=66). Despite equivalent levels of dementia, the discrepancy was smaller for patients with DLB than for patients with AD because of their greater visuospatial impairment (relative to normal control subjects) and smaller memory impairment. This pattern was maintained across mild and moderate levels of dementia.*

language processing. These differences in rate of decline occurred despite the two groups being equivalently impaired on all of these tests at their initial evaluation. This pattern of cognitive decline is consistent with the disproportionate decline in verbal fluency and visuospatial abilities displayed by autopsy-confirmed patients with DLB in the study by Salmon and colleagues (1998).

There is some evidence that the observed differences in the patterns of deficits exhibited by patients with DLB and AD are attenuated by the concomitant AD pathology that occurs in most patients with DLB. This is apparent when the performances of patients with pure AD are compared to those of DLB patients with or without significant concomitant AD pathology. The neuropsychological deficits exhibited by DLB patients without significant AD pathology (also known as patients with diffuse Lewy body disease or DLBD) were reported in a study by Salmon and colleagues (1996). These investigators retrospectively examined the test performance of five patients who presented with insidious cognitive decline that progressed to severe dementia and at autopsy were found to have subcortical and diffusely distributed cortical Lewy bodies with clinically insignificant AD pathology (AD pathology was absent in two cases and at a level comparable to that found in normal elderly individuals in the other three cases). When compared to patients with autopsy-confirmed pure AD, the DLBD patients showed similar levels of impairment on tests of language, attention and executive functions, but disproportionately severe deficits on tests of visuospatial or visuoconstructive ability (i.e. the WISC-R Block Design Test, the Clock Drawing Test) and psychomotor speed (i.e. Parts A and B of the Trail-Making Test). The memory performance of the patients with DLBD, in contrast, was less impaired than expected in relation to patients with AD. The discrepancy in the severity of visuospatial and memory deficits exhibited by the patients with DLBD was greater than the discrepancy displayed by patients with LBV (i.e. DLB with concomitant AD) in the study by Hamilton and colleagues (2004), and more distinct from the opposite pattern exhibited by patients with AD (see Figure 5.2).

The attenuation of the discrepancy in the severity of visuospatial and memory deficits exhibited by patients with LBV relative to those with DLBD suggests that the concomitant AD pathology that occurs in LBV worsens the memory impairment (as seen in the CVLT savings score in Figure 5.2) and reduces the saliency of the visuospatial deficit for a given level of global cognitive decline. Thus, the patterns of cognitive impairment are more distinct when comparing patients with DLBD to those with AD than when comparing patients with LBV to patients with AD. It should be noted, however, that both the cortical and subcortical Lewy body pathology present in DLB are likely to contribute importantly to the severity and nature of the dementia associated with the disease, whether AD pathology is present or not. Cortical features of the dementia such as impaired language, executive dysfunction and impaired visuospatial abilities may be mediated by the diffuse cortical Lewy body pathology that occurs in the disease, whereas cognitive deficits typical of subcortical dysfunction, such as impaired learning, decreased attention, impaired visuoconstructive abilities and psychomotor slowing (for a review, see Cummings, 1990), may be mediated by neuropathological changes in the substantia nigra and the corresponding depletion of dopaminergic input to the striatum (Perry et al, 1990a,b).

It is interesting to note that the cognitive abilities that appear to be disproportionately impaired in DLB are the same abilities that are mildly impaired in nondemented patients with PD. A number of studies have shown that compared to age-matched normal control subjects PD patients exhibit

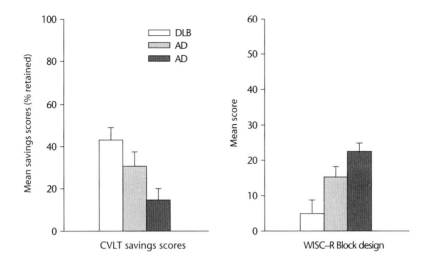

Figure 5.2 *The average scores achieved by patients with Alzheimer's disease (AD; n=24), patients with the Lewy body variant of AD (LBV; n=24) and patients with diffuse Lewy body disease (DLBD; n=5) on the retention savings score measure [(Long Delay Free Recall/Trial 5) × 100] from the California Verbal Learning Test (CVLT) and the WISC-R Block Design Test. The DLBD patients were less impaired than the AD patients on the episodic memory measure but more impaired on the measure of visuospatial ability. This dissociation with AD patients was more prominent for the DLBD patients than for patients with LBV.*

psychomotor slowing (Brown and Marsden, 1991) and have mild deficits in visuospatial abilities (Stern et al, 1993; Jacobs et al, 1995), verbal fluency (Jacobs et al, 1995), and other executive functions that are necessary to perform tasks such as the Wisconsin Card Sorting Test (Lees and Smith, 1983; Brown and Marsden, 1988), the interference condition of the Stroop Test (Brown and Marsden, 1991), dual-processing tasks (Brown and Marsden, 1991; Dalrymple-Alford et al, 1994), and tasks that require rapid shifts of attention (Filoteo et al, 1997).

As this brief review attests, studies of the neuropsychological features of DLB generally indicate that the disorder is characterized by a pattern of performance across tests of memory, executive function and visuospatial ability that is somewhat distinct from the pattern associated with pure AD. In the light of these differences, a number of studies have been designed to more closely examine the specific deficits exhibited by patients with DLB in each of these domains, and to compare and contrast these deficits to those of patients with AD. Studies that specifically focus on episodic memory, executive function and visuospatial ability in patients with DLB are reviewed in each of the following sections.

Episodic memory deficits in DLB

As previously mentioned, a number of studies have reported that the episodic memory deficits of patients with DLB are generally less severe than those of equally demented patients with AD (Salmon et al, 1996; Ballard et al, 1996; Graham et al, 1997; Walker et al, 1997; Shimomura et al, 1998; Connor et al, 1998; Heyman et al, 1999; Calderon et al, 2001). Few of these studies, however, have compared the specific components of episodic memory that are affected in the two disorders, or examined the relationship between these memory deficits and the underlying neuropathology. In one study that carefully addressed these issues, Hamilton and colleagues (2004) compared the performances of 24 patients with autopsy-confirmed DLB (all with LBV) and 24 patients with autopsy-confirmed AD on the CVLT and the WMS-R Logical Memory Test. Although the DLB and AD patients were equally demented as shown by equivalent scores on the Mattis DRS, they exhibited distinct patterns of performance on various components of the episodic memory measures (see Figure 5.3). The two groups were equally impaired in their ability to learn new verbal information on these tests, but the DLB patients exhibited better retention and recognition memory than patients with pure AD. These results substantiate the results of previous studies that used less rigorous memory tests with smaller samples of autopsy-confirmed (Salmon et al, 1996; Connor et al, 1998; Heyman et al, 1999) or clinically diagnosed patients (Ballard et al, 1996; Graham et al, 1997; Walker et al, 1997; Shimomura et al, 1998; Calderon et al, 2001).

The distinct patterns of memory performance exhibited by the DLB and AD patients on the CVLT and Logical Memory Test suggest that specific memory processes may be differentially impaired in the disorder. The severe learning deficit, rapid rate of forgetting of information, and severely impaired recognition memory exhibited by patients with AD is consistent with previous findings (Delis et al, 1991; Tröster et al, 1993) and suggests a primary impairment of encoding and storage in which information is unavailable even when retrieval support is provided by the recognition memory format (Delis et al, 1991). Despite similarly severe impairment in the learning and delayed recall

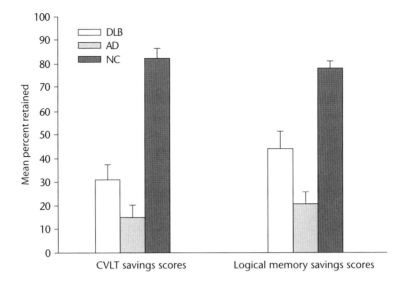

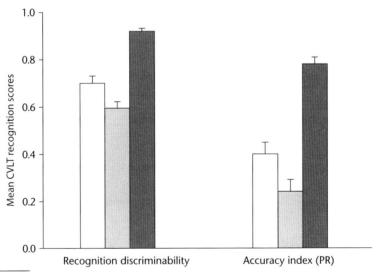

Figure 5.3 *The average scores achieved by normal control (NC) subjects (n=24), patients with Alzheimer's disease (AD; n=24) and patients with dementia with Lewy bodies (DLB; all with the Lewy body variant of AD; n=24) on various learning and memory measures from the California Verbal Learning Test (CVLT) and the WAIS-R Logical Memory Test. The DLB patients were less impaired than the AD patients on measures of retention [memory savings score = (total delayed recall/total immediate recall) × 100] and recognition memory (recognition discriminability and recognition accuracy index known as PR from the two-high threshold model). (Adapted from Hamilton et al, 2004).*

conditions when free recall was required, the patients with DLB had higher savings scores (i.e. the amount of information recalled after a delay as a percentage of the amount recalled immediately) and performed better on the recognition memory component of the CVLT compared to the AD patients. These differences in performance suggest that a deficit in retrieval plays a greater role in the memory impairment of patients with DLB than in that of patients with AD. While the pattern of deficits does not rule out the possibility that poor encoding contributes to memory impairment in the two disorders, it is clear that DLB patients have better retention than patients with AD when retrieval demands are reduced through the use of the recognition format.

The observed differences in the severity of impairment of specific memory processes in DLB and AD are consistent with the particular pathological changes that occur in the two disorders. As mentioned previously, a number of studies using neuropathologic (Lippa et al, 1994, 1998) or magnetic resonance imaging (Hashimoto et al, 1998; Barber et al, 2000, 2001) procedures have shown that the medial temporal lobe structures important for memory (e.g. hippocampus, entorhinal cortex, parahippocampal gyrus) are more severely affected in AD than in DLB. The extensive damage to these structures that occurs in AD is thought to mediate the severe amnesia that characterizes the disorder (Hyman et al, 1990). In contrast, damage to subcortical structures that are affected in Parkinson's disease and other disorders of the basal ganglia (e.g. Huntington's disease) are more affected in DLB than in AD. Damage to these structures has been implicated in a memory disorder characterized by a general deficit in the ability to initiate and carry out the systematic retrieval of successfully stored information (Martone et al, 1984; Butters et al, 1985, 1986; Moss et al, 1986; Delis et al, 1991). Thus, the less severe retention deficit and the greater impact of deficient retrieval processes in DLB than in AD is consistent with the combination of moderate medial temporal lobe damage and fronto-striatal dysfunction that occurs in the disease.

This interpretation of the basis of the episodic memory deficit exhibited by patients with DLB suggests that the distinction between their performance and that of AD patients would be even greater in that subset of DLB patients without concomitant AD pathology. Once the extensive medial temporal lobe damage associated with AD is removed, the deficient retrieval processes mediated by subcortical dysfunction in DLB may become more prominent. This appears to be the case when the CVLT performance of patients with DLBD is examined (Salmon et al, 1996). All five of the DLBD patients examined by

Salmon and colleagues (1996) scored 2–3 standard deviations below normal performance on key measures of the CVLT, but their performance differed from that typically observed in patients with AD. Whereas mildly demented AD patients usually exhibit severe impairment on CVLT measures of immediate learning and recall, retention, and recognition discriminability (Delis et al, 1991), the patients with DLBD exhibited only mild deficits in retention and recognition discriminability. This distinction can be clearly seen when the CVLT retention and recognition memory scores of the DLBD patients are directly compared to those of the AD patients from the study by Hamilton and colleagues (2004) (see Figure 5.4). It can also be seen that the discrepancy in the patterns of memory performance exhibited by the AD and DLB (all with LBV) patients in the Hamilton et al (2004) study are even more prominent when AD patients are compared to patients with DLBD.

It is interesting to note that the nature of the memory deficit associated with DLBD appears to reflect ineffective retrieval similar to that observed in

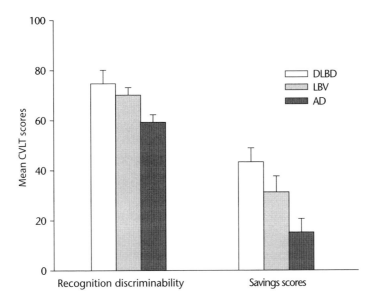

Figure 5.4   *The average scores achieved by patients with Alzheimer's disease (AD; n=24), patients with the Lewy body variant of AD (LBV; n=24) and patients with diffuse Lewy body disease (DLBD; n=5) on the recognition discriminability and retention savings score measures from the California Verbal Learning Test (CVLT). The DLBD patients were less impaired than the AD patients on both measures of episodic memory and this difference was more prominent than for patients with LBV.*

other patients with striatal dysfunction (Butters et al, 1986). Although ubiquitin-immunoreactive dystrophic neurites are often present in the CA2-3 region of the hippocampus in patients with DLBD (Dickson et al, 1991, 1994), the hippocampus and related structures (e.g. entorhinal cortex, parahippocampal gyrus) that are thought to underlie memory storage are generally less damaged than in AD (Lippa et al, 1994). This disparity leads to overall milder memory impairment in patients with DLBD than in those with AD, and to a pattern of deficits that is similar to that of patients with subcortical disorders (e.g. Parkinson's disease, Huntington's disease). Indeed, when the scores of the DLBD patients in the Salmon et al (1996) study were subjected to discriminant function equations that have been previously shown to effectively distinguish between patients with cortical (e.g. AD) and subcortical (e.g. Huntington's disease) dementia using key CVLT measures, four of the five DLBD patients were classified as 'subcortical' and only one as 'cortical'.

Deficits in executive function and attention in DLB

Studies that have examined the pattern of neuropsychological deficits associated with DLB often show that patients with the disorder have disproportionately severe deficits in executive functions and attention compared to equally demented patients with pure AD. This is evident on tests of attention such as the WAIS-R Digit Span subtest (Hansen et al, 1990) and the Cancellation Test (Noe et al, 2004), tests of initiation and systematic retrieval from semantic memory such as the Initiation/Perseveration subscale of the DRS (Connor et al, 1998; Aarsland et al, 2003) and the phonemic verbal fluency test (Hansen et al, 1990; Ballard et al, 1996; Galasko et al, 1998; Salmon et al, 1998), and tests of abstract reasoning such as the Raven Colored Progressive Matrices (Shimomura et al, 1998) or the WAIS-R Similarities subtest (Galasko et al, 1998).

These deficits were examined in detail in a series of studies carried out to compare the performances of clinically diagnosed DLB and AD patients on a microcomputer-based testing paradigm (i.e. the CANTAB) that allowed a detailed assessment of working memory, attention, and executive functions such as attentional set shifting, conditional pattern discrimination learning, and strategic thinking. In the first of these studies, Galloway and colleagues (Galloway et al, 1992) found that 7 patients with probable DLB and 10 patients with probable AD were equally impaired on a recognition memory test, but DLB patients required significantly more trials than patients with

AD to reach a learning criterion on a conditional pattern-location, paired-associates learning task. In a second study in this series, Sahgal and colleagues (1992a) showed that while the same AD and DLB subjects from the Galloway et al study were impaired on simultaneous and delayed matching to sample tasks, patients with probable DLB performed worse than those with probable AD only in the delayed condition. Sahgal and colleagues also showed in a third study (Sahgal et al, 1992b) that these same DLB and AD patients were equally impaired on a complex set-shifting task that required both intradimensional (i.e. from one set of lines to another) and extradimensional (i.e. from lines to colors) shifts of attention, but only the patients with DLB were impaired (relative to normal control subjects) on a visual search task that assessed the ability to focus attention. In a final study in this series, Sahgal and colleagues (1995) compared the performance of DLB and AD patients on a spatial working memory task that assessed both spatial memory and the ability to use an efficient search strategy. In this task, subjects were required to search through a number of boxes presented on a computer screen in order to locate a hidden 'token'. They were not to re-examine an empty box before finding the token on the current trial (i.e. a within-search error), nor were they to search a box in which the token had been found on a previous trial (i.e. a between-search error). The results showed that patients with probable DLB made more within-search and between-search errors than those with probable AD, but the groups did not differ in the search strategies they used to complete the task.

The prominent deficits in attention and executive functions exhibited by patients with DLB are consistent with the cortical and subcortical dysfunction that occurs in the disorder. These same cognitive deficits often occur in patients with basal ganglia dysfunction (e.g. Parkinson's disease and Huntington's disease) and have been attributed to the interruption of anatomically and functionally distinct circuits that link the frontal cortex with subcortical structures (for review, see Alexander, DeLong and Strick, 1986). These fronto-subcortical circuits may be affected in two ways in patients with DLB: by direct neocortical Lewy body pathology in the association areas of the frontal lobes and by substantia nigra pathology that interrupts dopaminergic projections to the striatum. When overlaid upon the pathological changes that occur in AD, the fronto-subcortical dysfunction of DLB may result in disproportionately severe deficits in executive function and attention.

Deficits in visuospatial abilities in DLB

A profound deficit in visuospatial and visuoconstructive abilities is one of the most consistent findings in studies examining the neuropsychological features of DLB. Numerous studies have shown that patients with DLB have disproportionately severe deficits in these abilities compared to equally demented patients with pure AD. The DLB patient's prominent visuospatial dysfunction has been shown using tests of visual perception (Mori et al, 2000; Calderon et al, 2001; Lambon Ralph et al, 2001), tests of visual search (Cormack et al, 2004), and tests that require drawing simple and complex two-dimensional figures (Hansen et al, 1990; Salmon et al, 1996; Gnanalingham et al, 1996, 1997; Galasko et al, 1998; Connor et al, 1998; Aarsland et al, 2003; Noe et al, 2004) or the construction of three dimensional objects (Hansen et al, 1990; Shimomura et al, 1998; Salmon et al, 2002; Hamilton et al, 2004).

In a study that examined visuoperceptual abilities, Calderon and colleagues (2001) found that 10 patients with probable DLB performed significantly worse than 9 patients with probable AD on tests of fragmented letter identification, discrimination of 'real' objects from non-objects, and segregation of overlapping figures. These particularly severe deficits in visuospatial and visuoperceptual abilities were apparent even though the DLB patients performed significantly better than the patients with AD on a verbal memory test and at the same level on tests of semantic memory (also see Lambon Ralph et al, 2001). Similar results were obtained by Mori and colleagues (2000) who found that 24 patients with probable DLB performed significantly worse than 48 equally demented patients with probable AD on tests of visual attention, size and form discrimination and visual figure-ground segregation. Mori and colleagues noted that DLB patients with visual hallucinations were more impaired than those without hallucinations on the figure-ground segregation test. Simard and colleagues (2003) reported a similar finding in which patients with probable DLB with visual hallucinations performed worse than those without hallucinations on the Benton Judgment of Line Orientation task.

A recent study focused upon the effects of DLB on the ability to carry out visual search (Cormack et al, 2004). Cormack and colleagues (2004) compared the performances of 15 patients with probable DLB and 18 patients with AD on visual search tasks that engaged either parallel or serial search processes. The parallel search task required subjects to quickly find a single red circle (target) within arrays of 2, 8, or 16 green circles (distracters). Normal individuals detect the target at a preattentive level in this task as the target appears to 'pop out' from the background distracters. The size of the distracter set has little influence on speed of detecting the target in this situation. The serial search task required subjects to quickly find a single red circle (target) within arrays of 2, 8 or 16 green circles and red squares (distracters). To perform this task, normal individuals must integrate extracted visual features using the sequential deployment of attention. Thus, the larger the number of distracters, the longer the serial search process takes. Because the parallel search process is thought to be mediated by occipitotemporal cortex and the serial search process by occipitoparietal cortex, the investigators hypothesized that parallel search might be prominently affected in patients with DLB due to their occipital and temporal cortex dysfunction while serial search might be impaired, but to a lesser degree, because of their additional mild parietal cortex damage. Patients with AD, in contrast, were not expected to be impaired on either search task because the integrity of their occipital cortex is largely maintained. The results of the study generally supported this hypothesis. The DLB patients showed a much greater deficit in parallel search (i.e. a failure of the 'pop-out' phenomenon) than did the patients with AD. However, the AD patients tended to show the expected sensitivity to the distracter set size in the serial search task while the DLB patients did not. Thus, the DLB patients were more impaired than the AD patients in both preattentive and feature integration conditions, with particularly striking deficits in preattentive parallel search processes. Performance on the parallel search task provided relatively good sensitivity (85%) and specificity (87%) for distinguishing patients with DLB from those with AD, but this finding needs to be replicated in larger samples.

The prominent deficits in visuoperceptual, visuospatial and visuoconstructional abilities exhibited by patients with DLB are consistent with the neuropathological changes that occur in the cortex of the occipital lobes. Some Lewy body pathology occurs in the occipital cortex (Kosaka and Isekil, 1996; Pellise et al, 1996; Rezaie et al, 1996; Gómez-Tortosa et al, 1999; Higuchi et al, 2000; Harding et al, 2002) of DLB patients, but white matter spongiform change with coexisting gliosis appears to be the most prominent feature of occipital lobe pathology associated with the disorder (Higuchi et al, 2000). This occipital pathology is accompanied by hypometabolism and decreased blood flow in primary visual and visual association cortex that is evident with positron emission tomography (PET) or single-photon emission computed tomography (SPECT) scanning (Albin et al, 1996; Ishii et al, 1998; Imamura et al, 1999, 2001; Higuchi et al, 2000; Lobotesis et al, 2001; Minoshima et al, 2001) relatively early in the course of the disorder. Because the occipital cortex is generally spared in AD, it is not surprising that functions that may be dependent upon these cortices, such as visuoperceptual and visuospatial abilities, are disproportionately impaired in patients with DLB.

Conclusions

Neuropsychological studies indicate that distinct features of the cognitive decline associated with DLB might aid in its clinical diagnosis and in differentiating the disorder from probable AD (See Table 5.1 for a summary). Although both DLB and AD result in global cognitive impairment with

Table 5.1 Summary of the relative patterns of cognitive deficits in mildly demented patients with Alzheimer's disease (AD) or dementia with Lewy bodies (DLB)

	DLB		AD
	DLBD	LBV	
Attention	Moderate	Moderate	Mild
Executive functions	Moderate/severe	Moderate/severe	Moderate
Psychomotor speed	Moderate/severe	Moderate	Mild
Language			
Confrontation naming	Mild	Mild	Mild
Semantic fluency	Moderate	Moderate	Moderate
Phonemic fluency	Moderate	Moderate	Mild
Memory			
Free recall	Mild/moderate	Moderate/severe	Severe
Recognition	Mild	Moderate	Severe
Retention	Mild	Moderate	Severe
Visuospatial abilities			
Constructional praxis	Severe	Moderate/severe	Mild
Visuoperception	Moderate/severe	Moderate/severe	Mild

LBV, Lewy body variant of AD (DLB patients with concomitant AD pathology); DLBD, diffuse Lewy body disease (DLB patients without concomitant AD pathology).

similar deficits in learning and language abilities, patients with DLB appear to have disproportionately severe deficits in visuospatial abilities, some aspects of attention and executive functions, and psychomotor speed. The nature of the memory deficits associated with DLB and AD are also somewhat distinct with DLB patients exhibiting milder deficits in retention and recognition memory than patients with AD. The apparent double dissociation between the severity of visuospatial and episodic memory deficits in the two groups suggests that the distinct patterns of performance cannot be easily attributed to differences in dementia severity or difficulty of the various cognitive tasks, but instead reflects a true difference in the brain-behavior relationships underlying DLB and AD.

The pattern of neuropsychological deficits exhibited by patients with DLB suggests that they are often as severely impaired as patients with AD in those cognitive abilities usually affected by AD pathology (e.g. aspects of episodic memory, language), but more impaired in those abilities thought to be additionally affected by subcortical (and possibly neocortical) Lewy body pathology (e.g. verbal fluency, psychomotor speed, visuospatial/constructional ability; Alexander et al, 1986). This suggests that both AD and Lewy body pathology contribute importantly to the cognitive manifestations of DLB. However, the specific neuropsychological processes and neuropathological factors that underlie the cognitive changes of DLB remain largely unknown and should be the focus of additional systematic clinicopathological study.

References

Aarsland D, Litvan I, Salmon D, Galasko D et al, Performance on the dementia rating scale in Parkinson's disease with dementia and dementia with Lewy bodies: comparison with progressive supranuclear palsy and Alzheimer's disease. J Neurol Neurosurg Psychiatry (2003) 74:1215–20.

Ala TA, Yang KH, Sung JH, Frey WH, Hallucinations and signs of parkinsonism help distinguish patients with dementia and cortical Lewy bodies from patients with Alzheimer's disease at presentation: A clinicopathological study. J Neurol Neurosurg Psychiatry (1997) 62:16–21.

Ala TA, Hughes LF, Kyrouac GA et al The Mini-Mental State exam may help in the differentiation of dementia with Lewy bodies and Alzheimer's disease. Int J Geriatr Psychiatry (2002) 17:503–9.

Albin RL, Minoshima S, D'Amato CJ et al, Fluoro-deoxyglucose positron emission tomography in diffuse Lewy body disease. Neurology (1996) 47:462–6.

Alexander GE, Delong MR, Strick PL, Parallel organization of functionally segregated circuits linking basal ganglia and cortex. Ann Rev Neurosci (1986) 9:357–81.

Armstrong RA, Cairns NJ, Lantos PL, The spatial patterns of Lewy bodies, senile plaques, and neurofibrillary tangles in dementia with Lewy bodies. Exp Neurol (1998) 150:122–7.

Ballard C, Patel A, Oyebode F, Wilcock G, Cognitive decline in patients with Alzheimer's disease, vascular dementia and senile dementia of the Lewy body type. Age Ageing (1996) 25:209–13.

Ballard C, O'Brien J, Gray A et al, Attention and fluctuating attention in patients with dementia with Lewy bodies and Alzheimer disease. Arch Neurol (2001) 58:977–82.

Barber R, Ballard C, McKeith IG et al, MRI volumetric study of dementia with Lewy bodies: a comparison with AD and vascular dementia. Neurology (2000) 54:1304–9.

Barber R, McKeith IG, Ballard C et al, A comparison of medial and lateral temporal lobe atrophy in dementia with Lewy bodies and Alzheimer's disease: magnetic resonance imaging volumetric study. Dement Geriatr Cogn Disord (2001) 12:198–205.

Beck BJ Neuropsychiatric manifestations of diffuse Lewy body disease. J Geriatr Psychiatry Neurol (1995) 8:189–96.

Brown RG, Marsden CD, An investigation of the phenomenon of 'set' in Parkinson's disease. Move Disord (1988) 3:152–61.

Brown RG, Marsden CD, Dual task performance and processing resources in normal subjects and patients with Parkinson's disease. Brain (1991) 114:215–31.

Butters N, Wolfe J, Martone M et al, Memory disorders associated with Huntington's Disease: Verbal recall, verbal recognition and procedural memory. Neuropsychologia (1985) 23:729–43.

Butters N, Wolfe J, Granholm E, Martone M, An assessment of verbal recall, recognition, and fluency abilities in patients with Huntington's disease. Cortex (1986) 22:11–32.

Byrne EJ, Lennox G, Lowe J et al, Diffuse Lewy body disease: Clinical features in 15 cases. J Neurol Neurosurg Psychiatry (1989) 52:709–17.

Calderon J, Perry RJ, Erzinclioglu SW et al, Perception, attention, and working memory are disproportionately impaired in dementia with Lewy bodies compared with Alzheimer's disease. J Neurol Neurosurg Psychiatry (2001) 70:157–64.

Cercy SP, Bylsma FW, Lewy body and progressive dementia: A critical review and meta-analysis. J Int Neuropsychol Soc (1997) 3:179–94.

Connor DJ, Salmon DP, Sandy TJ et al, Cognitive profiles of autopsy-confirmed Lewy body variant vs. pure Alzheimer's disease. Arch Neurol (1998) 55:994–1000.

Cormak F, Gray A, Ballard C, Tovee MJ, A failure of 'pop-out' in visual search tasks in dementia with Lewy bodies as compared to Alzheimer's and Parkinson's disease. Int J Geriatr Psychiatry (2004) 19:763–72.

Cummings JL Subcortical Dementia. (Oxford University Press: New York, 1990).

Dalrymple-Alford JC, Kalders AS, Jones RD, Watson RW, A central executive deficit in patients with Parkinson's disease. J Neurol Neurosurg Psychiatry (1994) 57:360–7.

Delis DC, Massman PJ, Butters N et al, Profiles of demented and amnesic patients on the California Verbal Learning Test: Implications for the assessment of memory disorders. Psychol Assess (1991) 3:19–26.

Dickson DW, Davies P, Mayeux R et al, Diffuse Lewy body disease: Neuropathological and biochemical studies of six patients. Acta Neuropathol (1987) 75:8–15.

Dickson DW, Ruan D, Crystal H et al, Hippocampal degeneration differentiates diffuse Lewy body disease (DLBD) from Alzheimer's disease: Light and electron microscopic immunocytochemistry of CA2-3 neurites specific to DLBD. Neurology (1991) 41:1402–9.

Dickson DW, Schmidt ML, Lee VM-Y et al, Immunoreactivity profile of hippocampal CA2/3 neurites in diffuse Lewy body disease. Acta Neuropathol (1994) 87:269–76.

Double KL, Halliday GM, McRitchie DA et al, Regional brain atrophy in ideopathic Parkinson's disease and diffuse Lewy body disease. Dementia (1996) 7:304–13.

Filoteo JV, Delis DC, Salmon DP et al, An examination of the nature of attentional deficits in patients with Parkinson's disease: Evidence from a spatial orienting task. J Int Neuropsychol Soc (1997) 3:337–47.

Förstl H, Burns A, Luthert P et al, The Lewy-body variant of Alzheimer's disease: Clinical and pathological findings. Br J Psychiatry (1993) 162:385–92.

Galasko D, Katzman R, Salmon DP et al, Clinical and neuropathological findings in Lewy body dementias. Brain Cogn (1996) 31:166–75.

Galasko D, Salmon DP, Lineweaver T et al, Neuropsychological measures distinguish patients with Lewy body variant from those with Alzheimer's disease. Neurology (1998) 50:A181. (Abstract)

Galloway PH, Sahgal A, McKeith IG et al, Visual pattern recognition memory and learning deficits in senile dementias of Alzheimer and Lewy body types. Dementia (1992) 3:101–7.

Gibb WRG, Esiri MM, Lees AJ, Clinical and pathological features of diffuse cortical Lewy body disease (Lewy body dementia). Brain (1985) 110:1131–53.

Gibb WRG, Luthert PJ, Janota I, Lantos PL, Cortical Lewy body dementia: Clinical features and classification. J Neurol Neurosurg Psychiatry (1989) 52:185–92.

Gnanalingham KK, Byrne EJ, Thornton A, Clock-face drawing to differentiate Lewy body and Alzheimer type dementia syndromes. Lancet (1996) 347:696–7.

Gnanalingham KK, Byrne EJ, Thornton A et al, Motor and cognitive function in Lewy body dementia: comparison with Alzheimer's and Parkinson's diseases. J Neurol Neurosurg Psychiatry (1997) 62:243–52.

Gómez-Tortosa E, Newell K, Irizarry MC et al, Clinical and quantitative pathologic correlates of dementia with Lewy bodies. Neurology (1999) 53:1284–91.

Gómez-Tortosa E, Irizarry MC, Gómez-Isla T, Hyman BT, Clinical and neuropathological correlates of dementia with Lewy bodies. Ann NY Acad Sci (2000) 920:9–15.

Graham C, Ballard C, Saad K, Variables which distinguish patients fulfilling clinical criteria for dementia with Lewy bodies from those with Alzheimer's disease. Int J Geriatr Psychiatry (1997) 12:314–18.

Hamilton JM, Salmon DP, Galasko D et al, A comparison of episodic memory deficits in neuropathologically-confirmed dementia with Lewy bodies and Alzheimer's disease. J Int Neuropsychol Soc (2004) 10:689–97.

Hansen L, Salmon D, Galasko D et al, The Lewy body variant of Alzheimer's disease: A clinical and pathologic entity. Neurology (1990) 40:1–8.

Hansen LA, Galasko D, Lewy body disease. Current Opin Neuro Neurosurg (1992) 5:889–94.

Harding AJ, Broe GA, Halliday GM, Visual hallucinations in Lewy body disease relate to Lewy bodies in the temporal lobe. Brain (2002) 125:391–403.

Hashimoto M, Kitagaki H, Imamura T et al, Medial temporal and whole-brain atrophy in dementia with Lewy bodies. Neurology (1998) 51:357–62.

Hely MA, Reid W, Halliday GM et al, Diffuse Lewy body disease: clinical features in nine cases without coexistent Alzheimer's disease. J Neurol Neurosurg Psychiatry (1996) 60:531–8.

Heyman A, Fillenbaum GG, Gearing M et al, Comparison of Lewy body variant of Alzheimer's disease with pure Alzheimer's disease: Consortium to establish a registry for Alzheimer's disease, part XIX. Neurology (1999) 52:1839–44.

Higuchi M, Tashiro M, Arai H et al, Glucose hypometabolism and neuropathological correlates in brains of dementia with Lewy bodies. Exp Neurol (2000) 162:247–56.

Hyman BT, Van Hoesen GW, Damasio AR, Memory-related neural systems in Alzheimer's disease: An anatomic study. Neurology (1990) 40:1721–30.

Imamura T, Ishii K, Hirono N et al, Visual hallucinations and regional cerebral metabolism in dementia with Lewy bodies (DLB). Neuroreport (1999) 10:1903–7.

Imamura T, Ishii K, Hirono N et al, Occipital glucose metabolism in dementia with Lewy bodies with and without Parkinsonism: a study using positron emission tomography. Dement Geriatr Cogn Disord (2001) 12:194–7.

Ince PG, Perry EK, Morris CM, Dementia with Lewy bodies: A distinct non-Alzheimer dementia syndrome? Brain Pathol (1998) 8:299–324.

Ishii K, Imamura T, Sasaki M et al, Regional cerebral glucose metabolism in dementia with Lewy bodies and Alzheimer's disease. Neurology (1998) 51:125–30.

Jacobs DM, Marder K, Cote LJ et al, Neuropsychological characteristics of preclinical dementia in Parkinson's disease. Neurology (1995) 45:1691–6.

Khachaturian ZS, Diagnosis of Alzheimer's disease. Arch Neurol (1985) 42:1097–105.

Kosaka K, Diffuse Lewy body disease in Japan. J Neurol (1990) 237:197–204.

Kosaka K, Iseki E, Dementia with Lewy bodies. Curr Opin Neurol (1996) 9:271–5.

Kosaka K, Yoshimura M, Ikeda K, Budka H, Diffuse type of Lewy body disease: Progressive dementia with abundant cortical Lewy bodies and senile changes of varying degree: A new disease? Clin Neuropathol (1984) 3:185–92.

Lambon Ralph MA, Powell J, Howard D et al, Semantic memory is impaired in both dementia with Lewy bodies and dementia of Alzheimer's type: a comparative neuropsychological study and literature review. J Neurol Neurosurg Psychiatry (2001) 70:149–56.

Lees AJ, Smith E, Cognitive deficits in the early stages of Parkinson's disease. Brain (1983) 137:221–4.

Lennox G, Lowe J, Landon M et al, Diffuse Lewy body disease: Correlative neuropathology using anti-ubiquitin immunocytochemistry. J Neurol Neurosurg Psychiatry (1989) 52:1236–47.

Lippa CF, Smith TW, Swearer JM, Alzheimer's disease and Lewy body disease: a comparative clinicopathological study. Ann Neurol (1994) 35:81–8.

Lippa CF, Johnson R, Smith TW, The medial temporal lobe in dementia with Lewy bodies: a comparative study with Alzheimer's disease. Ann Neurol (1998) 43:102–6.

Lobotesis K, Fenwick JD, Phipps A et al, Occipital hypoperfusion on SPECT in dementia with Lewy bodies but not AD. Neurology (2001) 56:643–9.

McKeith IG, Perry RH, Fairbairn AF et al, Operational criteria for senile dementia of Lewy body type (SDLT). Psychol Med (1992) 22:911–22.

McKeith IG, Galasko D, Kosaka K et al, Clinical and pathological diagnosis of dementia with Lewy bodies (DLB): Report of the Consortium on Dementia with Lewy Bodies (CDLB) International Workgroup. Neurology (1996) 47:1113–24.

McShane R, Gedling K, Reading M et al, Prospective study of relations between cortical Lewy bodies, poor eyesight, and hallucinations in Alzheimer's disease. J Neurol Neurosurg Psychiatry (1995) 59:185–8.

Martone M, Butters N, Payne M et al, Dissociations between skill learning and verbal recognition in amnesia and dementia. Arch Neurol (1984) 41:965–70.

Merdes AR, Hansen LA, Jeste DV et al, Influence of Alzheimer pathology on clinical diagnostic accuracy in dementia with Lewy bodies. Neurology (2003) 60:1586–90.

Minoshima S, Foster NL, Sima A et al, Alzheimer's disease versus dementia with Lewy bodies: Cerebral metabolic distinction with autopsy confirmation. Ann Neurol (2001) 50:358–65.

Mirra SS, Hart MN, Terry RD, Making the diagnosis of Alzheimer's disease. Arch Pathol Lab Med (1993) 117:132–44.

Mori E, Shimomura T, Fujimori M et al, Visuoperceptual impairment in dementia with Lewy bodies. Arch Neurol (2000) 57:489–93.

Moss MB, Albert MS, Butters N, Payne M, Differential patterns of memory loss among patients with Alzheimer's disease, Huntington's disease, and alcoholic Korsakoff's syndrome. Arch Neurol (1986) 43:239–46.

Noe E, Marder K, Bell KL et al, Comparison of dementia with Lewy bodies to Alzheimer's disease and Parkinson's disease with dementia. Movement Disorders (2004) 19:60–7.

Pellise A, Roig C, Barraquer-Bordas L, Ferrer I, Abnormal, ubiquinated cortical neurites in patients with diffuse Lewy body disease. Neurosci Lett (1996) 206:85–8.

Perry EK, Marshall E, Perry RH et al, Cholinergic and dopaminergic activities in senile dementia of Lewy body type. Alzheimer Dis Assoc Disord (1990a) 4:87–95.

Perry RH, Irving D, Blessed G et al, Senile dementia of the Lewy body type: A clinically and neuropathologically distinct form of Lewy body dementia in the elderly. J Neurol Sci (1990b) 95:119–39.

Perry RH, McKeith IG, Perry EK, (eds), Dementia with Lewy Bodies. Cambridge University Press: London (1996).

Reid RT, Sabbagh MN, Corey-Bloom J et al, Nicotinic receptor losses in dementia with Lewy bodies: comparisons with Alzheimer's disease. Neurobiol Aging (2000) 21:741–6.

Rezaie P, Cairns NJ, Chadwick A, Lantos PL, Lewy bodies are located preferentially in limbic areas in diffuse Lewy body disease. Neurosci Lett (1996) 212:111–14.

Sabbagh MN, Corey-Bloom J, Tiraboschi P et al, Neurochemical markers do not correlate with cognitive decline in the Lewy body variant of Alzheimer disease. Arch Neurol (1999) 56:1458–61.

Sahgal A, Galloway PH, McKeith IG, et al, Matching-to-sample deficits in patients with senile dementias of the Alzheimer and Lewy body types. Arch Neurol (1992a) 49:1043–6.

Sahgal A, Galloway PH, McKeith IG, et al, A comparative study of attentional deficits in senile dementias of Alzheimer and Lewy body types. Dementia (1992b) 3:350–4.

Sahgal A, McKeith IG, Galloway PH, et al, Do differences in visuospatial ability between senile dementias of the Alzheimer and Lewy body types reflect differences solely in mnemonic function? J Clin Exp Neuropsychol (1995) 17:35–43.

Salmon DP, Galasko D, Hansen LA, et al, Neuropsychological deficits associated with diffuse Lewy body disease. Brain Cogn (1996) 31:148–65.

Salmon DP, Lineweaver TT, Galasko D, Hansen L, Patterns of cognitive decline in patients with autopsy-verified Lewy body variant of Alzheimer's disease. J Int Neuropsychol Soc (1998) 4:228 (Abstract).

Salmon DP, Galasko D, Hamilton J, et al, Cognitive profiles differ across disease course in autopsy-proven dementia with Lewy bodies and Alzheimer's disease. Neurobiol Aging (2002) 23:S130 (Abstract).

Samuel W, Galasko D, Masliah E, Hansen LA, Neocortical Lewy body counts correlate with dementia in the Lewy body variant of Alzheimer's disease. J Neuropathol Exp Neurol (1996) 55:44–52.

Samuel W, Alford M, Hofstetter R, Hansen LA, Dementia with Lewy bodies versus pure Alzheimer's disease: Differences in cognition, neuropathology, cholinergic dysfunction and synapse density. J Neuropathol Exp Neurol (1997) 56:499–508.

Shimomura T, Mori E, Yamashita H et al, Cognitive loss in dementia with Lewy bodies and Alzheimer disease. Arch Neurol (1998) 55:1547–52.

Simard M, van Reekum R, Myran D, Visuospatial impairment in dementia with Lewy bodies and Alzheimer's disease: a process analysis approach. Int J Geriatr Psychiatry (2003) 18:387–91.

Soininen H, Helkala EL, Laulumaa V et al, Cognitive profile of Alzheimer patients with extrapyramidal signs: a longitudinal study. J Neural Transm (1992) 4:241–54.

Stern Y, Richards M, Sano M and Mayeux R, Comparison of cognitive changes in patients with Alzheimer's and Parkinson's disease. Arch Neurol (1993) 50:1040–5.

Tiraboschi P, Hansen LA, Alford M, et al, The decline in synapses and cholinergic activity is asynchronous in Alzheimer's disease. Neurology (2000) 55:1278–83.

Tiraboschi P, Hansen LA, Alford M et al, Early and widespread cholinergic losses differentiate dementia with Lewy bodies from Alzheimer disease. Arch Gen Psychiatry (2002) 59:946–51.

Tröster AI, Butters N, Salmon DP et al, The diagnostic utility of savings scores: Differentiating Alzheimer's and Huntington's diseases with Logical Memory and Visual Reproduction tests. J Clin Exp Neuropsychol (1993) 15:773–88.

Verghese J, Crystal HA, Dickson DW, Lipton RB, Validity of clinical criteria for the diagnosis of dementia with Lewy bodies. Neurology (1999) 53:1974–82.

Wagner MT, Bachman DL, Neuropsychological features of diffuse Lewy body disease. Arch Clin Neuropsychol (1996) 11:175–84.

Walker Z, Allen R, Shergill S, Katona C, Neuropsychological performance in Lewy body dementia and Alzheimer's disease. Br J Psychiatry (1997) 170:156–8.

Weiner MF, Risser RC, Cullum CM, et al, Alzheimer's disease and its Lewy body variant: A clinical analysis of postmortem verified cases. Am J Psychiatry (1996) 153:1269–73.

Yeatman R, McLean CA, Ames D, The clinical manifestations of senile dementia of Lewy body type: a case report. Aust NZ J Psychiatry (1994) 28:512–15.

chapter 6

Neuropsychiatric features of dementia with Lewy bodies

Liana G Apostolova and Jeffrey L Cummings

Neuropsychiatric symptoms are highly prevalent in some Lewy body (LB) disorders, including Parkinson's disease (PD), PD with dementia (PDD) and dementia with Lewy bodies (DLB). In the latter, early-onset neuropsychiatric features, most commonly hallucinations, delusions and delusional misidentifications, frequently predate the cognitive decline (Cercy and Bylsma, 1997). Detailed neuropsychiatric assessment is essential for the evaluation of all dementias. In DLB, neuropsychiatric assessment is critical since visual hallucinations (VH) are a core diagnostic feature (McKeith et al, 1992b, 1996). Psychotic symptoms and problematic behaviors result in patient distress, caregiver dissatisfaction, frequent hospitalization and early institutionalization (Steeley et al, 1990). Behavioral features also have prognostic implications: psychosis is associated with more rapid cognitive decline (Rosen and Zubenko, 1991). This chapter will focus on the neuropsychiatric symptoms in DLB and other LB spectrum disorders from a clinical, pathophysiological and therapeutic perspective.

Terminology and classification of DLB

For the purposes of this chapter, we divide neuropsychiatric symptoms into four major domains: (1) psychosis; (2) mood; (3) psychomotor; (4) neurovegetative (Table 6.1). The psychosis domain consists of hallucinations, delusions and delusional misidentifications. Mood abnormalities include anxiety, apathy, depression, euphoria, irritability and disinhibition. The psychomotor domain consists of agitation and aberrant motor behavior, and the

Table 6.1 Glossary of neuropsychiatric symptoms

Agitation	Excessive motor activity associated with a feeling of inner tension manifesting as verbal and physical aggression and active resistance to care or simply as pacing, fidgeting, hand wringing, pulling of clothes, inability to sit still (DSM-IV TR, 2000; Cummings, 2003)
Anxiety	The apprehensive anticipation of future danger or misfortune accompanied by a feeling of dysphoria or somatic symptoms of tension (DSM-IV TR, 1994)
Apathy	Lack of motivation, interest, empathy, enthusiasm and interpersonal involvement (Marin, 1990)
Delusion	A false, firmly sustained belief based on incorrect inference about external reality despite incontrovertible and obvious evidence to the contrary (DSM-IV TR, 1994)
Delusional misidentification	Delusional beliefs that real people or one's home are replaced by impostors, or that the mirror image of self is another person, or that TV or photo images are real – thought to result from visual misperception and false interpretation (Förstl et al, 1991)
Depression	Syndrome characterized by depressed mood, loss of interest or pleasure, appetite and/or sleep changes, feeling of worthlessness, difficulty concentrating, recurrent thoughts of death, psychomotor retardation or agitation (DSM-IV TR, 1994)
Disinhibition	Tactlessness and impulsivity (Cummings, 1998)
Euphoria	Persistent and unreasonable sense of wellbeing without the elevated mental and motor rate of mania (Yudofsky and Hales, 1992)
Hallucinations	Sensory perception that has a sense of reality but that occurs in the absence of stimulation of the relevant sensory organ (DSM-IV TR, 1994)
Irritability	Susceptibility to easily provoked anger or annoyance (DSM-IV TR, 1994)

neurovegetative domain of appetite and sleep changes (Table 6.2). Another approach divides the neuropsychiatric features in positive (e.g. hallucinations, delusions, agitation, irritability, abberant motor behavior, euphoria, anxiety and disinhibition) and negative behaviors (depression and apathy) (Table 6.2).

Table 6.2 Classification of neuropsychiatric symptoms

Domain	Positive behaviors	Negative behaviors
Psychotic	Hallucinations	
	Delusions	
	Delusional misidentifications	
Emotional	Anxiety	Apathy
	Euphoria	Depression
	Disinhibition	
	Irritability	
Psychomotor	Agitation	
	Aberrant motor behavior	
Neurovegetative	Increased appetite	Appetite loss
	Insomnia	Hypersomnia
	Parasomnia	Depressed consciousness
	Dyssomnia	

Neuropsychiatric symptoms in DLB

Neuropsychiatric symptoms occur in nearly all DLB patients (Ballard et al, 1996), most of whom experience more than one type of psychopathology. The prevalence is not influenced by the patient's age or gender (Del Ser et al, 2000). Complete remission over a 1-year period is infrequent at 28% for DLB, compared with 63% for AD and 33% for vascular dementia (VaD) (Ballard et al, 1996). The small remission rates are largely accounted for by persistent VH and are not influenced by age of onset, dementia severity, deafness, visual impairment or multiplicity of psychotic symptoms (Ballard et al, 1997a). The frequency and severity of individual behaviors assessed with the Neuropsychiatric Inventory (NPI) (Cummings et al, 1994) are presented in Figure 6.1.

Psychotic domain
Hallucinations
Hallucinations are exceedingly common in both pure (Lewy bodies only) and mixed (Lewy bodies and Alzheimer's type changes) DLB (Kosaka, 1990). Early in the disease course they are significantly more frequent in DLB compared with AD or PD (Klatka et al, 1996; Del Ser et al, 2001). Also unlike AD, 18% of the pure and 14% of the mixed DLB patients present with

(a)

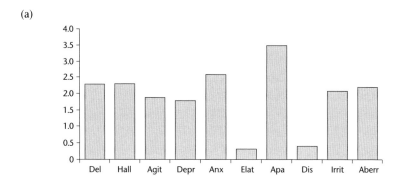

(b)

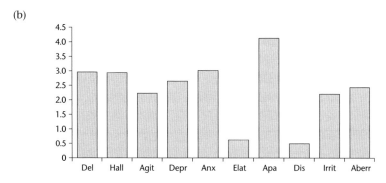

Figure 6.1 Frequency (a) and severity (b) of individual neuropsychiatric behaviors, assessed with the NLP, in DLB (N=120). Del, delusions; Hall, hallucinations; Agi, Agitation; Depr, depression; Anx, anxiety; Elat, elated mood; Apa, apathy; Dis, disinhibition; Irrit, irritability; Aberr, aberrant motor behavior. (Adapted from McKeith et al, 2000a; Del Ser et al, 2000).

hallucinations prior to dementia onset. In fact, the concomitant presence of Alzheimer changes on autopsy seemed to correlate with absence of psychopathology. In one meta-analysis of pathologically proven DLB, as many as 38% mixed and 21% pure DLB patients did not have documented neuropsychiatric symptoms (Cercy et al, 1997). While these absence rates appear high, one should keep in mind that collecting clinical data retrospectively might underestimate the true prevalence, since, unless specifically asked, most patients will not volunteer psychiatric history (Teunisse et al, 1996). Conversely, any prospective DLB study may report higher psychopathology prevalence rates as VH are a validated diagnostic criterion (McKeith et al, 2000a). Finally, another confounder is the patient's insight into his or her symptoms. Some DLB patients, especially of the mixed type (Del Ser et al, 2001), lack insight during the experience, but most gain it afterwards (McKeith and O'Brien, 1999).

VH are the most frequent neuropsychiatric symptom in DLB. The reported prevalence varies between 13% (Byrne et al, 1989) and 93% (Ballard et al, 1998), with means of 63% in cohorts from psychiatric and 27% from neurological services (Ballard et al, 1996, 1997b). Two large meta-analyses calculated VH to occur in 46–54% of DLB and 20–31% of AD patients respectively (Simmard et al, 2000; McKeith et al, 1999). VH are a presenting feature in 33–65% of DLB versus 8–25% of AD (McKeith et al, 1992b; Ballard et al, 1999) (Table 6.3).

VH in DLB are typically complex detailed brightly colored three-dimensional images of people and animals (McKeith et al, 1992b, 1996, 1999; Ballard et al, 1996). Less frequent themes are hallucinations of children, objects, insects, fire and birds (Ballard et al, 1996, 1997b). They are mostly of normal size, animated and complete. In half of the patients, they co-occur with auditory hallucinations (AH), such as speech or noise. The presence of AH along with VH persistence and multiplicity may help differentiate DLB from AD (Ballard et al, 1996, 1997a,b). VH may leave the patient indifferent or elicit various emotions, e.g. fear, amusement, anger (McKeith et al, 1992b, 1996).

A diurnal pattern with more (Ballard et al, 1997b) and/or more severe (McKeith et al, 1996) hallucinations in the evening and at night accentuates the impact of solitude, inactivity and poor lighting, and is evident in one-third of patients with DLB. Diminished useful field of vision is part of normal aging and results from decline in processing speed and the ability to sustain attention (Ball and Owsley, 1993) Coexisting visual impairment renders DLB patients unusually susceptible to VH. (McKeith et al, 1996) Hallucinators complain of poor eyesight more frequently than nonhallucinators (McShane et al, 1995). Visuoperception in DLB is further compromised by severe visuo-constructional and visuospatial deficits (Salmon and Galasko, 1996). The performance on elementary (size discrimination) and complex (form discrimination, overlapping figure identification and visual counting) visual tasks is compromised in DLB, with even greater impairment on the overlapping figure identification task in the hallucinating subgroup (Mori et al, 2000). In the closely related PD, VH are facilitated by impaired color and contrast discrimination (Diederich et al, 1998). Both VH and visuoperceptual impairment may relate to inferior temporal dysfunction (Collerton et al, 2003).

VH strongly predict LB pathology (Litvan et al, 1998), especially when they occur early in the disease course. Among 270 patients with AD and DLB, 93% of the hallucinators with Mini-Mental State Examination (MMSE) scores of 20

Table 6.3 Comparison of visual hallucinations in dementia with Lewy bodies (DLB), Alzheimer's disease (AD), and Parkinson's disease with dementia (PDD) and vascular dementia (VaD)

Feature	DLB (%)	AD (%)	PDD (%)	VaD (%)
Frequency	46[1]–54[2]	20[1]–31[2]	22[3]	8.5[4]
Presenting feature	33[5]–65[6]	8[5]–25[6]	—	—
Themes:				
People	93[7]–95[8]	75[8]	80[8]	—
Animals	46[8]–48[7]	13[8]	17[8]	
Children	0.1[8]–17[7]	13[8]	13[8]	
Objects	0.1[8]–15[7]	0[8]	7[8]	
Insects	0.05[8]	13[8]	0[8]	
Fire	0.03[8]–11[7]	0[8]	7[8]	
Birds	0.03[8]	13[8]	0[8]	
Size				
Normal size	84[8,9]	7[8,9]	—	—
Liliputian	11[8,9]	1[8,9]		
Enlarged	3[8,9]	0[8,9]		
Animation	76[8,9]	6[8,9]	—	—
Concurrent auditory hallucinations	24[9]–51[8]	0[8,9]	—	—
Completeness of the images	87[8,9]	88[8,9]	—	—
Multiplicity	22[9]–56[8]	3[8]	—	—
Persistence	44[9]–84[10]	37[10]	—	30[10]
Diurnal variation	32[8]	12.5[8]	—	—

References: [1]McKeith et al (1999); [2]Simmard et al (2000); [3]Fenelon et al (2003); [4]Leroi et al (2003); [5]McKeith et al (1992b); [6]Ballard et al (1999); [7]Aarsland et al (2001b); [8]Ballard et al (1997b); [9]Ballard et al (1996); [10]Ballard et al (1997a).

or higher had DLB pathology (Ballard et al, 1999) – an observation later confirmed by Rockwell et al (2000).

The relationship of hallucinations and cognition is obscure. McShane et al (1996) found a trend for persistent VH to predict faster cognitive decline. Del Ser et al (2000) described an association between NPI-4 (including delusions, hallucinations, depression and apathy) and lower MMSE scores. Yet Ballard et al (1999), using a different instrument, failed to show an increase in hallucinations, delusions or depression with respect to dementia progression. While it seems likely that as the disease progresses, more patients will develop VH, more studies are needed to convincingly resolve this question.

The role of antiparkinsonian agents as triggers or exacerbators of hallucinations is not fully substantiated. Some authors have observed a strong association (Klatka et al, 1996; Ballard et al, 2000), while a large study with 98 DLB, 48 PDD and 83 PD patients did not (Aarsland et al, 2001b).

As many as 35% of all DLB patients describe AH at disease onset (Ballard et al, 1999) The longitudinal prevalence for AH is 19–45% for DLB, compared with 4–13% for AD (Simard, 2000; McKeith et al, 1999; Ballard et al, 1999). AH and VH frequently coexist (McKeith et al, 1992b). As many as two-thirds of the DLB patients with AH will have VH. AH content is strongly influenced by VH (Ballard et al, 2001). AH remission rates in DLB and AD are similar. (Ballard et al, 1996, 2001).

Little is known about hallucinations in other modalities. Olfactory hallucinations occur in 7–12% and tactile hallucinations in 0–3% (Ballard et al, 1996; Simard et al, 2000; Aarsland et al, 2001b). Undeniably, a more detailed description is needed.

Delusions

Delusions are common in DLB. One meta-analysis calculated the mean prevalence at 49% compared with 31% in AD (Simard et al, 2000), with significant disparity only early in the course of the disease (Ballard et al, 1998). Delusions are slightly more prevalent in mixed compared with pure DLB (Cercy and Bylsma, 1997). The most common themes are delusional misidentification, followed by paranoid beliefs (theft, conspiracy, harassment, abandonment or infidelity), and phantom boarder (Klatka et al, 1996; Weiner et al, 1996; Hirono et al, 1999; Simard et al, 2000; Aarsland et al, 2001b). Nondelusional suspiciousness and paranoia are frequent (Weiner et al, 1996).

Delusional misidentifications help differentiate DLB from AD (Hirono et al, 1999). They occur in 33% of DLB patients (Simard et al, 2000). Mistaking TV images for in-the-home persons occurs in 19%, followed by Capgras syndrome (belief that a family member has been replaced by an impostor) in 10%, mistaking one's mirror image for another person in 9.5%, and delusion of their residence not being their home in 2.4% (Ballard et al, 1996).

The persistence rates for delusions do not help to differentiate DLB from AD (40% for DLB vs 44% for AD). However, delusional misidentifications seem to persist in 30% of DLB versus only 18% of AD patients (Ballard et al, 1997a, 2001). One study found a trend for correlation between delusions and cognition (Del Ser et al, 2000), while others did not (Ballard et al, 1999; Rockwell et al, 2000). A role for antiparkinsonian or anticholinergic agents in delusions is suggested by some (Ballard et al, 2000) but not others (Aarsland et al, 2001b; Ballard et al, 1996).

Mood domain

Depression

Depressive mood is a feature of many neurodegenerative disorders, with the highest frequencies being reported in PD (Cummings et al, 1988, 1992; Klatka et al, 1996). Major depression occurs in 24–29% of DLB versus 9–16% of AD patients (Simmard et al, 2000; McKeith et al, 1999). Depressive mood including minor depression is more frequent in pure (43%) compared with mixed (8%) DLB (Cercy and Bylsma, 1997). The likelihood of DLB versus AD pathology is 16 times greater when depression is present (Papka et al, 1998). While psychosis correlates with severity of depression in PDD (Aarsland et al, 1999a), such a correlation has not been validated for DLB. Depression is associated with decreased cognitive scores, and correlates with extrapyramidal symptoms (EPS) and levodopa use (Ballard et al, 1996).

Anxiety

Anxiety disorder meeting the Diagnostic and Statistical Manual of Mental Disorders (DSM) criteria is rare in DLB (Ballard et al, 1996), whereas feeling anxious is very common. Up to 84% of DLB patients appear or feel anxious (Rockwell et al, 2000); 38% have anxiety at disease onset (Ballard, 1999). Among three studies using the NPI, two found anxiety as one of the most prominent neuropsychiatric features (Hirono et al, 1999; Del Ser et al, 2000; McKeith and Burn, 2000c). Del Ser et al (2000) found anxiety to be more frequent than hallucinations and delusions in early DLB and to be as frequent in late DLB.

Other emotional disturbances

Only limited information is available on other emotional derangements in DLB. In the three studies utilizing the NPI, apathy emerged as the most common psychopathology in DLB. Irritability is also common, while euphoria and disinhibition are rare (Hirono et al, 1999; Del Ser et al, 2000; McKeith, 2000c; and see Figure 6.1).

Psychomotor domain

Agitation was very prevalent in two of the three NPI studies of DLB, while aberrant motor behavior was common in all (Hirono et al, 1999; Del Ser et al, 2000; McKeith, 2000c; and see Figure 6.1). Pure DLB may present with more aggressive behavior than does mixed DLB (Cercy et al, 1997).

Neurovegetative domain

DLB patients frequently display rapid eye movement (REM) sleep behavior disorder (RBD), characterized by loss of physiological skeletal muscle atonia during REM cycles and dream enactment. RBD predates dementia by an average of 9 years. It precedes the extrapyramidal features and VH in 50% and the fluctuations in 80% (Ferman, 1999, 2002). Several α-synucleinopathies, including PD and multiple system atrophy (MSA) as well as DLB, feature RBD. α-synuclein inclusions were present in all 10 neurodegenerative cases with RBD – pathologically confirmed as 9 DLB and 1 MSA. The positive predictive value for DLB in a demented patient with parkinsonism and RBD is 92% (Boeve et al, 1998, 2001). Hence RBD may be included in the revised diagnostic criteria for DLB (Ferman et al, 2002; Boeve et al, 2003a).

It has been suggested that VH in PD patients represent REM sleep intrusions into wakefulness (Arnulf et al, 2000). Whether REM intrusions partially or fully account for VH in DLB remains to be seen.

In addition to RBD, DLB patients also suffer from decreased sleep efficiency, increased upper airway resistance, obstructive sleep apnea/hypopnea and periodic limb movements of sleep (Boeve et al, 2003c).

While appetite changes are known to occur in DLB (Del Ser et al, 2000), no comprehensive data are yet available.

Pathological and pathophysiological correlates of neuropsychiatric symptoms in DLB

The cholinergic system sends massive regulatory afferents to the cerebral cortex (Mesulam et al, 1992). The hallucinogenic effect of anticholinergic compounds suggests that a cholinergic deficit may play a role in VH. Cholinergic neuronal hypocellularity of the substantia inominata (Hansen, 1990) and nucleus basalis is characteristic of DLB (Perry RH, 1990). In DLB, choline acetyltransferase (ChAT) activity in parietal, frontal and temporal neocortex is profoundly reduced (Hansen et al, 1990; Langlais et al, 1993; Perry et al, 1994; Tiraboshi et al, 2000), in contrast to the extreme ChAT deficits in AD archicortex (e.g. hippocampus) (Perry EK et al, 1993a). The deficits are more profound in hallucinators who evidence an 80% decline in cortical ChAT activity compared with 50% in nonhallucinators (Perry et al, 1990a, 1990b). Perry and Perry (1995) postulated that VH result from the inefficient cholinergic regulatory suppression of intrinsic cortical activation during perception and intrusion of irrelevant information from subconscious mental processes.

The hypocholinergic state in pure DLB, while associated with upregulation of postsynaptic muscarinic acetylcholine (ACh) receptors (mAChR) (Perry et al, 1990b), spares the nicotinic receptors (nAChRs) (Perry et al, 1990c). Delusions correlate with postsynaptic M_1 mAChR upregulation (especially BA 36) (Ballard et al, 2000), and hallucinations with decreased binding to nAChR (Perry et al, 1990c). Decreased α_7 nAChR binding in the temporal cortex contributes to both VH and delusional misidentifications (Court et al, 2001). Still the cholinergic deficit alone may not be sufficient to produce psychopathology.

Recently, dopamine has been linked to DLB psychosis. Neuronal loss in the substantia nigra, albeit not as severe as that in PD, occurs in DLB (Perry et al, 1990; Hansen et al, 1990). Dopamine uptake in the basal ganglia is more uniformly but less severely decreased compared with PD (Piggot, 1999). Basal ganglia levels of dopamine, tyrosine hydroxylase and homovanillic acid (HVA) diminish (Langlais, 1993; Weiner et al, 1996). Dopamine depletion in the caudate seems proportional to the neuronal loss of substantia nigra (Perry et al, 1990b). D_2 binding is decreased in DLB and increased in PD (Piggott, 1999). Sweet et al (2001) studied the dopamine receptor densities in psychotic DLB and AD patients and found increased D_1 and decreased D_2 and D_3 densities in DLB and increased D_3 density in AD. Dopamine and dopaminergic compounds may indirectly influence VH, increasing the dopaminergic/cholinergic imbalance.

A relatively hyperactive serotonin system is another putative contributor to psychopathology in DLB. Many serotonergic compounds such as lysergic acid diethylamide (LSD) induce hallucinations. DLB hallucinators demonstrate increased 5-hydroxyindoleacetic acid (5-HIAA)-to-ChAT and 5-HIAA-to-serotonin ratios (Perry EK et al, 1990c, 1993b), whereas nonhallucinators demonstrate low HVA and low 5-HIAA levels along with decreased S_2 (5-HT_2) receptor binding (Perry et al, 1990c; Cheng et al, 1991; Weiner, 1996). The relatively spared serotonergic system may trigger hallucinatory experiences in the hypocholinergic milieu of DLB (Perry et al, 1990c).

Norepinephrine (NE, noradrenaline), another monoamine, may also contribute to DLB psychopathology. In DLB, there is depletion of NE in the putamen (Langlais et al, 1993) and the neuronal loss in the locus ceruleus is more severe compared with AD (Perry et al, 1990; Hansen et al, 1990).

A few important associations between histopathology and psychosis have been described. Psychopathology corresponds to LB distribution in the limbic system (Burkhardt et al, 1988; Gomez-Tortosa et al, 1998). VH relate to amygdalar and parahippocampal LB density and (when present early in the course of disease) to parahippocampal and inferior temporal cortical LB density (Harding and Halliday, 2001; Harding et al, 2002). Cortical LB strongly correlate with early-onset VH, VH persistence and severity (McShane et al, 1995, 1996).

Neuroimaging correlates of neuropsychiatric features in DLB

Structural correlates of hallucinations in DLB have been studied with volumetric magnetic resonance imaging (MRI) methods. While decreased occipital-to-whole brain ratio is associated with hallucinations in AD (Holroyd et al, 2000), no occipital volume difference in DLB hallucinators compared with nonhallucinators has emerged (Midelkoop et al, 2001).

Functional neuroimaging techniques have been more revealing in studies of the pathophysiology of VH in DLB. Single-photon emission computed tomography (SPECT) and positron emission tomography (PET) find significant hypoactivity in primary and secondary visual cortices in DLB (Albin et al, 1996; Miller et al, 1996; Donnemiller et al, 1997; Imamura et al, 1997, 1999, 2001; Ishii et al, 1999; Lobotesis et al, 2001; Minoshima et al, 2001; Pasquier et al, 2002; Colloby et al, 2002). However, the temporal and parietal association cortices may generate the complex VH (Lee et al, 2000). Indeed, hallucinators show greater right posterior temporal and parietal glucose uptake than nonhallucinators (Imamura et al, 1999).

Therapy

Behavioral interventions

The initial approach to reducing psychopathology in patients with dementia is behavioral modification. The physician's therapeutic responsibility starts with the diagnostic visit, when educating the patient and the family about potential future psychiatric manifestations, identifying triggers and introducing behavioral approaches is fundamental. If symptoms develop, reassurance, compassion and targeted behavioral interventions are essential. Dysthymic and apathetic patients benefit from social, physical and mental activity. Anxiety calls for reassurance and introduction of coping strategies. The agitated, restless or disinhibited patient requires gentle yet firm redirection. VH may respond to increased sensory stimulation. Engaging the patient in activities and providing a night-light may bring substantial relief. Irrational delusions and hallucinations call for reassuring compassionate and nonconfrontational clarification.

Pharmacologic interventions

Acetylcholinesterase inhibitors

Acetylcholinesterase inhibitors (AChEIs) are known to ameliorate psychopathology and reduce difficult behaviors in dementia sufferers. The first AChEI reported to alleviate delusions and hallucinations in AD was physostigmine (Cummings et al, 1993). Two open-label tacrine trials showed improved cognition in both DLB and AD but did not look at psychopathology (Lebert et al, 1998; Querfurth et al, 2000), unlike one PD trial, where tacrine alleviated hallucinations and extrapyramidal symptoms (Hutchinson et al, 1996).

Rivastigmine provides cognitive and neuropsychiatric relief in DLB (Maclean et al, 2001; McKeith et al, 2000b,d) and improves mobility, activities of daily living and sleep (Maclean et al, 2001). A very robust response of apathy and anxiety and good response of delusions and hallucinations was demonstrated in a large randomized double-blind placebo-controlled study. The ratio of responders with at least 30% improvement on the NPI for rivastigmine compared with placebo was 2 : 1. The benefit disappeared after drug discontinuation (McKeith et al, 2000d). DLB patients treated with rivastigmine open-label for 1.8 years remained stable cognitively and neuropsychiatrically (Grace et al, 2001).

Reduction of psychiatric symptoms has been observed in many open-label donepezil studies (Shea et al, 1998; Kaufer et al, 1998; Samuel et al, 2000;

Lanctot and Herrmann, 2000). Worsening of extrapyramidal symptoms occurred in one-third of the patients in one trial (Shea et al, 1998). Such side-effects were not found in a PDD double-blind randomized trial (Aarsland et al, 2002).

Preliminary data from a 24-week multicenter open-label galantamine trial in DLB revealed a trend for improvement of the total NPI score and robust response of the NPI-4 subscore (including delusions, hallucinations, apathy and depression). No EPS worsening occurred (Edwards et al, 2004).

The side-effect profile of all AChEIs is similar. They may induce nausea, vomiting, gastrointestinal discomfort, diarrhea or anorexia. The occasional EPS worsening advises caution with AChEI initiation in DLB. The potential benefit outweighs the risks, and an AChEI trial is recommended in DLB (Swanberg and Cummings, 2002).

Antipsychotics

If resistant to AChEIs, the psychopathology in DLB is a challenging therapeutic target. Neuroleptic use in DLB is contraindicated. Adverse extrapyramidal effects have been reported in 81% of DLB versus 19% of AD patients. About half experienced severe reactions with sedation, confusion, rigidity and immobility, and three developed neuroleptic malignant syndrome. The mortality hazard ratio was 2.3 (McKeith et al, 1992a). This effect is likely mediated by reduced D_2 receptor density.

The atypical antipsychotics are generally safer with neuroleptic malignant syndrome being rare (McKeith et al, 1995). Clozapine (Chacko et al, 1993), risperidone (Allen et al, 1995; Kato et al, 2002), olanzapine (Walker et al, 1999; Cummings et al, 2002) and quietiapine (Davis and Baskys, 2002; Takahashi et al, 2003) successfully relieve psychotic symptoms in DLB. Nevertheless, even clozapine, despite its negligible D_2 affinity and strong D_4 antagonism, may cause confusion and behavioral changes (Burke et al, 1998). Therefore therapy with atypical antipsychotics should begin with very low doses under close supervision for cognitive or extrapyramidal side-effects (e.g. bradykinesia, rigidity, tremor, gait instability or falls) (Swanberg and Cummings, 2002). Some authors recommend that antipsychotics be introduced in inpatient settings (McKeith et al, 1995).

Antidepressants

The utility of antidepressants in DLB has not been studied. Similarly to AD, selective serotonin reuptake inhibitors (SSRIs) may help depression in DLB

(Swanberg and Cummings, 2002). Psychiatric side-effects such as anxiety, confusion, hallucinations, euphoria and aggression, along with dyskinesias, akathisia, parkinsonism and sexual dysfunction, have been reported. Gastrointestinal side-effects such as nausea, vomiting and diarrhea (Spigset, 1999) may exacerbate the adverse effect profile of AChEIs.

Other therapeutic interventions
RBD is classically treated with clonazepam. In general, the benzodiazepines are best avoided in the setting of dementia due to increased risk of confusion, sedation or unpredictable agitation. An intriguing open-label melatonin trial for RBD including seven DLB patients delivered promising results (Boeve et al, 2003b).

Neuropsychiatric features of other Lewy body spectrum disorders

The LB spectrum also includes MSA, PD, PDD, pantothenate kinase deficiency (PKAN), primary autonomic failure and LB dysphagia. Many authors feel that PD, PDD and DLB are essentially a pathological continuum sharing brain-stem, hypothalamic and nucleus basalis α-synuclein inclusions and clinical features such as extrapyramidal symptoms, psychopathology and cognitive changes. α-synuclein immunostaining has revealed cortical LB in virtually all PD patients (Hurtig et al, 2000). Moreover, cortical LB correlate with cognitive decline (Harding et al, 2001), especially their entorhinal and anterior cingulate distribution (Kovari et al, 2003).

Dementia is very prevalent among people with PD (Cummings et al, 1988, 1992). Ten years into PD, 38% of patients have dementia, and in another 4 years an additional 13% become demented (Hughes et al, 2000). Compared with normal aging, PD raises the risk for dementia sixfold (Aarsland et al, 2001a).

Sixty-one percent of PD patients experience at least one psychiatric symptom (Aarsland et al, 1999b). Hallucinations, typically with preserved insight, have a longitudinal prevalence of 46%. In addition to complex VH (22%), the delusional feeling of another's presence is very common (Fenelon et al, 2000). AH occur in 10% of PD patients (Inzelberg et al, 1998; Fenelon et al, 2000). Age, disease stage and duration, cognitive impairment, sleep disturbance, concomitant depression, and poor eyesight are independent risk factors for PD psychopathology (Sanchez-Ramos et al, 1996; Inzelberg et al, 1998;

Aarsland et al, 1999a,b; Fenelon et al, 2000; Holroyd et al, 2001). The risk of hallucinations increases fourfold in the presence of dementia (Aarsland et al, 2001b). Conversely, hallucinations relate to an increased risk for cognitive decline (Goetz and Stebbins, 1995). Delusions occur in 16% of all PD patients and are more prevalent in those with dementia (Klatka et al, 1996; Aarsland et al, 2001b). Both dementia and psychosis have higher prevalence in institutionalized cohorts (Aarsland et al, 1996, 1999b). Anxiety occurs in 20%, agitation and apathy in 16.5%, and irritability and aberrant motor behavior in about 10% each. There is no association between psychopathology and levodopa intake (Aarsland et al, 1999a).

Few studies have called attention to neuropsychiatric symptoms in other LB disorders. MSA patients exhibit less depression (Pilo et al, 1996; Fetoni et al, 1999) but more emotional blunting compared with PD patients (Fetoni et al, 1999). PKAN may lead to severe depression (Morphy et al, 1989; Sachs et al, 1966), aggression, anxiety, psychosis with AH (Oner et al, 2003) and irritability (Wigboldus and Bryun, 1968). A recent large study reported clinical data on 123 PKAN patients (Hayflick et al, 2003). Among the 23 with late-onset atypical PKAN, 6 had significant personality changes, impulsivity, aggressive behavior, depression and emotional lability. All of them had *PKAN2* gene mutation. Atypical patients lacking *PKAN2* mutation were devoid of psychopathology. More prospective studies are needed to expand our currently limited understanding of the psychopathology of these rare LB spectrum disorders and to address various therapeutic modalities.

Summary

Neuropsychiatric symptoms, most notably VH, are fundamental for the diagnosis of DLB. Early recognition and therapy are vital for the wellbeing of patients, families and professional aids and for prevention of recurrent hospitalizations and early institutionalization. AChEIs can be considered as first-line treatment for both their cognitive and their neuropsychiatric benefits. Cautious use of an atypical antipsychotic and an SSRI may be required in some patients. Typical antipsychotics should be avoided for their unacceptably high risk of severe side-effects. Ongoing and future scientific efforts will help clarify the various aspects of DLB psychopathology and provide more therapeutic modalities.

References

Aarsland D, Tandberg E, Larsen JP, Cummings JL, Frequency of dementia in Parkinson disease. Arch Neurol (1996) 53:538–42.

Aarsland D, Larsen JP, Cummings JL, Laake K, Prevalence and clinical correlates of psychotic symptoms in Parkinson disease: a community-based study. Arch Neurol, (1999a) 56:595–601.

Aarsland D, Larsen JP, Lim NG et al, Range of neuropsychiatric disturbances in patients with Parkinson's disease. J Neurol Neurosurg Psychiatry (1999b) 67:492–6.

Aarsland D, Andersen K, Larsen JP et al, Risk of dementia in Parkinson's disease: a community-based, prospective study. Neurology (2001a) 56:730–6.

Aarsland D, Ballard C, Larsen JP, McKeith I, A comparative study of psychiatric symptoms in dementia with Lewy bodies and Parkinson's disease with and without dementia. Int J Geriatr Psychiatry (2001b) 16:528–36.

Aarsland D, Laake K, Larsen JP, Janvin C, Donepezil for cognitive impairment in Parkinson's disease: a randomised controlled study. J Neurol Neurosurg Psychiatry (2002) 72:708–12.

Albin RL, Minoshima S, D'Amato CJ et al, Fluoro-deoxyglucose positron emission tomography in diffuse Lewy body disease. Neurology (1996) 47:462–6.

Allen RL, Walker Z, D'Ath PJ, Katona CL, Risperidone for psychotic and behavioural symptoms in Lewy body dementia. Lancet (1995) 346:185.

Arnulf I, Bonnet AM, Damier P et al, Hallucinations, REM sleep and Parkinson's disease: a medical hypothesis. Neurology (2000) 55:281–8.

Ball K, Owsley C, The useful field of view test: a new technique for evaluating age-related declines in visual function. J Am Optom Assoc (1993) 64:71–9.

Ballard C, Lowery K, Harrison R, McKeith IG, Noncognitive symptoms in Lewy body dementia. In: Perry RH, McKeith IG, Perry EK, eds, Dementia with Lewy Bodies (1st edn) (Cambridge University Press: Cambridge, UK, 1996) 67–84.

Ballard C, O'Brien J, Coope B et al, A prospective study of psychotic symptoms in dementia sufferers: psychosis in dementia. Int Psychogeriatr (1997a) 9:57–64.

Ballard C, McKeith I, Harrison R et al, A detailed phenomenological comparison of complex visual hallucinations in dementia with Lewy bodies and Alzheimer's disease. Int Psychogeriatr (1997b) 9:381–8.

Ballard CG, O'Brien J, Lowery K et al, A prospective study of dementia with Lewy bodies. Age Ageing (1998) 27:631–6.

Ballard C, Holmes C, McKeith I et al, Psychiatric morbidity in dementia with Lewy bodies: a prospective clinical and neuropathological comparative study with Alzheimer's disease. Am J Psychiatry (1999) 156:1039–45.

Ballard C, Piggott M, Johnson M et al, Delusions associated with elevated muscarinic binding in dementia with Lewy bodies. Ann Neurol (2000) 48:868–76.

Ballard CG, O'Brien JT, Swann AG et al, The natural history of psychosis and depression in dementia with Lewy bodies and Alzheimer's disease: persistence and new cases over 1 year of follow-up. J Clin Psychiatry (2001) 62:46–9.

Boeve BF, Silber MH, Ferman TJ et al, REM sleep behavior disorder and degenerative dementia: an association likely reflecting Lewy body disease. Neurology (1998) 51:363–70.

Boeve BF, Silber MH, Ferman TJ et al, Association of REM sleep behavior disorder and neurodegenerative disease may reflect an underlying synucleinopathy. Mov Disord (2001) 16:622–30.

Boeve BF, Silber MH, Parisi JE et al, Synucleinopathy pathology and REM sleep behavior disorder plus dementia or parkinsonism. Neurology (2003a) 6:40–5.

Boeve BF, Silber MH, Ferman TJ, Melatonin for treatment of REM sleep behavior disorder in neurologic disorders: results in 14 patients. Sleep Med (2003b) 4:281–4.

Boeve BF, Ferman TJ, Silber MH et al, Sleep disturbances in dementia with Lewy bodies involve more than REM sleep behavior disorder. Presented at the 55th Annual meeting of the American Academy of Neurology, Honolulu, HI (2003c).

Burke WJ, Pfeiffer RF, McComb RD, Neuroleptic sensitivity to clozapine in dementia with Lewy bodies. J Neuropsychiatry Clin Neurosci (1998) 10:227–9.

Burkhardt CR, Filley CM, Kleinschmidt-DeMasters BK et al, Diffuse Lewy body disease and progressive dementia. Neurology (1988) 38:1520–8.

Byrne EJ, Lennox G, Lowe J, Godwin-Austen RB, Diffuse Lewy body disease: clinical features in 15 cases. J Neurol Neurosurg Psychiatry (1989) 52:709–17.

Cercy SP, Bylsma FW, Lewy bodies and progressive dementia: a critical review and meta-analysis. J Int Neuropsychol Soc (1997) 3:179–94.

Chacko RC, Hurley RA, Jankovic J, Clozapine use in diffuse Lewy body disease. J Neuropsychiatry Clin Neurosci (1993) 5:206–8.

Cheng AV, Ferrier IN, Morris CM et al, Cortical serotonin-S2 receptor binding in Lewy body dementia, Alzheimer's and Parkinson's diseases. J Neurol Sci (1991) 106:50–5.

Collerton D, Burn D, McKeith I, O'Brien J, Systematic review and meta-analysis show that dementia with Lewy bodies is a visual-perceptual and attentional-executive dementia. Dement Geriatr Cogn Disord (2003) 16:229–37.

Colloby SJ, Fenwick JD, Williams ED et al, A comparison of ^{99m}Tc-HMPAO SPET changes in dementia with Lewy bodies and Alzheimer's disease using statistical parametric mapping. Eur J Nucl Med Mol Imaging (2002) 29:615–22.

Court JA, Ballard CG, Piggott MA et al, Visual hallucinations are associated with lower alpha bungarotoxin binding in dementia with Lewy bodies. Pharmacol Biochem Behav (2001) 70:571–9.

Cummings JL, The dementias of Parkinson's disease: prevalence, characteristics, neurobiology, and comparison with dementia of the Alzheimer type. Eur Neurol (1988) 28(Suppl 1):15–23.

Cummings JL, Depression and Parkinson's disease: a review. Am J Psychiatry (1992) 149: 443–54.

Cummings JL, The Neuropsychiatry of Alzheimer's Disease and Related Dementias (1st edn) (Martin Dunitz: London, 2003).

Cummings JL, Back C, The cholinergic hypothesis of neuropsychiatric symptoms in Alzheimer's disease. Am J Geriatr Psychiatry (1998) 6:S64–S78.

Cummings JL, Gorman DG, Shapira J, Physostigmine ameliorates the delusions of Alzheimer's disease. Biol Psychiatry (1993) 33:536–41.

Cummings JL, Mega M, Gray K et al, The Neuropsychiatric Inventory: comprehensive assessment of psychopathology in dementia. Neurology (1994) 44: 2308–14.

Cummings JL, Street J, Masterman D, Clark WS, Efficacy of olanzapine in the treatment of psychosis in dementia with Lewy bodies. Dement Geriatr Cogn Disord (2002) 13:67–73.

Davis P, Baskys A, Quetiapine effectively reduces psychotic symptoms in patients with Lewy body dementia: an advantage of the unique pharmacological profile? Brain Aging (2002) 2:49–53.

Del Ser T, McKeith I, Anand R et al, Dementia with Lewy bodies: findings from an international multicentre study. Int J Geriatr Psychiatry (2000) 15:1034–45.

Del Ser T, Hachinski V, Merskey H, Munoz DG, Clinical and pathologic features of two groups of patients with dementia with Lewy bodies: effect of coexisting Alzheimer-type lesion load. Alzheimer Dis Assoc Disord (2001) 15:31–44.

DSM-IV TR, Diagnostic and Statistical Manual of Mental Disorders (4th edn), Text Revision (American Psychiatric Association: Washington DC, 2000).

Diederich NJ, Goetz CG, Raman R et al, Poor visual discrimination and visual hallucinations in Parkinson's disease. Clin Neuropharmacol (1998) 21:289–95.

Donnemiller E, Heilmann J, Wenning GK, et al, Brain perfusion scintigraphy with ^{99m}Tc-HMPAO or ^{99m}Tc-ECD and ^{123}I-β-CIT single-photon emission tomography in dementia of the Alzheimer-type and diffuse Lewy body disease. Eur J Nucl Med (1997) 24:320–5.

Edwards KR, Hershey L, Wray L et al, Efficacy and safety of galantamine in patients with dementia with Lewy bodies: a 12–week interim analysis. Dement Geriatr Cogn Disord (2004) 17(Suppl 1):40–8.

Fenelon G, Mahieux F, Huon R, Ziegler M, Hallucinations in Parkinson's disease: prevalence, phenomenology and risk factors. Brain (2000) 123:733–45.

Ferman TJ, Boeve BF, Smith GE et al, REM sleep behavior disorder and dementia: cognitive differences when compared with AD. Neurology (1999) 52:951–7.

Ferman TJ, Boeve BF, Smith GE et al, Dementia with Lewy bodies may present as dementia and REM sleep behavior disorder without parkinsonism or hallucinations. J Int Neuropsychol Soc (2002) 8:907–14.

Fetoni V, Soliveri P, Monza D et al, Affective symptoms in multiple system atrophy and Parkinson's disease: response to levodopa therapy. J Neurol Neurosurg Psychiatry (1999) 66:541–4.

Förstl H, Burns A, Jacoby R, Levy R, Neuroanatomical correlates of clinical misidentification and misperception in senile dementia of the Alzheimer type. J Clin Psychiatry (1991) 52:268–71.

Goetz CG, Stebbins GT Mortality and hallucinations in nursing home patients with advanced Parkinson's disease. Neurology (1995) 45:669–71.

Gomez-Tortosa E, Ingraham AO, Irizarry MC, Hyman BT, Dementia with Lewy bodies. J Am Geriatr Soc (1998) 46:1449–58.

Grace J, Daniel S, Stevens T, Shankar KK et al, Long-term use of rivastigmine in patients with dementia with Lewy bodies: an open-label trial. Int Psychogeriatrics (2001) 13:199–205.

Hansen L, Salmon D, Galasko D et al, The Lewy body variant of Alzheimer's disease: a clinical and pathological entity. Neurology (1990) 40:1–8.

Harding AJ, Halliday GM, Cortical Lewy body pathology in the diagnosis of dementia. Acta Neuropathol (Berl) (2001) 102:355–63.

Harding AJ, Broe GA, Halliday GM, Visual hallucinations in Lewy body disease relate to Lewy bodies in the temporal lobe. Brain (2002) 125:391–403.

Hayflick SJ, Westaway SK, Levinson B et al, Genetic, clinical, and radiographic delineation of Hallervorden–Spatz syndrome. N Engl J Med (2003) 348:33–40.

Hirono N, Mori E, Tanimukai S et al, Distinctive neurobehavioral features among neurodegenerative dementias. J Neuropsychiatry Clin Neurosci (1999) 11: 498–503.

Holroyd S, Shepherd ML, Downs JH 3rd, Occipital atrophy is associated with visual hallucinations in Alzheimer's disease. J Neuropsychiatry Clin Neurosci (2000) 12:25–8.

Holroyd S, Currie L, Wooten GF, Prospective study of hallucinations and delusions in Parkinson's disease. J Neurol Neurosurg Psychiatry (2001) 70:734–8.

Hughes TA, Ross HF, Musa S et al, A 10–year study of the incidence of and factors predicting dementia in Parkinson's disease. Neurology (2000) 54:1596–602.

Hurtig HI, Trojanowski JQ, Galvin J et al, Alpha-synuclein cortical Lewy bodies correlate with dementia in Parkinson's disease. Neurology (2000) 54:1916–21.

Hutchinson M, Fazzini E, Cholinesterase inhibition in Parkinson's disease. J Neurol Neurosurg Psychiatry (1996) 61: 324–5.

Imamura T, Ishii K, Sasaki M et al, Regional cerebral glucose metabolism in dementia with Lewy bodies and Alzheimer's disease: a comparative study using positron emission tomography. Neurosci Lett (1997) 235:49–52.

Imamura T, Ishii K, Hirono N et al, Visual hallucinations and regional cerebral metabolism in dementia with Lewy bodies (DLB). Neuroreport (1999) 10:1903–7.

Imamura T, Ishii K, Hirono N et al, Occipital glucose metabolism in dementia with Lewy bodies with and without Parkinsonism: a study using positron emision tomography. Dement Geriatr Cogn Disord (2001) 12:194–7.

Inzelberg R, Kipervasser S, Korczyn AD, Auditory hallucinations in Parkinson's disease. J Neurol Neurosurg Psychiatry (1998) 64:533–5.

Ishii K, Yamaji S, Kitagaki H et al, Regional cerebral blood flow difference between dementia with Lewy bodies and AD. Neurology (1999) 53:413–16.

Kato K, Wada T, Kawakatsu S, Otani K, Improvement of both psychotic symptoms and Parkinsonism in a case of dementia with Lewy bodies by the combination therapy of risperidone and L-DOPA. Prog Neuropsychopharmacol Biol Psychiatry (2002) 26:201–3.

Kaufer DI, Catt KE, Lopez OL, DeKosky ST, Dementia with Lewy bodies: response of delirium-like features to donepezil. Neurology (1998) 51:1512.

Klatka LA, Louis ED, Schiffer RB, Psychiatric features in diffuse Lewy body disease: a clinicopathologic study using Alzheimer's disease and Parkinson's disease comparison groups. Neurology (1996) 47:1148–52.

Kosaka K, Diffuse Lewy body disease in Japan. J Neurol (1990) 237:197–204.

Kovari E, Gold G, Herrmann FR et al, Lewy body densities in the entorhinal and anterior cingulate cortex predict cognitive deficits in Parkinson's disease. Acta Neuropathol (Berl) (2003) 106:83–8.

Lanctot KL, Herrmann N, Donepezil for behavioural disorders associated with Lewy bodies: a case series. Int J Geriatr Psychiatry (2000)15:338–45.

Langlais PJ, Thal L, Hansen L et al, Neurotransmitters in basal ganglia and cortex of Alzheimer's disease with and without Lewy bodies. Neurology (1993) 43: 1927–34.

Lebert F, Pasquier F, Souliez L, Petit H, Tacrine efficacy in Lewy body dementia. Int J Geriatr Psychiatry (1998) 13:516–19.

Lee HW, Hong SB, Seo DW et al, Mapping of functional organization in human visual cortex: electrical cortical stimulation. Neurology 2000 Feb 22; 54(4):849–54. PMID 10690975

Leroi I, Voulgari A, Breitner JC, Lyketsos CG, The epidemiology of psychosis in dementia. Am J Geriatr Psychiatry (2003) 11:83–91.

Litvan I, MacIntyre A, Goetz CG et al, Accuracy of the clinical diagnoses of Lewy body disease, Parkinson disease, and dementia with Lewy bodies: a clinicopathologic study. Arch Neurol (1998) 55:969–78.

Lobotesis K, Fenwick JD, Phipps A et al, Occipital hypoperfusion on SPECT in dementia with Lewy bodies but not AD. Neurology (2001) 56:643–9.

Maclean LE, Collins CC, Byrne EJ, Dementia with Lewy bodies treated with rivastigmine: effects on cognition, neuropsychiatric symptoms, and sleep. Int Psychogeriatr (2001) 13:277–88.

McKeith I, Fairbairn A, Perry R et al, Neuroleptic sensitivity in patients with senile dementia of Lewy body type. BMJ (1992a) 305:673–6.

McKeith IG, Perry RH, Fairbairn AF et al, Operational criteria for senile dementia of Lewy body type (SDLT). Psychol Med (1992b) 22:911–22.

McKeith IG, Ballard CG, Harrison RW, Neuroleptic sensitivity to risperidone in Lewy body dementia. Lancet (1995) 346:699.

McKeith IG, Galasko D, Kosaka K et al, Consensus guidelines for the clinical and pathologic diagnosis of dementia with Lewy bodies (DLB): report of the consortium on DLB international workshop. Neurology (1996) 47:1113–24.

McKeith IG, O'Brien J. Dementia with Lewy bodies. Aust NZ J Psychiatry (1999) 33:800–8.

McKeith IG, Ballard CG, Perry RH et al, Prospective validation of consensus criteria for the diagnosis of dementia with Lewy bodies. Neurology (2000a) 54:1050–8.

McKeith IG, Grace JB, Walker Z et al, Rivastigmine in the treatment of dementia with Lewy bodies: preliminary findings from an open trial. Int J Geriatr Psychiatry (2000b) 15:387–92.

McKeith IG, Burn D, Spectrum of Parkinson's disease, Parkinson's dementia, and Lewy body dementia. Dementia (2000c) 18:865–83.

McKeith I, Del Ser T, Spano P et al, Efficacy of rivastigmine in dementia with Lewy bodies: a randomised, double-blind, placebo-controlled international study. Lancet (2000d) 356:2031–6.

McShane R, Gedling K, Reading M et al, Prospective study of relations between cortical Lewy bodies, poor eyesight, and hallucinations in Alzheimer's disease. J Neurol Neurosurg Psychiatry (1995) 59:185–8.

McShane R, Keene J, Gedling K, Hope T, Hallucinations, cortical Lewy body pathology, cognitive function and neuroleptics use in dementia. In: Perry RH, McKeith IG, Perry EK, eds, Dementia with Lewy Bodies (1st edn) (Cambridge University Press: Cambridge, 1996) 85–98.

Marin RS, Differential diagnosis and classification of apathy. Am J Psychiatry (1990) 147:22–30.

Mesulam MM, Hersh LB, Mash DC, Geula C, Differential cholinergic innervation within functional subdivisions of the human cerebral cortex: a choline acetyltransferase study. J Comp Neurol (1992) 318:316–28.

Middelkoop HA, van der Flier WM, Burton EJ et al, Dementia with Lewy bodies and AD are not associated with occipital lobe atrophy on MRI. Neurology (2001) 57:2117–20.

Miller BL, Urrutia LE, Cornford M, Mena I, The clinical and functional imaging characteristics of parkinsonian dementia. In Perry RH, McKeith IG, Perry EK, eds, Dementia with Lewy Bodies (1st edn) (Cambridge University Press: Cambridge, UK, 1996) 114–31.

Minoshima S, Foster NL, Sima AA et al, Alzheimer's disease versus dementia with Lewy bodies: cerebral metabolic distinction with autopsy confirmation. Ann Neurol (2001) 50:358–65.

Mori E, Shimomura T, Fujimori M et al, Visuoperceptual impairment in dementia with Lewy bodies. Arch Neurol (2000) 57:489–93.

Morphy MA, Feldman JA, Kilburn G, Hallervorden–Spatz disease in a psychiatric setting. J Clin Psychiatry (1989) 50:66–8.

Oner O, Oner P, Deda G, Icagasioglu D, Psychotic disorder in a case with Hallervorden–Spatz disease. Acta Psychiatr Scand (2003)108:394–7.

Papka M, Rubio A, Schiffer RB, Cox C, Lewy body disease: can we diagnose it? J Neuropsychiatry Clin Neurosci (1998) 10:405–12.

Pasquier J, Michel BF, Brenot-Rossi I et al, Value of ^{99m}Tc-ECD SPECT for the diagnosis of dementia with Lewy bodies. Eur J Nucl Med Mol Imaging (2002) 29:1342–8.

Perry EK, Perry RH, Acetylcholine and hallucinations: disease-related compared to drug-induced alterations in human consciousness. Brain Cogn (1995) 28: 240–58.

Perry EK, Kerwin J, Perry RH et al, Cerebral cholinergic activity is related to the incidence of visual hallucinations in senile dementia of Lewy body type. Dementia (1990a) 1:2–4.

Perry EK, Marshall E, Perry RH et al, Cholinergic and dopaminergic activities in senile dementia of Lewy body type. Alzheimer Dis Assoc Disord (1990b) 4:87–95.

Perry EK, Marshall E, Kerwin J et al, Evidence of a monoaminergic-cholinergic imbalance related to visual hallucinations in Lewy body dementia. J Neurochem (1990c) 55:1454–6.

Perry EK, Irving D, Kerwin JM et al, Cholinergic transmitter and neurotrophic activities in Lewy body dementia: similarity to Parkinson's and distinction from Alzheimer disease. Alzheimer Dis Assoc Disord (1993a) 7:69–79.

Perry EK, Marshall E, Thompson P et al, Monoaminergic activities in Lewy body dementia: relation to hallucinosis and extrapyramidal features. J Neural Transm Park Dis Dement Sect (1993b) 6:167–77.

Perry EK, Haroutunian V, Davis KL et al, Neocortical cholinergic activities differentiate Lewy body dementia from classical Alzheimer's disease. Neuroreport (1994) 5:747–9.

Perry RH, Irving D, Blessed G et al, Senile dementia of Lewy body type. A clinically and neuropathologically distinct form of Lewy body dementia in the elderly. J Neurol Sci (1990) 95:119–39.

Piggott MA, Striatal dopaminergic markers in dementia with Lewy bodies, Alzheimer's and Parkinson's diseases: rostrocaudal distribution. Brain (1999) 122:1449–68.

Pilo L, Ring H, Quinn N, Trimble M, Depression in multiple system atrophy and in idiopathic Parkinson's disease: a pilot comparative study. Biol Psychiatry (1996) 39:803–7.

Querfurth HW, Allam GJ, Geffroy MA et al, Acetylcholinesterase inhibition in dementia with Lewy bodies: results of a prospective pilot trial. Dement Geriatr Cogn Disord (2000) 11:314–21.

Rockwell E, Choure J, Galasko D et al, Psychopathology at initial diagnosis in dementia with Lewy bodies versus Alzheimer disease: comparison of matched groups with autopsy-confirmed diagnoses. Int J Geriatr Psychiatry (2000) 15:819–23.

Rosen J, Zubenko GS, Emergence of psychosis and depression in the longitudinal evaluation of Alzheimer's disease. Biol Psychiatry (1991) 29: 224–32.

Sachs OW, Aguilar MJ, Brown MJ, Hallervorden–Spatz disease: its pathogenesis and place among the axonal dystrophies. Acta Neuropathologica (1966) 6:164–74.

Salmon DP, Galasko D, Neuropsychological aspects of Lewy body dementia. In: Perry RH, McKeith IG, Perry EK, eds, Dementia with Lewy Bodies (1st edn) (Cambridge University Press: Cambridge, 1996) 99–113.

Samuel W, Caligiuri M, Galasko D et al, Better cognitive and psychopathologic response to donepezil in patients prospectively diagnosed as dementia with Lewy bodies: a preliminary study. Int J Geriatr Psychiatry (2000) 15: 794–802.

Sanchez-Ramos JR, Ortoll R, Paulson GW, Visual hallucinations associated with Parkinson disease. Arch Neurol (1996) 53:1265–8.

Shea C, MacKnight C, Rockwood K, Donepezil for treatment of dementia with Lewy bodies: a case series of nine patients. Int Psychogeriatr (1998) 10: 229–38.

Simard M, van Reekum R, Cohen T, A review of the cognitive and behavioral symptoms in dementia with Lewy bodies. J Neuropsychiatry Clin Neurosci (2000) 12:425–50.

Spigset O, Adverse reactions of selective serotonin reuptake inhibitors: reports from a spontaneous reporting system. Drug Saf (1999) 20:277–87.

Steele C, Rovner B, Chase GA, Folstein M, Psychiatric symptoms and nursing home placement of patients with Alzheimer's disease. Am J Psychiatry (1990) 147: 1049–51.

Swanberg MM, Cummings JL, Benefit–risk considerations in the treatment of dementia with Lewy bodies. Drug Saf (2002) 25:511–23.

Sweet RA, Hamilton RL, Healy MT et al, Alterations of striatal dopamine receptor binding in Alzheimer disease are associated with Lewy body pathology and antemortem psychosis. Arch Neurol (2001) 58:466–72.

Takahashi H, Yoshida K, Sugita T et al, Quetiapine treatment of psychotic symptoms and aggressive behavior in patients with dementia with Lewy bodies: a case series. Prog Neuropsychopharmacol Biol Psychiatry (2003) 27:549–53.

Teunisse RJ, Cruysberg JR, Hoefnagels WH et al, Visual hallucinations in psychologically normal people: Charles Bonnet's syndrome. Lancet (1996) 347:794–7.

Tiraboschi P, Hansen LA, Alford M et al, Cholinergic dysfunction in diseases with Lewy bodies. Neurology (2000) 54:407–11.

Walker Z, Grace J, Overshot R et al, Olanzapine in dementia with Lewy bodies: a clinical study. Int J Geriatr Psychiatry (1999) 14:459–66.

Weiner MF, Risser RC, Cullum CM et al, Alzheimer's disease and its Lewy body variant: a clinical analysis of postmortem verified cases. Am J Psychiatry (1996) 153:1269–73.

Wigboldus JM, Bryun GW, Hallervorden–Spatz disease. In: Vinken PJ, Bryun GW eds, Handbook of Clinical Neurology Diseases of the Basal Ganglia (Elsevier: Amsterdam, 1968) Vol. 6, 604–31.

Yudofsky SC, Hales RE eds, American Psychiatric Press Textbook of Neuropsychiatry (2nd edn) (American Psychiatric Press: Arlington, 1992).

chapter 7

Neurology of dementia with Lewy bodies

David J Burn

Introduction

Although cognitive impairment and neuropsychiatric features are central to the diagnosis of dementia with Lewy bodies (DLB), neurological impairments are also an integral component of the condition (McKeith et al, 2004). Of the neurological abnormalities detected upon examination of the DLB patient, extrapyramidal signs (EPS), manifesting as parkinsonism, are dominant. Reflecting this importance, spontaneous (i.e. not drug-induced) parkinsonism is a core diagnostic feature for DLB (McKeith et al, 1996). Debate continues as to whether the parkinsonian syndrome of DLB differs significantly from that seen in Parkinson's disease (PD). In addition to parkinsonian features, other neurological abnormalities, such as an eye movement disorder, have also been reported in DLB. This chapter will review the neurology of DLB, with particular emphasis upon the extrapyramidal syndrome and its relationship to PD.

Frequency of extrapyramidal signs in DLB

Estimates of the frequency of parkinsonian features at presentation in DLB range between 10% and 78% (McKeith and Burn, 2000). The proportion of DLB cases with EPS at some stage of their illness varies from 40% to 100% (Gnanalingham et al, 1997; Louis et al, 1997; McKeith et al, 1992), with differences likely to represent ascertainment bias, use of neuroleptic agents and variable definitions of clinical phenomenology. In contrast to the cognitively unimpaired PD patient, eliciting unambiguous parkinsonian signs in DLB may be fraught with difficulty and may trap the unwary or inexperienced doctor. Thus, in the demented patient, paratonic rigidity (Gegenhalten) may be mistaken for parkinsonian (lead-pipe) rigidity, a frontal (apraxic, cortical) gait for a parkinsonian gait, and slowed apraxic movements for true parkinsonian bradykinesia (Kurlan et al, 2000). The inclusion of such cortically mediated signs would artificially inflate the true frequency of EPS in DLB.

In a review of 75 case reports of DLB, published between 1961 and 1991, Lennox (1992) determined the frequency of parkinsonism to be 90%, with 50% of patients having three or more of rigidity, tremor, bradykinesia, gait disorder and flexed posture. Two cross-sectional studies comprising 218 DLB patients have reported frequencies for EPS of 68% and 92% (Aarsland et al, 2001; Del Ser et al, 2000).

EPS are therefore a frequent, but not invariable, clinical finding in DLB (Table 7.1). Indeed, an absence of EPS may be the main reason for misdiagnosis of DLB (McKeith et al, 2000). Pathologically, an increased cortical neurofibrillary burden in otherwise-typical DLB cases has been associated with a reduced clinical diagnostic accuracy for DLB and a tendency towards fewer EPS (Merdes et al, 2003).

Table 7.1 Frequency of parkinsonian signs recorded in series of DLB patients and response to levodopa treatment

Reference	No. of cases	Percentage with EPS	Study design	Response to levodopa
Lennox (1992)	75	89	Review	NS
Louis et al (1997)	31	92	Retro and Pro/P+	70% of 10
Gnanalingham et al (1997)	16	100	Xs/P−	100% of 12
Ballard et al (1997)	35	66	Xs/P±	NS
Imamura et al (1999)	15	53	Xs/P−	NS
Del Ser et al (2000)	120	92	Xs/P−	NS
Aarsland et al (2001)	98	68	Xs/ P±	NS
Rojo et al (2002)	40	92	Xs/P−	66% of 19

NS, not stated; Retro, retrospective; Pro, prospective; Xs, cross-sectional; P+/−/±, pathological data available/not available/from some cases only, respectively.

The phenomenology of the extrapyramidal syndrome in DLB

One of the first reports of EPS in DLB compared the parkinsonian features of 8 patients with pathologically confirmed DLB with 20 patients with PD (Louis and Fahn, 1996). Four of seven DLB cases had rigidity noted (57%), compared with 75% of the PD group, a nonsignificant difference. Bradykinesia was recorded in seven out of eight (86%) DLB cases. Tremor was present in six of seven DLB patients and was specifically noted to be a rest tremor in two of the seven. A response to levodopa was described in four DLB patients for whom adequate information was available, although the doses required were not stated.

The same authors subsequently compared EPS in 31 DLB and 34 PD pathologically confirmed cases (Louis et al, 1997). Clinical information was obtained prospectively in some patients. In contrast with their previous report, the DLB group had an older mean age of disease onset than the PD group. Interestingly, those DLB patients presenting with parkinsonism were, on average, 10 years younger than the DLB patients presenting with neuropsychiatric features (60.0 versus 70.9 years). Of the DLB patients, 92% had at least one sign of parkinsonism, with 92% having either rigidity or bradykinesia. A tremor of any sort and a specific rest tremor were recorded in 76% and 55%, respectively. These compared with 88% and 85%, respectively, of the PD group. Myoclonus was documented in 18.5% of DLB patients but none of the PD group. A trial of levodopa was used in 42% DLB patients, with a clinical response recorded in 7 of 10 (70%). The dose of levodopa required and the precise nature of the response were not stated. In attempting to differentiate DLB from PD on the basis of the parkinsonian syndrome, the authors concluded that patients with DLB were 10 times more likely to have one of four clinical features (myoclonus, absence of rest tremor, no perceived need to treat with levodopa and no response to levodopa). The positive predictive value for having DLB with any one of these features was 85.7% (sensitivity 66.7% and specificity 85.7%).

Gnanalingham et al (1997) reported a comparison of clinical features, including EPS, in 16 DLB, 15 PD and 25 Alzheimer disease (AD) patients. Nine of 16 DLB patients (56%) presented with EPS. Greater rigidity and lower scores on a finger-tapping test were noted more frequently in the DLB patients, compared with the PD group, while resting tremor and left/right asymmetry were less common. Since the PD patients were diagnosed according to UK

Parkinson's Disease Brain Bank criteria, and disease asymmetry forms part of these criteria, the latter observation is, of course, a potential tautology. Twelve of 16 (75%) DLB patients had received levodopa at some stage of their disease, and 10 were taking antiparkinsonian drugs at the time of the study. All cases were noted to have been 'responsive', although the degree of motor improvement and the drug dosages required were not stated.

An international multicenter study reported parkinsonism to be present in 92.4% of 120 DLB patients (Del Ser et al, 2000). There was a small but statistically significant difference between male and female patients on a five-item UPDRS subscale (UPDRS-5), with male DLB patients being more severely affected. UPDRS-5 comprises rest tremor, action tremor, bradykinesia, facial expression and rigidity, and is independent of cognitive impairment (Ballard et al, 1997). In the multicenter study, older DLB patients tended to have higher UPDRS scores, although the difference was not statistically significant. Cases with severe cognitive impairment (MMSE < 18) had significantly more severe EPS than those with less cognitive decline using the full UPDRS part III, but when this relationship was re-examined using UPDRS-5, there was no difference between the groups. Patients with more severe dementia may thus have had difficulty understanding and executing some of the instructions, as discussed above. Severity of parkinsonism may therefore be independent of cognitive decline. In common with previous studies, bradykinesia was the most frequent EPS recorded, in 93.3% of the sample. DLB patients were less likely to have tremor of any sort, but if present it was usually symmetrical.

Most recently, Aarsland et al (2001) compared EPS in 98 DLB and 130 PD patients. The DLB group was older at the time of assessment and had a shorter duration of disease compared with the PD patients. Of the DLB patients, 67 (68%) had EPS. More severe action tremor, rigidity, bradykinesia, difficulty arising from a chair, greater facial impassivity and gait disturbance were noted in the DLB group.

The extrapyramidal features reported for DLB in comparison with PD are summarized in Table 7.2. It is important to note that these findings have not all been reliability reproduced.

Table 7.2 Parkinsonian features reported for DLB in relation to PD

Features more common in DLB than in PD
- Rigidity
- Severe facial impassivity
- Postural instability
- Myoclonus

Features less common in DLB than in PD
- Rest tremor
- Asymmetry
- Good levodopa response ± perceived need to treat with levodopa

The spectrum of parkinsonism in PD with and without dementia and DLB

Does the parkinsonian syndrome associated with DLB differ fundamentally from that seen in PD? Given the neuropathological and neurochemical similarities common to both disorders (particularly involvement of the nigrostriatal dopaminergic system), this seems highly improbable, and, while clinical series may describe higher or lower frequencies of certain EPS in DLB compared with PD, there are no *absolute* discriminating features. The pattern of EPS in DLB does, however, seem to show an axial bias (i.e. greater postural instability and facial impassivity), with a tendency towards less tremor, consistent with greater 'nondopaminergic' motor involvement. According to the classification proposed by Jankovic et al (1990), derived from items in UPDRS parts II and III, the postural instability–gait difficulty (PIGD) phenotype of parkinsonism is over-represented in DLB (Burn et al, 2003). This phenotype is also over-represented in PD patients with dementia (PDD), while tremor dominant and PIGD subtypes are more evenly distributed in nondemented PD patients.

The EPS in PD, PDD and DLB are therefore likely to be a spectrum, with a shift towards greater nondopaminergic motor system involvement through PD to DLB. This is consistent with previous studies reporting motor features mediated by nondopaminergic pathways (speech, posture and balance) to correlate more closely with incident dementia in PD than tremor, rigidity and bradykinesia (Foltynie et al, 2002). Degeneration within cholinergic brainstem nuclei, such as the pedunculopontine nucleus, may contribute significantly to the nondopaminergic clinical features.

Progression of parkinsonism in DLB

The progression of parkinsonism in DLB over a 12-month period has been contrasted with EPS noted in AD and vascular dementia patients (Ballard et al, 2000). Unsurprisingly, significant parkinsonism was more frequent in DLB cases (71%) than in patients with AD (7%) or vascular dementia (10%). The degree of cognitive impairment had no influence on the occurrence of EPS. DLB patients with established parkinsonism had an annual increase in severity, assessed using UPDRS, of 9%, a figure comparable with the increase reported for PD. Progression was, however, more rapid in DLB patients with early parkinsonism (49% increase in motor UPDRS score in 1 year) – an observation also in common with PD.

Treatment of parkinsonism in DLB

For the reasons cited above, there does not seem to be any fundamental difference between the extrapyramidal syndrome of PD, PDD and DLB. Although parkinsonism may not be present in all DLB cases at presentation, it develops in the majority during the course of their illness. PDD and DLB therefore differ in that – almost without exception – PD patients develop dementia while taking antiparkinsonian drugs, yet the DLB patient evolves EPS in the face of pre-existing cognitive impairment. Parkinsonism varies between mild and not requiring specific treatment, to severe and incapacitating. In the latter case, and after excluding that the problem is not drug-induced, levodopa preparations are the drugs of choice, although these need to be introduced more cautiously than in the de novo PD patient. Recent data suggest that levodopa is reasonably well tolerated in DLB, but there is also evidence that these patients show a suboptimal response to dopaminergic treatment (Bonelli et al, 2003; Molloy et al, 2004). Of 18 DLB patients given long-term levodopa treatment in one series, two withdrew prematurely with gastrointestinal symptoms, while only two patients had to stop medication with worsening confusion (Molloy et al, 2004). In another study, 20 DLB patients underwent a standardized levodopa test (200/50 mg soluble levodopa/benserazide) during practically defined 'off', in comparison with PDD and PD groups. A less than 20% improvement in motor UPDRS score during the levodopa test was noted in 47% of DLB patients, compared with 55% of PDD and no PD cases, while, in contrast, a greater than 40% improvement in UPDRS was seen in only 18% of DLB and PDD cases, compared with 40% of the PD group (Bonelli et al, 2003). Possible (and not mutually exclusive) explanations for this hyporesponsiveness include intrinsic striatal pathology (Duda et al, 2002), reduced levels of dopamine D_3 receptors (Joyce et al, 2002) or a greater preponderance of cholinergically mediated motor features (Burn et al, 2003).

Other work suggests that gait impairment in DLB may be more responsive to levodopa, compared with upper limb dysfunction (S Molloy, personal communication). Thus, of 14 DLB patients, 64% showed a decrease in step–time product of greater than 20% after levodopa, compared with 54% PD and 71% PDD patients. This observation is not incompatible with other recent data for PD patients with freezing of gait (Bartels et al, 2003) or falls (Schaafsma et al, 2003), suggesting that freezing of gait is an independent motor symptom that has a different pathophysiological basis to bradykinesia, rigidity and postural instability, and that may improve with levodopa.

Future therapeutic approaches for the management of parkinsonism associated with DLB should include larger, double-blinded trials of levodopa administration and the exploration of novel nondopaminergic therapies, such as adenosine A_{2A} antagonists (Bara-Jimenez et al, 2003). Drugs acting via nondopaminergic neurotransmitter systems may offer an improved therapeutic index for the treatment of motor problems without exacerbating neuropsychiatric problems.

Other neurological features

Postural instability, leading to falls, is both an early and a common feature of DLB. A retrospective clinical analysis of pathologically confirmed cases of PD and DLB showed that falls occurred at some point in the disease duration in 91% of 11 and 79% of 14 cases, respectively (Wenning et al, 1999). The mean latency to onset of recurrent falls was, however, much shorter in the DLB group at 48 months, compared with 118 months in the PD group. In a prospective study, multiple falls (defined as more than five falls) occurred in 37% of 30 DLB patients and in only 6% of 35 AD patients (Ballard et al, 1999). The falls often resulted in injury. Other than having DLB, multiple falls were associated with parkinsonism, previous falls, greater impairment of activities of daily living and greater age.

A cross-sectional study of 245 subjects has compared the prevalence, type and severity of gait disorders in DLB, AD, vascular dementia, PD with and without dementia, and healthy age-matched controls (Allan et al, 2003). Gait disorders occurred most commonly in PDD (95.7%), DLB (81.5%) and vascular dementia (74.4%), and were significantly less common in AD (37.5%). A gait disorder present in early dementia (MMSE > 20) was diagnostic of non-AD dementia (DLB, PDD and vascular dementia), with a sensitivity of 80% and specificity of 100%.

Multifocal action myoclonus, which occurs in approximately 15% of DLB patients, is clinically more severe than that associated with PD, although it has the same electrophysiological characteristics. The balance of evidence favors a cortical origin for the myoclonus (Caviness et al, 2003). Since myoclonus also occurs in AD, it could be speculated that concomitant cortical Alzheimer-type pathology could influence the presence and severity of myoclonus in DLB.

Certain aspects of saccadic eye movements (rapid eye movements that shift the fovea to a visual target) are abnormal in DLB (Mosimann et al, 2003). Thus, mean saccadic latency is significantly increased and mean gain of the first saccade is reduced in DLB patients compared with AD and normal controls, while both DLB and AD patients make more errors in an antisaccade task compared with normal controls. The pathophysiological basis for these changes is uncertain, but is likely to reflect both cortical and subcortical pathology.

A supranuclear gaze paresis has also been described in DLB (Fearnley et al, 1991; de Bruin et al, 1992; Brett et al, 2002). Thus, the patient is unable to look up or down to command, yet, when the head is passively flexed and extended with the eyes fixed on an object in front of them, vertical gaze is seen to be intact. In combination with cognitive impairment and falls, this sign may cause diagnostic confusion with Steele–Richardson–Olszewski syndrome (progressive supranuclear palsy). It is, of course, important to establish that an apparent supranuclear gaze palsy is not due to inattention or oculomotor apraxia.

Rare neurological features described in DLB include an alien limb (Santacruz et al, 1996), chorea and dystonia (Lennox and Lowe, 1997). Whether the chorea and dystonia were drug-induced in these cases is open to question.

Conclusions

Neurological abnormalities are common in DLB and are dominated by parkinsonism. The assessment of extrapyramidal and other signs in a cognitively impaired DLB patient may be difficult. In particular, it is important not to overinterpret cortical problems such as apraxia or paratonic rigidity as representing parkinsonism, since this could lead to the inappropriate prescription of antiparkinsonian medications. The parkinsonism of DLB does not differ fundamentally from that seen in PD, although axial features, with postural instability, tend to be over-represented. More work is needed to establish the rate of progression and the response to treatment of the extrapyramidal syndrome in DLB. Further study of more subtle neurological features, such as saccadic eye movement abnormalities and myoclonus, may be of help in the differential diagnosis of DLB and could also shed further light upon the temporal and spatial evolution of the pathophysiological process.

References

Aarsland D, Ballard C, McKeith I et al, Comparison of extrapyramidal signs in dementia with Lewy bodies and Parkinson's disease. J Neuropsychiatry Clin Neurosci (2001) 13:374–9.

Allan LM, Burn DJ, McKeith IG et al, Use of the Tinetti scales to assess gait and balance in dementia with Lewy bodies. Third International Workshop on Dementia with Lewy Bodies and Parkinson's Disease Dementia. Newcastle upon Tyne, UK, 2003.

Ballard C, McKeith I, Burn D et al, The UPDRS scale as a means of identifying extrapyramidal signs in patients suffering from dementia with Lewy bodies. Acta Neurol Scand (1997) 96:366–71.

Ballard CG, Shaw F, Lowery K et al, The prevalence, assessment and associations of falls in dementia with Lewy bodies and Alzheimer's disease. Dement Geriatr Cogn Disord (1999) 10:97–103.

Ballard C, O'Brien J, Swann A et al, One year follow-up of parkinsonism in dementia with Lewy bodies. Dement Geriatr Cogn Disord (2000) 11:219–22.

Bara-Jimenez W, Sherzai A, Dimitrova T et al, Adenosine A_{2A} receptor antagonist treatment of Parkinson's disease. Neurology (2003) 61:293–6.

Bartels AL, Balash Y, Gurevich T et al, Relationship between freezing of gait (FOG) and other features of Parkinson's: FOG is not correlated with bradykinesia. J Clin Neurosci (2003) 10:584–8.

Bonelli S-B, Steffelbauer M, Wolf E et al, Levodopa responsiveness in dementia with Lewy bodies, Parkinson's disease with and without dementia. Third International Workshop on Dementia with Lewy Bodies and Parkinson's Disease Dementia. Newcastle upon Tyne, UK, 2003.

Brett FM, Henson C, Staunton H, Familial diffuse Lewy body disease, eye movement abnormalities, and distribution of pathology. Arch Neurol (2002) 59:464–7.

Burn DJ, Rowan EN, Minnett T et al, Extrapyramidal features in Parkinson's disease with and without dementia and dementia with Lewy bodies: a cross-sectional comparative study. Mov Disord (2003) 18:884–9.

Caviness JN, Adler CH, Caselli RJ, Electrophysiology of the myoclonus in dementia with Lewy bodies. Neurology (2003) 60:523–4.

de Bruin VM, Lees AJ, Daniel SE, Diffuse Lewy body disease presenting with supranuclear gaze palsy, parkinsonism, and dementia: a case report. Mov Disord (1992) 7:355–8.

Del Ser T, McKeith I, Anand R et al, Dementia with Lewy bodies: findings from an international multicentre study. Int J Geriatr Psychiatry (2000) 15:1034–45.

Duda JE, Giasson BI, Mabon ME et al, Novel antibodies to synuclein show abundant striatal pathology in Lewy body diseases. Ann Neurol (2002) 52:205–10.

Fearnley JM, Revesz T, Brooks DJ et al, Diffuse Lewy body disease presenting with a supranuclear gaze palsy. J Neurol Neurosurg Psychiatry (1991) 54:159–61.

Foltynie T, Brayne C, Barker RA, The heterogeneity of idiopathic Parkinson's disease. J Neurol (2002) 249:138–45.

Gnanalingham KK, Byrne EJ, Thornton A et al, Motor and cognitive function in Lewy body dementia: comparison with Alzheimer's and Parkinson's disease. J Neurol Neurosurg Psychiatry (1997) 62:243–52.

Imamura T, Hirono N, Hashimoto M et al, Clinical diagnosis of dementia with Lewy bodies in a Japanese dementia registry. Dement Geriat Cogn Disord (1999) 10:210–16.

Jankovic J, McDermott M, Carter J et al, Variable expression of Parkinson's disease: a baseline analysis of the DATATOP cohort. Neurology (1990) 40:1529–34.

Joyce JN, Ryoo HL, Beach TB et al, Loss of response to levodopa in Parkinson's disease and co-occurrence with dementia: role of D3 and not D2 receptors. Brain Res (2002) 955:138–52.

Kurlan R, Richard IH, Papka M, Marshall F, Movement disorders in Alzheimer's disease: more rigidity of definitions is needed. Mov Disord (2000) 15:24–9.

Lennox G, Lewy body dementia. Baillières Clin Neurol (1992) 1:653–76.

Lennox GG, Lowe JS, Dementia with Lewy bodies. Baillières Clin Neurol (1997) 6:147–66.

Louis ED, Fahn S, Pathologically diagnosed diffuse Lewy body disease and Parkinson's disease: Do the parkinsonian features differ? Adv Neurol (1996) 69:311–14.

Louis ED, Klatka LA, Liu Y, Fahn S, Comparison of extrapyramidal features in 31 pathologically confirmed cases of diffuse Lewy body disease and 34 pathologically confirmed cases of Parkinson's disease. Neurology (1997) 48:376–80.

McKeith IG, Burn DJ, Spectrum of Parkinson's disease, Parkinson's dementia, and Lewy body dementia. In: DeKosky ST, ed, Neurologic Clinics: Dementia (Saunders: Philadelphia, 2000) Vol 18: 865–83.

McKeith IG, Perry RH, Fairbairn AF et al, Operational criteria for senile dementia of Lewy body type (SDLT). Psychol Med (1992) 22:911–22.

McKeith IG, Galasko D, Kosaka K et al, Consensus guidelines for the clinical and pathological diagnosis of dementia with Lewy bodies (DLB): report of the consortium on DLB international workshop. Neurology (1996) 47:1113–24.

McKeith IG, Ballard CG, Perry RH et al, Prospective validation of consensus criteria for the diagnosis of dementia with Lewy bodies. Neurology (2000) 54:1050–8.

McKeith I, Mintzer J, Aarsland D et al, Dementia with Lewy bodies. Lancet Neurol (2004) 3:19–28.

Merdes AR, Hansen LA, Jeste DV et al, Influence of Alzheimer pathology on clinical diagnostic accuracy in dementia with Lewy bodies. Neurology (2003) 60:1586–90.

Molloy S, O'Brien JT, McKeith IG, Burn DJ, The motor response to levodopa in dementia with Lewy bodies: a comparison to Parkinson's disease with and without dementia. J Neurol Neurosurg Psychiatry (2004) in press.

Mosimann UP, Felblinger J, Müri R et al, Saccadic eye movements in dementia with Lewy bodies. Int Psychogeriatrics (2003) 18: 349–50.

Rojo A, Aguilar M, Navas I, Quintana S, Parkinsonism and the response to treatment in dementia with Lewy bodies (DLB). Mov Disord (2002) 17:S257–S258.

Santacruz P, Torner L, Cruz-Sánchez F et al, Corticobasal degeneration syndrome: a case of Lewy body variant of Alzheimer's disease. Int J Geriatr Psychiatry (1996) 11:559–64.

Schaafsma JD, Giladi N, Balash Y et al, Gait dynamics in Parkinson's disease: relationship to Parkinsonian features, falls and response to levodopa. J Neurol Sci (2003) 212:47–53.

Wenning GK, Ebersbach G, Verny M et al, Progression of falls in postmortem-confirmed parkinsonian disorders. Mov Disord (1999) 14:947–50.

-

chapter 8

Autonomic dysfunction in dementia with Lewy bodies

Rose Anne Kenny and Louise M Allan

Background

The autonomic or 'involuntary' nervous system (ANS) is responsible for the control of many bodily functions of which we are not usually aware, such as heart rate, blood pressure, body temperature, saliva and tear production, pupil size, gut motility, and sphincter control. It is one of the most fundamental homeostatic mechanisms within mammalian physiology, and can be disturbed in many disease processes. Despite a dearth of published research, it seems reasonable to postulate that dysautonomia will be common in neurodegenerative causes of dementia, as several neurodegenerative conditions are known to cause autonomic dysfunction. In particular, autonomic failure has long been associated with Parkinson's disease (Martignoni et al, 1995; Koike and Takahashi, 1997; Chaudhuri, 2001), which many investigators now believe to be part of a spectrum of 'Lewy body disorders' including Parkinson's disease (PD), Parkinson's disease with dementia (PDD), dementia with Lewy bodies (DLB) and pure autonomic failure (Hishikawa et al, 2003). If this is the case, one might expect that DLB would also be associated with autonomic failure. Furthermore, DLB has been associated with underactivity of the cholinergic nervous systems (Perry et al, 1990). Acetylcholine is essential for parasympathetic and preganglionic sympathetic neurotransmission. This chapter will review the evidence for the association of autonomic dysfunction with DLB. As most previous research has focused on cardiovascular autonomic function and the neurocardiovascular instability syndromes, the majority of the chapter will be devoted to this area.

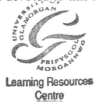

For ease of reference, the sympathetic and parasympathetic divisions of the ANS are shown in Figure 8.1.

Symptoms of autonomic dysfunction

The importance of the ANS is often only appreciated when it is not functioning adequately. Patients with orthostatic intolerance due to generalized autonomic failure have a recognizable pattern of symptoms and aggravating factors that relate to the severity of autonomic failure (Low et al, 1995) (Table 8.1). The commonest symptoms of autonomic failure are orthostatic dizziness, syncope and fatigue. Syncope and falls in older adults are often indistinguishable and in fact are manifestations of similar pathophysiological processes. Up to one-third of cognitively normal older adults have retrograde amnesia for witnessed loss of consciousness (Kenny and Traynor, 1991). Falls in the elderly can therefore be due to unrecognized syncope. Orthostatic hypotension can present with falls alone in the elderly (Ward and Kenny, 1996).

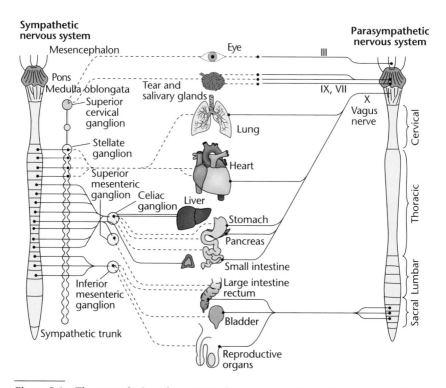

Figure 8.1   *The sympathetic and parasympathetic nervous systems. (From Jänig, 1995.)*

Table 8.1 Symptoms of autonomic failure

Symptoms of orthostatic hypotension	Other autonomic symptoms
Light-headedness or dizziness	Bloating, nausea and vomiting
Syncope	Dry mouth
Falls	Dry eyes
Weakness	Loss of sweating or excessive sweating
Fatigue	Sensitivity to glare
Head and neck pain (coat-hanger pain)	Diarrhea and constipation
Vertigo	Urinary retention
Pallor	Erectile dysfunction
Clamminess	
Blurred vision	
Palpitations	
Tremulousness	
Cognitive difficulties	
Anxiety	
Provoking factors	
Standing	
Physical exertion	
Warm environment	
Time of day	
Meals	

There are few published data regarding autonomic symptoms in DLB. Both syncope and falls are included as supporting features in the diagnostic criteria for DLB (McKeith et al, 1996) and could be caused by underlying autonomic dysfunction. Falls are a common feature of DLB (Ballard et al, 1998, 1999; Del Ser et al, 2000). Orthostatic dizziness has been reported as an early symptom of DLB in 3 cases in a series of 8 patients (Kuzuhara and Yoshimura, 1993), and syncope has been reported as the initial symptom of DLB in 2 of a series of 11 DLB patients (Watanabe et al, 2001). In a retrospective examination for autonomic symptoms in the case notes of a series of cases of DLB, urinary incontinence and constipation were the most commonly documented autonomic symptoms, occurring in 97% and 83% respectively, whereas syncope occurred in 28% (Horimoto et al, 2003; Jellinger et al, 2003). However, retrospective studies are notoriously unreliable for the detection of falls and syncope, and detection of other autonomic symptoms relies upon an initial index of suspicion when taking the history. Prospective studies have suggested that urinary incontinence occurs earlier in DLB than in Alzheimer's disease (AD) (Del Ser et al, 1996, 2001). A scale for assessment of autonomic symptoms in PD has been devised and has demonstrated higher scores in PD patients than in age-matched healthy controls (Berrios et al, 1995). We have used this scale (which contains 12 key autonomic symptoms rated on a scale of 0–3) in our prospective series of dementia patients, and have found significant correlation of the scale with a sensitive measure of autonomic function (heart-rate variability). Autonomic symptom scores in DLB were significantly higher than in age-matched controls or AD. There is clearly a need for further research in this area. The use of symptom scales may be a cheap and effective tool to aid screening for the potential diagnosis of DLB, and may also reveal the scale of this problem in contributing to the symptomatic burden of DLB, both for patients and for carers.

Laboratory evaluation of autonomic function

The detection of an autonomic neuropathy requires a formal laboratory evaluation of autonomic function. Several methods are available, which will be discussed below.

Clinical autonomic function tests

Clinical autonomic function testing usually focuses upon the neurocardiovascular system, as this can be investigated non-invasively. Commonly used tests include the measurement of orthostatic changes in blood pressure and heart rate, the cardiovascular responses to the Valsalva manouver (expiration against a closed glottis), respiratory sinus arrhythmia during respiration at a controlled frequency, response to a cold stimulus (cold pressor test) and isometric exercise (Figures 8.2–8.4) (Anonymous, 1996a). Abnormalities in more than three of these tests are usually taken as an indication of clinically significant autonomic failure (Ewing et al, 1985). Alternatively, a composite scoring system may be used, which has been shown to correlate with severity of disease and prognosis in other common causes of autonomic neuropathy (Low, 1993). Low's group have retrospectively reviewed the autonomic function tests in patients with DLB referred to their laboratory over a 5-year period, and have found that autonomic dysfunction was common, with severity intermediate between PD and multisystem atrophy (MSA) (Watkul et al, 2003). There are currently no prospective studies of autonomic function in DLB using standard clinical autonomic function tests.

(a)

(b)

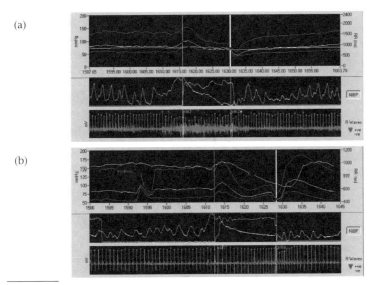

Figure 8.2 *Valsalva manouver: (a) DLB patient; (b) healthy control. In each example the upper trace shows systolic and diastolic blood pressure (red), mean blood pressure (yellow) and R–R intervals (white) against time. The central trace shows respiration (green) and expiratory pressure (white), indicating adequate compliance with the manouver. The lower trace shows the surface ECG (red) and markers of the start and end of the Valsalva manouver (green). In the DLB patient (a), a marked fall in blood pressure during the Valsalva manouver, absence of blood pressure overshoot following the manouver and poor heart rate response are demonstrated.*

(a)

(b)

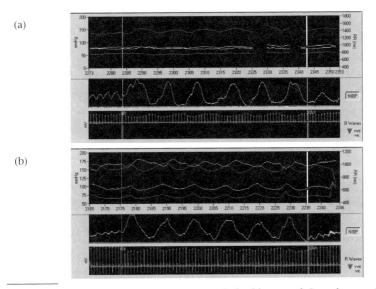

Figure 8.3 *Deep breathing: (a) DLB patient; (b) healthy control. In each example the upper trace shows systolic and diastolic blood pressure (red), mean blood pressure (yellow) and R–R intervals (white) against time. The central trace shows six cycles of deep respiration (green), indicating adequate compliance with the manouver. The lower trace shows the surface ECG (red) and markers of the start and end of the manouver (green). In the DLB patient (a), a poor heart-rate response is demonstrated.*

(a)

(b)

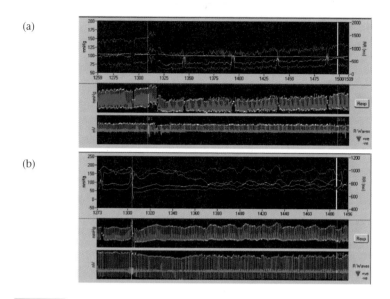

Figure 8.4 *Active stand: (a) DLB patient; (b) healthy control. In each example the upper trace shows systolic and diastolic blood pressure (red), mean blood pressure (yellow) and R–R intervals (white) against time. The central trace shows the analog output of non-invasive blood pressure monitoring (digital photoplethysmography). The lower trace shows the surface ECG (red) and markers of the start and end of the manouver (green). In the DLB patient (a), marked orthostatic hypotension and a poor heart-rate response are demonstrated.*

Heart-rate variability

Heart-rate variability is a non-invasive method of assessing autonomic function that has been used extensively as a research tool, although it is less suitable for clinical use (Figure 8.5) (Akselrod et al, 1981; Anonymous, 1996b). It requires less cooperation from the subject than other autonomic function tests and is suitable for use in patients with dementia. Power-spectral analysis of heart-rate variability produces power bands, or spectra, which vary according to the tone of modulating autonomic activity (Malliani et al, 1991). High-frequency changes in heart rate are abolished by atropine and thus are thought to represent the rapid activity of the parasympathetic nervous system, whereas low-frequency variation in heart rate is thought to reflect both sympathetic and parasympathetic activity. Very low-frequency variability is thought to be due to a combination of factors, including thermoregulation. The technique is sensitive for the detection of early autonomic neuropathy, as shown in diabetic patients (Bellavere et al, 1992).

We have found that heart-rate variability in the low-frequency band and the very low frequency band is reduced in DLB when compared with controls

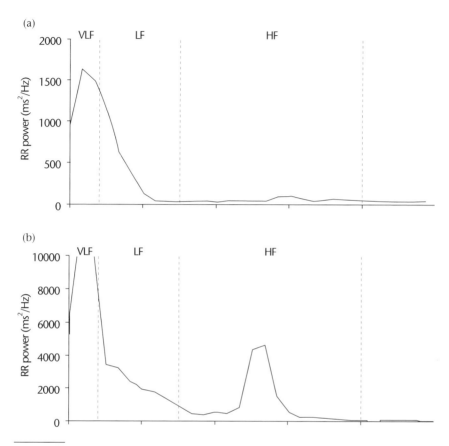

Figure 8.5 *Power spectrum of heart-rate variability in (a) a patient with Parkinson's disease with dementia and (b) a healthy control. VLF, very low frequency (<0.04 Hz); LF, low frequency (0.04–0.15 Hz); HF, high frequency (0.15–0.4 Hz). Total power and power in each band are much reduced in the patient compared with the healthy control. (Note the difference in the vertical-axis scales.)*

(Allan et al, 2003). In the same study, we found a reduction in heart-rate variability in all frequency bands in PD patients both with and without dementia. There were no significant differences between DLB and PDD. This corroborates the recent view that DLB is part of a continuous spectrum of Lewy body disorders, which include PD and PDD.

The finding of reduced heart-rate variability in DLB has clinical significance because reduced heart-rate variability has been shown to be a risk factor for increased mortality after myocardial infarction (Kleiger et al, 1987; Zuaretti et al, 1996) and for increased all-cause mortality in an elderly population (Tsuji et al, 1994). This may be because of an excess of sudden deaths due to arrhythmias, and it has been postulated that this is a potential therapeutic target in cardiovascular disease (Routledge et al, 2002). Dementia has long been recognized to be associated with an excess of all-cause mortality, but the causes of the excess deaths are not well understood (Dewey and Sab, 2001). In a pilot study, we have also shown that cholinesterase inhibitors can cause a further reduction in heart-rate variability in dementia patients with AD and DLB (McLaren et al, 2003). The role of autonomic dysfunction in mortality rates in dementia subtypes and the contribution of cholinesterase inhibition to mortality and autonomic symptomatology clearly need further study.

Cardiac ^{123}I-MIBG scintigraphy

m-Iodobenzylguanidine (MIBG) is a physiological analog of norepinephrine (noradrenaline), which has previously been used as a non-invasive method of screening for local myocardial sympathetic nerve damage in various cardiac and neurological diseases. There are now several studies confirming that cardiac uptake of ^{123}I-MIBG is reduced in idiopathic PD both with and without autonomic failure (Orimo et al, 1999, 2002; Yoshita, 2000). Two studies have shown that cardiac uptake of ^{123}I-MIBG is also markedly reduced in DLB but not AD (Watanabe et al, 2001; Yoshita et al, 2001) (Figure 8.6). Both groups postulate that cardiac uptake of MIBG is a more reliable marker of DLB than an orthostatic test. One group has reported better sensitivity and specificity of this test for distinguishing between AD and DLB when directly compared with FP-CIT single-photon emission computed tomography (SPECT) (Yoshita and Yamada, 2003). It remains to be seen whether alternative non-invasive clinical autonomic function tests might be an equally good marker of the diagnosis.

Other autonomic function tests

Other methods of evaluation of autonomic function include quantitative sudomotor axon testing, thermoregulatory sweat testing, sympathetic skin response, microneurography, pupillography, measurement of tear production, nocturnal penile tumescence studies and sphincter electromyography. One group has reported a very high prevalence of lower urinary tract signs in DLB in comparison with PDD, PD and AD (Ransmayr et al, 2003), but there are no other laboratory studies of noncardiovascular autonomic function in DLB.

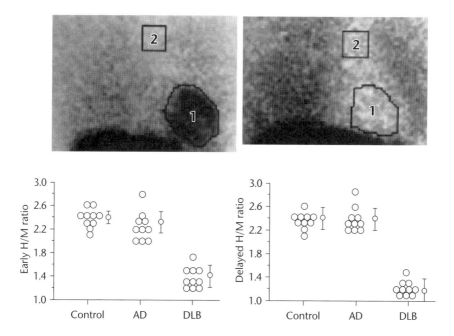

Figure 8.6 *Examples of cardiac* [123]*I-MIBG uptake in a patient with AD (left) and a patient with DLB (right). (From Watanabe et al, 2001).*

Neurocardiovascular instability

Neurocardiovascular instability (NCVI) is defined as age-related changes in blood pressure and heart-rate behavior, predominantly resulting in hypotension and bradyarrhythmia (Kenny et al, 2002). The commonest manifestations of NCVI are orthostatic hypotension, carotid sinus syndrome, postprandial hypotension and vasovagal syndrome. Older adults are more susceptible to NCVI because of age-related physiological changes in the cardiovascular system, autonomic nervous system and humoral control of blood pressure, in addition to polypharmacy. Most patients with dementia are in this susceptible age group, and therefore it is important to remember that NCVI in dementia patients is not always due to underlying autonomic dysfunction. However, if DLB is associated with autonomic dysfunction, one might expect that the prevalence of NCVI would be higher in DLB than in other dementias. Neurocardiovascular instability has been shown to be present in 70% of cognitively impaired fallers and is over-represented in those patients who benefit from multifactorial interventions for prevention of falls (Shower et al, 2003). This suggests that neurocardiovascular instability may be a risk factor for falls in DLB that is amenable to intervention. This may be relatively more important than other risk factors such as gait and balance instability, environmental hazard modification, and visual impairment.

Orthostatic hypotension

In patients with autonomic failure, the most troubling of the symptoms described are orthostatic dizziness and syncope. These symptoms are frequently due to orthostatic hypotension (OH). It seems likely that cognitive difficulties and falls in DLB could be exacerbated by OH. The prevalence of OH in DLB has not been clearly established. Its prevalence in any elderly population depends upon the methodology employed to determine whether it is present, the comorbidities of the participants, and the number and type of medications they are taking. There is some evidence comparing the prevalence of OH in DLB with that in AD, but no studies comparing DLB with healthy age-matched controls, PD with and without dementia, or vascular dementia. The standard definition of OH is a fall in systolic blood pressure of 20 mmHg or to a level below 90 mmHg, or a fall in diastolic blood pressure of 10 mmHg, within 3 minutes of standing (Anonymous, 1996c). None of the studies that have assessed OH in DLB have used this definition.

In a prospective study of 30 patients with DLB, the prevalence of OH was 40% of all patients, 38% of patients who were not taking any medications that could have caused OH, and 29% of patients who had no history of hypertension or ECG evidence of ischemic heart disease (Ballard et al, 1998). OH was also found to occur in 32% of 35 patients with AD, and the difference in prevalence was not significant. This study used the definition of OH as a fall in systolic blood pressure of more than 20 mmHg during 2 minutes of standing. Non-invasive beat-to-beat photoplethysmography was used to determine the blood pressure, which is a highly sensitive method.

Watanabe et al (2001) used a definition of OH as a fall of 30 mmHg in systolic pressure or 15 mHg in diastolic pressure upon standing for an unspecified period of time. In a series of 11 patients, OH was present in 7 (63%), of whom 4 also displayed syncope on standing. No control group was studied. Yoshita et al (2001) studied a series of 14 DLB patients, of whom 13 had OH (93%), using a definition of OH as a fall in systolic blood pressure of 20 mmHg or diastolic blood pressure of 10 mm Hg within 10 minutes of standing. The prolonged length of the stand may have accounted for the extremely high prevalence in this study, and indeed some would argue that hypotension occurring beyond the first 3 minutes should be classified as a vasovagal response. Yoshita et al (2001) did include a control group of 14 AD patients, only 4 of whom had OH. The method of blood pressure measurement is not given in either of these studies.

In case series of Londos et al (2000) in which the diagnosis of DLB was retrospectively applied, 17 AD and 18 DLB cases underwent orthostatic testing. There were no differences in the prevalence of OH between DLB and AD, as this was high in both groups. However, the maximal drop in blood pressure on orthostasis was higher in the DLB group than the AD group (32.4 ± 12.6 mmHg vs 24.2 ± 11.5 mmHg). The DLB patients were also more likely to have received treatment that could exacerbate OH, leading Londos et al (2000) to caution against polypharmacy in this group. As this was a retrospective study, the exact role of culprit medications in this series could not be established.

The role of medications in exacerbation of OH in DLB is unclear. A peripherally acting cholinesterase inhibitor (pyridostigmine) has been reported to be a useful treatment for OH in a group of patients without dementia (Singer et al, 2003). However, in a pilot study, we have found that the administration of donepezil exacerbates OH, and causes the development of de novo OH in some patients (Allan et al, 2000). Levodopa can exacerbate OH in PD (Kujawa et al, 2000).

The evidence so far therefore suggests that, although it is important to consider OH in dementia, particularly when planning treatment, the presence of OH is not sufficiently specific to discriminate between AD and DLB. The significance of the severity or duration of OH is also unclear. There is some evidence that a fall in systolic blood pressure of greater than 30 mmHg on standing is associated with a greater risk of significant white matter hyperintensities in basal ganglia and deep white matter on magnetic resonance imaging (MRI) (Ballard et al, 2000), but longitudinal studies are required to elucidate this further.

There are several nonpharmacological interventions for OH, including avoidance of precipitating factors for low blood pressure, physical countermanouvers (Bouvette et al, 1996), elevation of the head of the bed at night (Ten Harkel et al, 1992) and application of graduated pressure with support garments (Denq et al, 1997). Recommended pharmacological interventions include fludrocortisone (Hussain et al, 1996), midodrine (Low et al, 1997; Wright et al, 1998), desmopressin (DDAVP) and octreotide (Bordet et al, 1994). All drug treatment for OH requires frequent monitoring for supine hypertension, electrolyte imbalance and congestive heart failure.

Carotid sinus hypersensitivity and carotid sinus syndrome

Carotid sinus reflex sensitivity (Figure 8.7) is assessed by measuring heart-rate and blood-pressure responses to carotid sinus massage. The recommended duration of carotid sinus massage is from 5 to 10 seconds. Carotid sinus hypersensitivity (CSH) is present if carotid sinus massage produces asystole exceeding 3 seconds (cardioinhibitory – Figure 8.8), or a fall in systolic blood pressure exceeding 50 mmHg in the absence of cardioinhibition (vasodepressor) or a combination of the two (mixed) (Kenny et al, 2000) (Figures 8.9 and 8.10). Complications resulting from carotid sinus massage include cardiac arrhythmias and neurological sequelae. Persistent neurological complications are reported to occur in 0.04% (Munro et al, 1994; Davies and Kenny, 1998; Richardson et al, 2000). Carotid sinus massage should not be performed in patients who have had a recent cerebrovascular event or myocardial infarction, i.e. within 3 months of events. In one-third of patients, a diagnostic response is only achieved during upright carotid sinus massage (Parry et al, 2000).

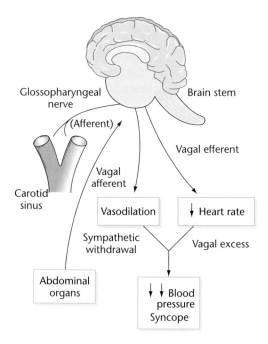

Figure 8.7 *Anatomy of the carotid sinus reflex.*

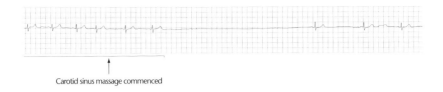

Carotid sinus massage commenced

Figure 8.8 *An example of cardioinhibitory carotid sinus hypersensitivity. A period of asystole of over 6 seconds is recorded.*

In two prospective studies, the prevalence of cardioinhibitory CSH in DLB was 41% and 31% respectively (Ballard et al, 1998; Kenny et al, 2004). This was significantly higher than in AD (28% and 11% respectively). Vasodepressor CSH occurred in 10% of cases, and was not significantly more common than in AD. However, the magnitude of blood-pressure fall was significantly greater in DLB patients than in AD patients (Kenny et al, 2004). In the DLB patients, the magnitude of blood-pressure fall on CSM correlated with the severity of deep white matter hyperintensities on MRI (Kenny et al, 2004).

Carotid sinus syndrome (CSS) is diagnosed in subjects with otherwise unexplained recurrent syncope who have CSH. The syndrome is an important but frequently overlooked cause of syncope and presyncope in older subjects. The symptoms are usually precipitated by mechanical stimulation of the carotid

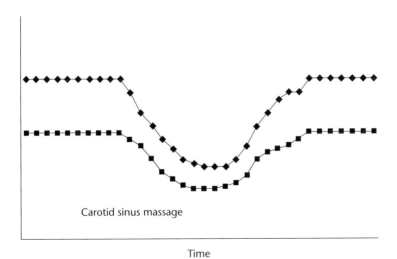

Carotid sinus massage

Time

Figure 8.9 *Vasodepressor carotid sinus hypersensitivity: a fall in blood pressure of over 50 mmHg in response to carotid sinus massage.*

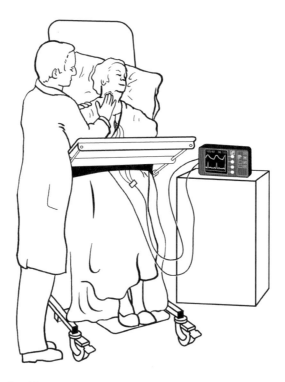

Figure 8.10   *Tilt table. (From Kenny et al, 2002.)*

sinus, i.e. by head turning, tight neckwear, neck pathology and vagal stimuli such as prolonged standing. Other recognized triggers for symptoms are post-prandial state, straining, looking or stretching upwards, exertion, defecation, and micturition (Kenny, 2002). The prevalence of CSS in DLB is unknown and difficult to assess because of the overlap between syncope and falls in older adults. Ballard et al (1999) did not show increased risk of recurrent falls in patients with CSH, but this may have been due to the short follow-up period of this study. Syncope after the use of cholinesterase inhibitors has been reported (NICE, 2001). We have reported a case with CSS in which syncopal symptoms started after cholinesterase treatment was commenced. Insertion of a cardiac pacemaker cured syncopal symptoms and allowed the patient to resume cholinesterase treatment (Newby et al, 2004).

Dual-chamber cardiac pacing is the treatment of choice in patients with symptomatic cardioinhibitory CSS. With appropriate pacing, syncope is abolished in 85–90% of patients with cardioinhibition (Morley et al, 1982;

Madigan et al, 1984; Brignole et al, 1992). Patients with non-accidental falls who have cardioinhibitory CSH also benefit from cardiac pacing (Kenny et al, 2001). Treatment of vasodepressor CSS is less successful, due to poor understanding of its pathophysiology. Fludrocortisone, a mineralocorticoid widely used in the treatment of OH, has been used in the treatment of vasodepressor CSS with good results but its use is limited in the longer term by adverse effects (da Costa et al, 1993).

Vasovagal syncope

CSH can coexist with other hypotensive disorders such as vasovagal syncope and OH in patients with cognitive impairment (Shaw et al, 2003). Only one study has examined vasovagal syncope in DLB patients. Ballard et al (1998) showed a positive response to a prolonged passive head-up tilt in 7% of their patients with DLB.

A number of drugs are reported to be useful in alleviating vasovagal symptoms, including β-blockers, disopyramide, fludrocortisone, fluoxetine, sertraline and midodrine. Elastic support hose, relaxation techniques (biofeedback) and conditioning using repeated head-up tilt as therapy are useful adjuvant therapies. Permanent cardiac pacing is beneficial in some patients, who have recurrent syncope and cardioinhibitory responses (Parry and Kenny, 1999; Brignole et al, 2001).

Hypotension and hypertension

A strong relationship between supine hypertension and OH has been reported among unmedicated, institutionalized older subjects (Lipsitz, 1989), and has also been reported in patients with autonomic neuropathy (Goldstein et al, 2003) (Figure 8.11). There have been several longitudinal studies suggesting that midlife hypertension is associated with dementia (Skoog et al, 1996) but that systemic blood pressure falls before the onset of dementia in later life (Guo et al, 1996). In a large dementia case series in which diagnoses of DLB or AD were retrospectively applied, Londos et al (2000) found that blood pressure did decline with advancing dementia in both diagnoses, but significant hypotension (systolic blood pressure <120 mmHg) was more prevalent in late DLB than in late AD (40% vs 31%). This effect was independent of age. The DLB patients were more likely to have taken culprit medications associated with hypotension. This is a potential confounding factor, which draws attention to

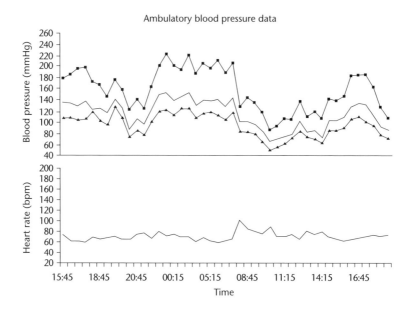

Figure 8.11 *Twenty-four-hour blood pressure with supine hypertension and orthostatic hypotension. Note the high blood pressure during night-time hours when the patient is supine, and the hypotension on arising in the morning, which is commonly associated with dizziness, syncope and falls.*

the need for prospective studies to elucidate whether DLB is associated with supine hypertension or hypotension. The management of patients who have supine hypertension and OH is very difficult, as antihypertensive treatments exacerbate OH and treatment for OH will exacerbate supine hypertension.

Neuropathology

There is emerging neuropathological evidence that Lewy bodies (LBs) are widespread in the autonomic nervous system in the Lewy body disorders (Hague et al, 1997; Iwanaga et al, 1999; Arai et al, 2000; Hishikawa et al, 2003). LBs and α-synuclein staining have been reported in the locus ceruleus, substantia nigra, preganglionic parasympathetic cells and sympathetic ganglia at autopsy in cases of pure autonomic failure (Hague et al, 1997; Wakabayashi et al, 1999; Arai et al, 2000). There are similar findings in PD (Wakabayashi et al, 1993). LBs are not confined to the cardiovascular autonomic nervous system, having been found in the enteric nervous system (Wakabayashi et al, 1990, 1993). In one study, a series of cases with confirmed neocortical LB disease at autopsy all showed parkinsonism, dementia and autonomic failure in life, as did many with limbic-type disease (Hishikawa et al, 2003). Those with brainstem-type disease had autonomic failure without dementia. However, only three of the cases were deemed to have presented with a clear diagnosis of DLB during life. This was a retrospective study, and autonomic failure was diagnosed from case notes rather than formal autonomic function tests, which is very unreliable, as previously noted. Further prospective clinicopathological studies comparing patients with DLB, PDD, PD and pure autonomic failure are currently ongoing.

Summary

In summary, there is now sufficient evidence to suggest that autonomic dysfunction may be a significant and adverse feature of DLB. However, there are no prospective or longitudinal studies with sufficient formal evaluation of autonomic function to confirm this conclusively. Future work should prioritize autonomic dysfunction, as there are potential clinical implications in terms of falls, syncope and serious injury, in addition to possible adverse effects on progression and mortality.

References

Akselrod S, Gordon D, Ubel FA et al, Power spectrum analysis of heart rate fluctuation: a quantitative probe of beat-to-beat cardiovascular control. Science (1981) 213:220–2.

Allan L, Ballard C, McLaren A, Kenny R, Neurocardiovascular instability in neurodegenerative dementia. Clin Neuropsychol Assess (2000) 1:50.

Allan LM, Ballard CJ, Allen J et al, Autonomic dysfunction is present in dementia with Lewy bodies. Abstract JAGS (In Press).

American Academy of Neurology, Assessment: Clinical autonomic testing report of the Therapeutics and Technology Assessment Subcommittee of the American Academy of Neurology. Neurology (1996a) 46:873–80.

Arai K, Kato N, Kashiwado K, Hattori T, Pure autonomic failure in association with human alpha-synucleinopathy. Neurosci Lett (2000) 296:171–3.

Ballard CG, O'Brien J, Lowery K et al, A prospective study of dementia with Lewy bodies. Age Ageing (1998) 27:631–6.

Ballard CG, Shaw F, Lowery K et al. The prevalence, assessment and associations of falls in dementia with Lewy bodies and Alzheimer's disease. Dement Geriatr Cogn Disord (1999) 10:97–103.

Ballard C, O'Brien J, Barber B et al, Neurocardiovascular instability, hypotensive episodes, and MRI lesions in neurodegenerative dementia. Ann NY Acad Sci (2000) 903:442–5.

Ballard C, Shaw F, McKeith I, Kenny R, High prevalence of neurovascular instability in neurodegenerative dementias. Neurology (1998) 51:1760–2.

Bellavere F, Balzani I, De Masi G et al, Power spectral analysis of heart-rate variations improves assessment of diabetic cardiac autonomic neuropathy. Diabetes (1992) 41: 633–40.

Berrios GE, Campbell C, Politynska BE, Autonomic failure, depression and anxiety in Parkinson's disease. Br J Psychiatry (1995) 166:789–92.

Bordet R, Benhadjali J, Libersa C, Destee A, Octreotide in the management of orthostatic hypotension in multiple system atrophy: pilot trial of chronic administration. Clin Neuropharmacol (1994) 17:380–3.

Bouvette CM, McPhee BR, Opfer-Gehrking TL, Low PA, Role of physical counter-maneuvers in the management of orthostatic hypotension: efficacy and biofeedback augmentation. Mayo Clin Proc (1996) 71:847–53.

Brignole M, Menozzi C, Lolli G, et al, Long-term outcome of paced and nonpaced patients with severe carotid sinus syndrome. American Journal of Cardiology (1992) 69(12), 1039–43.

Brignole M, Alboni P, Benditt D et al, Task Force on Syncope, European Society of Cardiology. Part 2. Diagnostic tests and treatment: summary of recommendations. Europace (2001) 3:261–8.

Chaudhuri KR, Autonomic dysfunction in movement disorders. Curr Opin Neurol (2001) 14:505–11.

Consensus statement on the definition of orthostatic hypotension, pure autonomic failure, and multiple system atrophy. J Neurol Sci (1996c) 144:218–19.

da Costa D, McIntosh S, Kenny RA, Benefits of fludrocortisone in the treatment of symptomatic vasodepressor carotid sinus syndrome. Br Heart J (1993) 69: 308–10.

Davies AJ, Kenny RA, Frequency of neurologic complications following carotid sinus massage. Am J Cardiol (1998) 81:1256–7.

Del Ser T, Hachinski V, Merskey H, Munoz DG, Clinical and pathologic features of two groups of patients with dementia with Lewy bodies: effect of coexisting Alzheimer-type lesion load. Alzheimer Dis Assoc Disord (2001) 15:31–44.

Del-Ser T, Munoz DG, Hachinski V, Temporal pattern of cognitive decline and incontinence is different in Alzheimer's disease and diffuse Lewy body disease. Neurology (1996) 46:682–6.

Del Ser T, McKeith I, Anand R et al, Dementia with Lewy bodies: findings from an international multicentre study. Int J Geriatr Psychiatry (2000) 15:1034–45.

Denq JC, Opfer-Gehrking TL, Giuliani M et al, Efficacy of compression of different capacitance beds in the amelioration of orthostatic hypotension. Clin Autonom Res (1997) 7:321–6.

Dewey ME, Saz P, Dementia, cognitive impairment and mortality in persons aged 65 and over living in the community: a systematic review of the literature. Int J Geriatr Psychiatry (2001) 16:751–61.

Ewing DJ, Martyn CN, Young RJ, Clarke BF, The value of cardiovascular autonomic function tests: 10 years experience in diabetes. Diabetes Care (1985) 8(5):491–8.

Goldstein DS, Pechnik S, Holmes C, et al, Association between supine hypertension and orthostatic hypotension in autonomic failure. Hypertension (2003) 42:136–42.

Guo Z, Viitanen M, Fratiglioni L, Winblad B, Low blood pressure and dementia in elderly people: the Kungsholmen project. BMJ (1996) 312:805–8.

Hague K, Lento P, Morgello S et al, The distribution of Lewy bodies in pure autonomic failure: autopsy findings and review of the literature. Acta Neuropathol (1997) 94:192–6.

Hishikawa N, Hashizume Y, Yoshida M, Sobue G, Clinical and neuropathological correlates of Lewy body disease. Acta Neuropathol (2003) 105:341–50.

Horimoto Y, Matsumoto M, Akatsu H et al, Autonomic dysfunctions in dementia with Lewy bodies. J Neurol (2003) 250:530–3.

Hussain RM, McIntosh SJ, Lawson J, Kenny RA, Fludrocortisone in the treatment of hypotensive disorders in the elderly. Heart (1996) 76:507–9.

Iwanaga K, Wakabayashi K, Yoshimoto M et al, Lewy body-type degeneration in cardiac plexus in Parkinson's and incidental Lewy body diseases. Neurology (1999) 52:1269–1271.

Jellinger KA, Horimoto Y, Matsumoto M et al, Neuropathological spectrum of synucleinopathies, Autonomic dysfunctions in dementia with Lewy bodies. Movement Disorders (2003) 18(Suppl 6):530–3.

Kenny RA, Neurally mediated syncope. Clin Geriatr Med (2002) 18:191–210.

Kenny RA, Traynor G, Carotid sinus syndrome – clinical characteristics in elderly patients. Age Ageing (1991) 20:449–54.

Kenny RA, O'Shea D, Parry SW, The Newcastle protocols for head-up tilt table testing in the diagnosis of vasovagal syncope, carotid sinus hypersensitivity, and related disorders. Heart (2000) 83:564–9.

Kenny RA, Richardson DA, Steen N et al, Carotid sinus syndrome: a modifiable risk factor for nonaccidental falls in older adults (SAFE PACE). J Am Coll Cardiol (2001) 38:1491–6.

Kenny RA, Kalaria R, Ballard C, Neurocardiovascular instability in cognitive impairment and dementia. Ann NY Acad Sci (2002) 977:183–95.

Kenny RA, Shaw F, O'Brien JT et al, Carotid sinus syndrome is common in dementia with Lewy bodies and correlated with deep white matter lesions. J Neurol Neurosurg Psychiatry (2004) 75:966–71.

Kleiger RE, Miller JP, Bigger JT, Moss AJ, Decreased heart rate variability and its association with increased mortality after acute myocardial infarction. Am J Cardiol (1987) 59: 256–62.

Koike Y, Takahashi A, Autonomic dysfunction in Parkinson's disease. Eur Neurol (1997) 38(Suppl 2): 8–12.

Kujawa K, Leurgans S, Raman R et al, Acute orthostatic hypotension when starting dopamine agonists in Parkinson's disease. Arch Neurol (2000) 57:461–3.

Kuzuhara S, Yoshimura M, Clinical and neuropathological aspects of diffuse Lewy body disease in the elderly. Adv Neurol (1993) 60:464–9.

Lipsitz LA, Altered blood pressure homeostasis in advanced age: clinical and research implications. J Gerontol (1989) 44:M179–83.

Londos E, Passant U, Gustafson L, Blood pressure and drug treatment in clinically diagnosed Lewy body dementia and Alzheimer's disease. Arch Gerontol Geriatrics (2000) 30:35–46.

Low PA, Composite autonomic scoring scale for laboratory quantification of generalized autonomic failure. Mayo Clin Proc (1993) 68:748–52.

Low PA, Opfer-Gehrking TL, McPhee BR et al, Prospective evaluation of clinical characteristics of orthostatic hypotension. Mayo Clinic Proceedings (1995) 70(7): 617–22.

Low PA, Gilden JL, Freeman R et al, Efficacy of midodrine vs placebo in neurogenic orthostatic hypotension. A randomized, double-blind multicenter study. Midodrine Study Group. JAMA (1997) 277:1046–51.

McKeith IG, Galasko D, Kosaka K et al, Consensus guidelines for the clinical and pathologic diagnosis of dementia with Lewy bodies (DLB): report of the consortium on DLB international workshop. Neurology (1996) 47:1113–24.

McLaren AT, Allen J, Murray A et al, Cardiovascular effects of donepezil in patients with dementia. Dementia Geriatr Cogn Disord, (2003) 15:83–8.

Madigan NP, Flaker GC, Curtis JJ et al, Carotid sinus hypersensitivity: beneficial effects of dual-chamber pacing. Am J Cardiol (1984) 53:1034–40.

Malliani A, Pagani M, Lombardi F, Cerutti S, Cardiovascular neural regulation explored in the frequency domain. Circulation (1991) 84:482–92.

Martignoni E, Pacchetti C, Godi L et al, Autonomic disorders in Parkinson's disease. J Neural Transm Suppl (1995) 45:11–19.

Morley CA, Perrins EJ, Grant P et al, Carotid sinus syncope treated by pacing, analysis of persistent symptoms and role of atrioventricular sequential pacing. Br Heart J (1982) 47:411–8.

Munro NC, McIntosh S, Lawson J et al, Incidence of complications after carotid sinus massage in older patients with syncope. J Am Geriatr Soc (1994) 42:1248–51.

Newby VJ, Kenny RA et al, Cholinesterase inhibitors and cardiac syncope, Int J Geriatr Psychiatry (in press) (2004).

NICE (National Institute for Clinical Excellence), Guidance for the Use of Donepezil, Rivastigmine and Galantamine for the Treatment of Alzheimer's Disease (NICE: London, 2001).

Orimo S, Ozawa E, Nakade S et al, [123]I-*meta*-iodobenzylguanidine myocardial scintigraphy in Parkinson's disease. J Neurol Neurosurg Psychiatry (1999) 67:189–94.

Orimo S, Oka T, Miura H et al, Sympathetic cardiac denervation in Parkinson's disease and pure autonomic failure but not in multiple system atrophy. J Neurol Neurosurg Psychiatry (2002) 73:776–7.

Parry SW, Kenny RA, The management of vasovagal syncope. QJM (1999) 92:697–705.

Parry SW, Richardson DA, O'Shea D et al, Diagnosis of carotid sinus hypersensitivity in older adults: carotid sinus massage in the upright position is essential. Heart (2000) 83:22–3.

Perry EK, Marshall E, Perry RH et al, Cholinergic and dopaminergic activities in senile dementia of Lewy body type. Alzheimer Dis Assoc Disord (1990) 4:87–95.

Ransmayr G, Kiss G, Holliger S et al, Lower urinary tract signs in dementia with Lewy bodies compared to Parkinson's and Alzheimer's disease. In: Proceedings of 3rd International Workshop on Dementia with Lewy Bodies and Parkinson's Disease Dementia, Newcastle upon Tyne (2003).

Richardson DA, Bexton R, Shaw FE et al, Complications of carotid sinus massage – a prospective series of older patients. Age Ageing (2000) 29:413–17.

Routledge HC, Chowdhary S, Townend JN, Heart rate variability – a therapeutic target? J Clin Pharmacy Therap (2002) 27:85–92.

Shaw FE, Bond J, Richardson DA et al, Multifactorial intervention after a fall in older people with cognitive impairment and dementia presenting to the Accident and Emergency Department: randomised controlled trial. BMJ (2003) 326:73.

Singer W, Opfer-Gehrking TL, McPhee BR et al. Acetylcholinesterase inhibition: a novel approach in the treatment of neurogenic orthostatic hypotension. J Neurol Neurosurg Psychiatry (2003) 74:1294–8.

Skoog I, Lernfelt B, Landahl S, et al, 15-year longitudinal study of blood pressure and dementia. Lancet (1996) 347:1141–5.

Task Force of the European Society of Cardiology and the North American Society of Pacing and Electrophysiology. Heart rate variability: standards of measurement, physiological interpretation and clinical use. Circulation (1996b) 93:1043–65.

Ten Harkel AD, Van Lieshout JJ, Wieling W, Treatment of orthostatic hypotension with sleeping in the head-up tilt position, alone and in combination with fludrocortisone. J Intern Med (1992) 232:139–45.

Tsuji H, Venditti FJ, Manders ES et al, Reduced heart rate variability and mortality risk in an elderly cohort. The Framingham Heart Study. Circulation (1994) 90:878–83.

Wakabayashi K, Takahashi H, Ohama E, Ikuta F. Parkinson's disease: an immunohistochemical study of Lewy body-containing neurons in the enteric nervous system. Acta Neuropathol (1990) 79:581–3.

Wakabayashi K, Takahashi H, Ohama E et al, Lewy bodies in the visceral autonomic nervous system in Parkinson's disease. Adv Neurol (1993) 60:609–12.

Wakabayashi K, Hayashi S, Morita T et al, Neurofibrillary tangles in the peripheral sympathetic ganglia of non-Alzheimer elderly individuals. Clin Neuropathol (1999) 18:171–5.

Ward C, Kenny RA, Reproducibility of orthostatic hypotension in symptomatic elderly. Am J Med (1996) 100(4):418–22.

Watanabe H, Ieda T, Katayama T et al, (2001) Cardiac ¹²³I-*meta*-iodobenzylguanidine (MIBG) uptake in dementia with Lewy bodies: comparison with Alzheimer's disease. J Neurol Neurosurg Psychiatry 70:781–3.

Watkul PT, Boeve BF, Bennarroch E et al, Autonomic dysfunction in dementia with Lewy bodies. In: Proceedings of 3rd International Workshop on Dementia with Lewy Bodies and Parkinson's Disease Dementia, Newcastle upon Tyne, UK (2003).

Wright RA, Kaufmann HC, Perera R et al, A double-blind, dose-response study of midodrine in neurogenic orthostatic hypotension. Neurology (1998) 51:120–4.

Yoshita M, Loss of ¹²³I-*meta*-iodobenzylguanidine uptake by the heart in Parkinson's disease. J Nucl Med (2000) 41:1442.

Yoshita M, Yamada M, Occipital cerebral hypoperfusion and cardiac sympathetic dysfunction in dementia with Lewy bodies and dementia of the Alzheimer's type. In: Proceedings of 3rd International Workshop on Dementia with Lewy Bodies and Parkinson's Disease Dementia, Newcastle upon Tyne, UK (2003).

Yoshita M, Taki J, Yamada M, A clinical role for [¹²³I]MIBG myocardial scintigraphy in the distinction between dementia of the Alzheimer's-type and dementia with Lewy bodies. J Neurol Neurosurg Psychiatry (2001) 71:583–8.

Zuanetti G, Neilson JM, Latini R et al, Prognostic significance of heart rate variability in post-myocardial infarction patients in the fibrinolytic era. The GISSI-2 results. Gruppo Italiano per lo Studio della Sopravvivenza nell' Infarto Miocardico. Circulation (1996) 94:432–6.

chapter 9

Neuroimaging

John O'Brien and Sean Colloby

Introduction

Neuroimaging changes have not been well investigated in dementia with Lewy bodies (DLB), and even less in Parkinson's disease dementia (PDD), compared with other dementias such as Alzheimer's disease (AD) and vascular dementia (VaD), where they have even gained a place in diagnostic classifications. However, both structural (mainly magnetic resonance imaging (MRI)) and functional (mainly perfusion/metabolic and dopaminergic single-photon emission computed tomography (SPECT) and positron emission tomography (PET)) imaging investigations in DLB and PDD have revealed important information about these two disorders. They have enhanced our understanding regarding similarities with and differences from other dementias, provided insights about neurobiological mechanisms of key symptoms, and offered putative diagnostic markers for these disorders.

Structural imaging changes in DLB and PDD

An initial report of eight subjects who were diagnosed as having AD during life but had Lewy body pathology at postmortem found more pronounced frontal lobe atrophy on computed tomography (CT) than in pure AD cases (Förstl et al, 1993). However, subsequent, larger, studies using MRI have failed to replicate this finding (Harvey et al, 1999; Barber et al, 2000). Instead, the main structural imaging change emerging as characteristic of DLB is of relative preservation of the hippocampus and medial temporal lobe compared with AD (Hashimoto et al, 1998; Harvey et al, 1999; Barber et al, 2000), possibly helping to explain the preservation of mnemonic function in such cases. This can be detected using simple visual ratings of hippocampal atrophy and has been confirmed by volumetric region of interest studies (Figure 9.1).

Although hippocampal volume is significantly reduced, by around 15% compared with controls, the reduction is considerably less than that seen in AD, with some 40% of cases having no evidence of any atrophy. Based on an autopsy examination of four cases, Harvey et al (1999) suggested that temporal lobe atrophy on MRI might be a marker of concurrent tangle pathology in DLB, although clearly larger studies are needed to examine this issue further.

More general measures of atrophy have also been examined in DLB, with subjects having a similar degree of ventricular enlargement to those with AD (Barber et al, 2000), while the rate of volume loss over time using serial MRI is also comparable (around 1.5–2% per year in AD and DLB, compared with 0.5% in controls) (O'Brien et al, 2001). White matter lesions are known to be increased in AD, and may contribute along with degenerative pathology to the severity of cognitive impairment. A similar increase has been described in DLB cases (Barber et al, 1999), although effects on cognitive function have not yet been determined. One difference between AD and DLB is the demonstration of a 12% reduction in putamen volume in DLB – something that is not seen in AD (Cousins et al, 2003). This may be related to greater intrinsic striatal pathology in DLB than in either Parkinson's disease (PD) (where putamen volume is usually reported to be normal) or AD. Since occipital hypoperfusion has been demonstrated using functional imaging in DLB (see below),

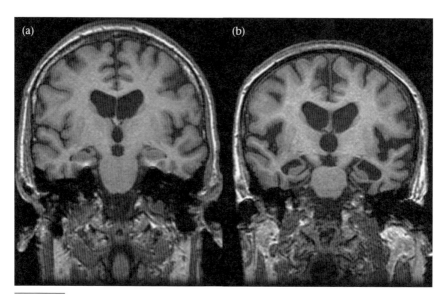

Figure 9.1   *Coronal MRI scan showing (a) a DLB subject and (b) an AD subject. Note the relative preservation of the hippocampus and medial temporal lobe in DLB compared with AD.*

structural imaging investigations of the occipital lobe have now been performed, and a detailed region-of-interest (ROI) study found no evidence of occipital atrophy in DLB (Middelkoop et al, 2001).

As well as visual rating and volumetric methods of analysis, unbiased voxel-based methods have also been applied to DLB. Burton et al (2002) reported the first study using voxel-based morphometry in DLB. This method has some methodological advantages over previous techniques, since it is not operator-dependent and examines changes in all parts of the brain, rather than only in predetermined regions. Burton et al (2002) showed gray matter loss in temporal and frontal lobes and in insular cortex in DLB compared with controls. Compared with AD, DLB subjects showed relative preservation of gray matter volume in the medial temporal lobe, hippocampus and amygdala, again strongly confirming previous studies that had used visual ratings and volumetric analysis.

In PDD, hippocampal atrophy on MRI has been reported, but the few studies to date have produced inconsistencies. For example, Laakso et al (1996) found hippocampal atrophy in PDD to be even greater than in AD, while opposite results were reported in another study (Camicioli et al, 2003), which also found hippocampal atrophy in nondemented people with PD correlating with impaired episodic memory. Studies using more sensitive serial MRI techniques have shown significantly greater annual brain volume loss in non-demented PD patients compared with controls. Voxel-based morphometry has been used to demonstrate atrophy of the frontal lobe in PD, which extends to temporal, occipital and parietal lobes in PDD (Burton et al, 2004). Interestingly, no significant differences were found between PDD and DLB, supporting the notion that they are closely related, if not identical, conditions.

In summary, the limited evidence available suggests that DLB, like AD, is associated with generalized atrophy, increased white matter change and progressive volume loss over time. The main defining feature of DLB and PDD is relative preservation of the hippocampus and medial temporal lobe. PD is associated with frontal gray matter loss and mild hippocampal atrophy; when dementia develops, other structures, including the parieto-occipital cortex, become involved. No structural imaging changes have been demonstrated that separate DLB from PDD.

Functional imaging changes in DLB and PDD

Functional imaging includes techniques such as magnetic resonance spectroscopy (MRS), which assesses metabolic changes in brain, functional MRI (fMRI), which looks at changes in brain function under resting conditions or cognitive activation, SPECT and PET.

MRS

A review of 15 studies in PD using MRS found a 5% decrease in *N*-acetylaspartate (NAA)/creatine (a marker of neuronal integrity) in the lentiform nucleus in PD, which contrasted with a greater (15%) reduction in some other parkinsonism conditions such as progressive supranuclear palsy (Firbank et al, 2002). Several cortical regions have also been investigated in PD, with studies reporting reductions in NAA/creatine concentrations in the temporoparietal (Firbank et al, 2002) and posterior cingulate (Camicioli et al, 2004) regions compared with normal controls. In AD, proton MRS consistently reveals reduced cortical NAA (10%) in most regions examined, with slightly greater loss (15%) in the temporal lobes. In many studies, increases in myoinositol are also seen (Firbank et al, 2002). There have been very few MRS studies in DLB. Molina et al. (2002) studied 12 DLB patients and 11 age-matched healthy controls, finding lower mean NAA/creatine, glutamate/glutamine/creatine and choline/creatine ratios in the white matter but no differences in gray matter. Relatively normal cortical NAA contrasts with findings of gray matter loss on structural MRI (Burton et al, 2002). Kantarci et al (2004) studied 20 DLB subjects and found, in contrast to AD and frontotemporal dementia (FTD), that NAA was preserved in posterior cingulate in DLB. In contrast, the Cho-Cr ratio was decreased in DLB (as well as in AD) leading the authors to suggest this was a marker of cholinergic deficit. Clearly MRS may make an important contribution to understanding pathophysiology, and perhaps differential diagnosis in DLB. Further studies are required.

fMRI

Activation studies with fMRI represent a powerful tool in the study of functional anatomy and offer the opportunity to study regional cerebral function under different conditions with the analysis of associated task specific changes in blood oxygen level-dependent (BOLD) signal. Compared with controls, cortical reductions in activation in non-demented PD subjects have been shown using various motor tasks in the sensorimotor (Elsinger et al,

2003) and primary motor (Tambasco et al, 2000) areas, while others (Haslinger et al, 2001) have reported hypo-activation in supplementary motor areas accompanied by hyper-activation in both the primary and premotor cortices. Cognitive function has also been assessed, with one study reporting significant intensity reductions during a working-memory paradigm in striatofrontal sites in PD patients with cognitive impairment compared with those patients who were not cognitively impaired (Lewis et al, 2003). There is no literature at present describing the functional anatomy in DLB or PDD using fMRI.

PET and SPECT: perfusion and metabolic studies

There have been several studies investigating PET and SPECT changes in DLB. PET studies of glucose metabolism and SPECT investigations using blood flow markers such as ^{99m}Tc-HMPAO have demonstrated many similarities to the patterns seen in AD (Donnemiller et al, 1997; Varma et al, 1997; Defebvre et al, 1999; Ishii et al, 1999; Lobotesis et al, 2001; Minoshima et al, 2001). Pronounced biparietal hypoperfusion is seen, together with variable deficits in frontal and temporal lobes, which again are usually symmetric. Bilateral parietal hypoperfusion in DLB is even more extensive than in AD cases matched for age and dementia severity (Colloby et al, 2002), particularly in Brodmann area 7, an area that mediates important aspects of visuospatial function. Pronounced hypoperfusion in this area may underpin the pronounced visuospatial impairments characteristic of DLB, although further studies correlating imaging changes with detailed neuropsychology are required.

In contrast to AD, a very consistent finding from functional imaging studies in DLB is of a profound occipital hypometabolism on PET and hypoperfusion on SPECT (Donnemiller et al, 1997; Ishii et al, 1999; Lobotesis et al, 2001; Colloby et al, 2002). Hypometabolism appears to affect primary visual cortex as well as visual association areas (Brodmann areas 17–19) (Figure 9.2). In contrast, temporal lobe perfusion is relatively preserved, paralleling the findings from structural imaging studies described above. Some studies have suggested that these changes might be of sufficient magnitude to assist with in vivo diagnosis; for example, Minoshima et al (2001) reported a sensitivity of 90% and a specificity of 80% for occipital hypometabolism in separating DLB from AD, although only 11 DLB cases were studied. However, a larger SPECT study (Lobotesis et al, 2001) showed that while occipital hypoperfusion had reasonable specificity (86%) for distinguishing DLB from AD and controls, its

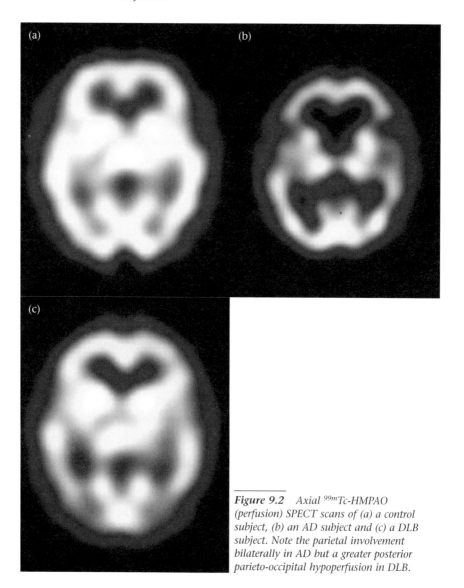

Figure 9.2 *Axial ^{99m}Tc-HMPAO (perfusion) SPECT scans of (a) a control subject, (b) an AD subject and (c) a DLB subject. Note the parietal involvement bilaterally in AD but a greater posterior parieto-occipital hypoperfusion in DLB.*

sensitivity was lower (68%). Whether such occipital changes are related to the occurrence of visual hallucinations remains unclear, some groups finding an association while others do not (Lobotesis et al, 2001, Minoshima et al, 2001).

Metabolic and perfusion changes in PDD appear similar to those in DLB. One difficulty in interpreting PET and SPECT studies lies in defining what changes simply can be accounted for as a result of underlying brain atrophy, and which are additional and specifically related to impaired functioning independent of atrophy. Firbank et al (2003) undertook both MRI and perfusion (^{99m}Tc-HMPAO) SPECT scans in subjects with AD, PD, DLB and PDD compared with healthy controls. Using a voxel-based approach, they identified regions that showed a reduction in perfusion on SPECT not related to associated structural brain changes. AD subjects showed a perfusion deficit in the midline parietal region, involving the posterior cingulate as well as the precuneus. In contrast, those with PDD and DLB had deficits that were more posterior and superior, affecting precuneus and inferior lateral parietal regions. Perfusion deficits were in areas associated with visual processing, and the authors speculated that they may be associated with the visuospatial perception deficits that are present in persons with DLB and PDD. As with structural imaging, no clear differences were seen between DLB and PDD.

PET and SPECT: studies of the dopaminergic system

Several PET tracers, including [^{18}F]fluoro-L-dopa, [^{11}C]-2-β-carbomethoxy-3-β-4-fluorophenyltropane (β-CIT-FE) and [^{18}F]2β-carbomethoxy-3β-(4-iodo-phenyl)-N-(3-fluoropropyl)-N-tropane (FP-CIT) have been developed to assess various aspects of dopaminergic function. All have identified striatal abnormalities, particularly in the putamen, especially in early-stage PD using both voxel-based (Ito et al, 1999; Lucignani et al, 2002; Ma et al, 2002) and ROI methods of analysis (Rinne et al, 2001). Similarly, SPECT tracers such as ^{123}I-β-CIT and ^{123}I-FP-CIT have been used to measure striatal dopamine transporter binding in PD. Studies using these SPECT ligands generally have used visual or semiquantitative methods to demonstrate significant reductions in striatal binding in PD compared with normal controls (Booij et al, 1997, 1999; Seibyl et al, 1998; Habraken et al, 1999; Benamer et al, 2000; Varrone et al, 2001; Sjoholm et al, 2002; Walker et al, 2002b; O'Brien et al, 2004). Importantly, in studies of early cases, bilateral striatal changes are seen despite the presence of unilateral clinical features (Tissingh et al, 1998), showing that imaging can detect abnormalities well before they cause clinical symptoms. Postsynaptic D_2 receptor status has also been investigated using tracers such as [^{123}I]iodobenzamide (IBZM) and [^{123}I]iodobenzofuran (IBF), where striatal binding appears to be preserved (Brucke et al, 1991; Tatsch et al, 1991; Oyanagi et al, 2002) or even upregulated (Laulumaa et al, 1993) in PD. This suggests that in PD only presynaptic nerve fibers are affected, at least in the early stages of the illness.

One of the main uses of dopaminergic imaging clinically is to help distinguish patients with PD from other disorders that may cause diagnostic confusion, especially essential tremor (ET). ET is a condition most commonly misdiagnosed with PD, where up to 25% of cases are initially diagnosed as having PD (Benamer et al, 2000). Dopamine transporter imaging has been successful in differentiating ET from PD using ^{123}I-β-CIT (Asenbaum et al, 1998) and ^{123}I-FP-CIT (Benamer et al, 2000; Marek et al, 2000), with subjects with ET having levels of striatal uptake within normal limits. Such studies have found the sensitivity and specificity for clinical diagnosis of distinguishing parkinsonism from ET to be 95% and 93% respectively (Benamer et al, 2000), while others have reported the sensitivity in diagnosing parkinsonism to be 98% with a specificity of 83% for ET and healthy controls (Marek et al, 2000). However, it is important to note that similar changes to PD on dopaminergic imaging are seen in other parkinsonian syndromes such as progressive supranuclear palsy, multisystem atrophy and corticobasal degeneration.

Studies of dopamine transporter binding in DLB have also demonstrated reductions in striatal uptake compared with patients with AD using ^{123}I-β-CIT (Donnemiller et al, 1997). However, one disadvantage with CIT is that imaging has to be delayed 24 hours post-injection. ^{123}I-FP-CIT, which has faster imaging kinetics, is now commercially available, and has reduced the post-injection delay to 3.5–4 hours. Using this SPECT ligand, Walker et al (2002a) conducted a study involving 27 DLB patients, 19 with PD, 17 with AD and 16 controls, and showed a significant reduction in uptake in the caudate and putamen, distinguishing DLB and PD from AD and controls. Importantly, imaging changes showed a stronger correlation with autopsy diagnosis than the clinical diagnosis in a subset of 10 cases for which postmortem results were available. O'Brien et al (2004) studied 164 older subjects (33 controls, 34 with AD, 23 with DLB, 38 with PD and 36 with PDD) using ^{123}I-FP-CIT SPECT. They found significant reductions ($p<0.001$) in ^{123}I-FP-CIT binding in the caudate, anterior and posterior putamen in DLB subjects compared with AD subjects and controls (Figure 9.3). Transporter loss in DLB was of similar magnitude to that seen in PD, but with a lower rostrocaudal (caudate–putamen) gradient ($p=0.001$), while the greatest loss in all three areas was seen in those with PDD. In terms of diagnostic accuracy, both ROI analysis and visual ratings provided good separation between DLB and AD (sensitivity 78%, specificity 94% and positive predictive value 90%), but not between DLB/PD/PDD. Using IBZM, Walker et al (1997) found that DLB patients showed lower uptake in the caudate and putamen compared with AD and controls, although this did not reach statistical significance.

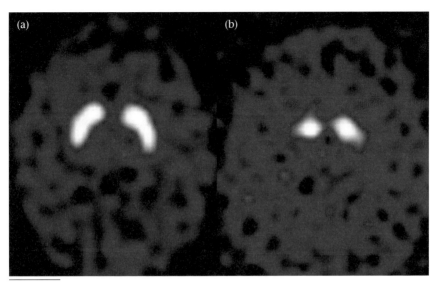

Figure 9.3 *[123]I-FP-CIT SPECT scans showing (a) an AD subject and (b) a DLB subject. Notice the profound reduction in uptake in the basal ganglia in DLB compared with AD (where uptake is normal).*

PET and SPECT: studies of other neurotransmitter systems

Both AD and DLB are associated with reduced levels of activity of the enzyme acetylcholinesterase (AChE) (Perry et al, 1980). AChE activity was investigated using PET among patients with PDD, AD, PD and controls (Bohnen et al, 2003). Patients with PDD were found to have the lowest level of activity, followed by those with PD, AD and controls, although AD patients showed a greater loss of activity in the medial temporal lobes. Using a marker of the vesicular acetylcholine transporter, significant differences between AD subjects and controls as well as between PD subjects with and without dementia have been found (Kuhl et al, 1996), although cases with DLB were not specifically examined. Cholinergic imaging has been relatively underutilized to date and may have a valuable role to play in detecting early cholinergic deficits at a presymptomatic stage.

In summary, current evidence suggests that metabolic and blood flow changes in DLB share several similarities with AD, although differences include greater biparietal hypoperfusion, occipital hypoperfusion (which is normal in AD) and relative preservation of temporal lobe activity. Loss of the dopamine transporter can also be demonstrated in DLB and PDD. However, the diagnostic utility of such changes in clinical practice remains to be fully determined.

References

Asenbaum S, Pirker W, Angelberger P et al, I-123 β-CIT and SPECT in essential tremor and Parkinson's disease. J Neurol Trans (1998) 105:1213–28.

Barber R, Scheltens P, Gholkar A et al, White matter lesions on magnetic resonance imaging in dementia with Lewy bodies, Alzheimer's disease, vascular dementia, and normal aging. J Neurol Neurosurg Psychiatry (1999) 67:66–72.

Barber R, Ballard C, McKeith IG et al, MRI volumetric study of dementia with Lewy bodies: a comparison with AD and vascular dementia. Neurology (2000) 54: 1304–9.

Benamer TS, Patterson J, Grosset DG et al, Accurate differentiation of parkinsonism and essential tremor using visual assessment of [^{123}I]-FP-CIT SPECT imaging: the [^{123}I]-FP-CIT study group. Mov Disord (2000) 15:503–10.

Bohnen NI, Kaufer DI, Ivanco LS et al, Cortical cholinergic function is more severely affected in parkinsonian dementia than in Alzheimer disease: an in vivo positron emission tomographic study. Arch Neurol (2003) 60:1745–8.

Booij J, Tissingh G, Boer GJ et al, [^{123}I]FP-CIT SPECT shows a pronounced decline of striatal dopamine transporter labelling in early and advanced Parkinson's disease. J Neurol Neurosurg Psychiatry (1997) 62:133–40.

Booij J, Hemelaar TG, Speelman JD et al, One-day protocol for imaging of the nigro-striatal dopaminergic pathway in Parkinson's disease by [^{123}I]FPCIT SPECT. J Nucl Med (1999) 40:753–61.

Brucke T, Podreka I, Angelberger P et al, Dopamine-D2 receptor imaging with spect – studies in different neuropsychiatric disorders. J Cereb Blood Flow Metab (1991) 11:220–8.

Burton EJ, Karas G, Paling SM et al, Patterns of cerebral atrophy in dementia with Lewy bodies using voxel-based morphometry. Neuroimage (2002) 17:618–30.

Burton EJ, McKeith IG, Burn DJ et al, Cerebral atrophy in Parkinson's disease with and without dementia: a comparison with Alzheimer's disease, dementia with Lewy bodies and controls. Brain (2004) 127:791–800.

Camicioli R, Moore MM, Kinney A et al, Parkinson's disease is associated with hippocampal atrophy. Mov Disord (2003) 18:784–90.

Camicioli RM, Korzan JR, Foster SL et al, Posterior cingulate metabolic changes occur in Parkinson's disease patients without dementia. Neurosci Lett (2004) 354:177–80.

Colloby SJ, Fenwick JD, Williams ED et al, A comparison of ^{99m}Tc-HMPAO SPET changes in dementia with Lewy bodies and Alzheimer's disease using statistical parametric mapping. Eur J Nucl Med (2002) 29:615–22.

Cousins DA, Burton EJ, Burn D et al, Atrophy of the putamen in dementia with Lewy bodies but not Alzheimer's disease: an MRI study. Neurology (2003) 61:1191–5.

Defebvre LJ, Leduc V, Duhamel A et al, Technetium HMPAO SPECT study in dementia with Lewy bodies, Alzheimer's disease and idiopathic Parkinson's disease. J Nucl Med (1999) 40:956–62.

Donnemiller E, Heilmann J, Wenning GK et al, Brain perfusion scintigraphy with ^{99m}Tc-HMPAO or ^{99m}Tc-ECD and ^{123}I-β-CIT single-photon emission tomography in dementia of the Alzheimer-type and diffuse Lewy body disease. Eur J Nucl Med (1997) 24:320–5.

Elsinger CL, Rao SM, Zimbelman JL et al, Neural basis for impaired time reproduction in Parkinson's disease: an fMRI study. J Int Neuropsychol Soc (2003) 9:1088–98.

Firbank MJ, Harrison RM, O'Brien JT, A comprehensive review of proton magnetic resonance spectroscopy studies in dementia and Parkinson's disease. Dement Geriatr Cogn Disord (2002) 14:64–76.

Firbank MJ, Colloby SJ, Burn DJ et al, Regional cerebral blood flow in Parkinson's disease with and without dementia. Neuroimag (2003) 20:1309–19.

Förstl H, Burns A, Luthert P et al, The Lewy-body variant of Alzheimer's disease. Clinical and pathological findings. Br J Psychiatry (1993) 162:385–92.

Habraken JB, Booij J, Slomka P et al, Quantification and visualization of defects of the functional dopaminergic system using an automatic algorithm. J Nucl Med (1999) 40:1091–7.

Harvey GT, Hughes J, McKeith IG et al, Magnetic resonance imaging differences between dementia with Lewy bodies and Alzheimer's disease: a pilot study. Psychol Med (1999) 29:181–7.

Hashimoto M, Kitagaki H, Imamura T et al, Medial temporal and whole-brain atrophy in dementia with Lewy bodies: a volumetric MRI study. Neurology (1998) 51:357–62.

Haslinger B, Erhard P, Kampfe N et al, Event-related functional magnetic resonance imaging in Parkinson's disease before and after levodopa. Brain (2001) 124:558–70.

Ishii K, Yamaji S, Kitagaki H et al, Regional cerebral blood flow difference between dementia with Lewy bodies and AD. Neurology (1999) 53:413–16.

Ito K, Morrish PK, Rakshi JS et al, Statistical parametric mapping with F-18-dopa PET shows bilaterally reduced striatal and nigral dopaminergic function in early Parkinson's disease. J Neurol Neurosurg Psychiatry (1999) 66:754–8.

Kantarci K, Petersen RC, Boeve BF et al, 1H MR spectroscopy in common dementias. Neurology (2004) 63(8):1393–8.

Kuhl DE, Minoshima S, Fessler JA et al, In vivo mapping of cholinergic terminals in normal aging, Alzheimer's disease, and Parkinson's disease. Ann Neurol (1996) 40:399–410.

Laakso MP, Partanen K, Riekkinen P et al, Hippocampal volumes in Alzheimer's disease, Parkinson's disease with and without dementia, and in vascular dementia: an MRI study. Neurology (1996) 46:678–81.

Laulumaa V, Kuikka JT, Soininen H et al, Imaging of D_2-dopamine receptors of patients with Parkinson's disease using single-photon emission computed-tomography and Iodobenzamide I-123. Arch Neurol (1993) 50:509–12.

Lewis SJ, Dove A, Robbins TW et al, Cognitive impairments in early Parkinson's disease are accompanied by reductions in activity in frontostriatal neural circuitry. J Neurosci (2003) 23:6351–6.

Lobotesis K, Fenwick JD, Phipps A et al, Occipital hypoperfusion on SPECT in dementia with Lewy bodies but not AD. Neurology (2001) 56:643–9.

Lucignani G, Gobbo C, Moresco RM et al, The feasibility of statistical parametric mapping for the analysis of positron emission tomography studies using C-11-2-β-carbomethoxy-3-β-(4-fluorophenyl)-tropane in patients with movement disorders. Nucl Med Comm (2002) 23:1047–55.

Ma Y, Dhawan V, Mentis M et al, Parametric mapping of F-18 FPCIT binding in early stage Parkinson's disease: a PET study. Synapse (2002) 45:125–33.

Marek K, Seibyl J, Holloway R et al, A multicenter assessment of dopamine transporter imaging with DOPASCAN/SPECT in parkinsonism. Neurology (2000) 55:1540–7.

Middelkoop HA, van der Flier WM, Burton EJ et al, Dementia with Lewy bodies and AD are not associated with occipital lobe atrophy on MRI. Neurology (2001) 57:2117–20.

Minoshima S, Foster NL, Sima AA et al, Alzheimer's disease versus dementia with Lewy bodies: cerebral metabolic distinction with autopsy confirmation. Ann Neurol (2001) 50:358–65.

Molina JA, Garcia-Segura JM, Benito-Leon J et al, Proton magnetic resonance spectroscopy in dementia with Lewy bodies. Eur Neurol (2002) 48:158–63.

O'Brien JT, Paling S, Barber R et al, Progressive brain atrophy on serial MRI in dementia with Lewy bodies, AD, and vascular dementia. Neurology (2001) 56:1386–8.

O'Brien JT, Colloby S, Fenwick J et al, Dopamine transporter loss visualized with FP-CIT SPECT in the differential diagnosis of dementia with Lewy bodies. Arch Neurol (2004) 61:919–25.

Oyanagi C, Katsumi Y, Hanakawa T et al, Comparison of striatal dopamine D2 receptors in Parkinson's disease and progressive supranuclear palsy patients using I-123 iodobenzofuran single-photon emission computed tomography. J Neuroimaging (2002) 12:316–24.

Perry EK, Perry RH, Tomlinson BE et al, Coenzyme A-acetylating enzymes in Alzheimer's disease: possible cholinergic 'compartment' of pyruvate dehydrogenase. Neurosci Lett (1980) 18:105–10.

Rinne JO, Nurmi E, Ruottinen HM et al, F-18 FDOPA and F-18 CFT are both sensitive PET markers to detect presynaptic dopaminergic hypofunction in early Parkinson's disease. Synapse (2001) 40:193–200.

Seibyl JP, Marek K, Sheff K et al, Iodine-123-β-CIT and iodine-123-FPCIT SPECT measurement of dopamine transporters in healthy subjects and Parkinson's patients. J Nucl Med (1998) 39:1500–8.

Sjoholm H, Sundsfjord J, Mellgren SI, β-CIT-SPECT combined with UPDRS appears to distinguish different parkinsonian conditions. Acta Neurol Scand (2002) 105:5–7.

Tambasco N, Lalli F, Rossi A et al, Activation of cortical motor areas in Parkinson's disease – A functional magnetic resonance study. Riv Neuroradiol (2000) 13:105–9.

Tatsch K, Schwarz J, Oertel WH, Kirsch CM, Spect imaging of dopamine D2-receptors with I-123 Ibzm – initial experience in controls and patients with Parkinson's syndrome and Wilson's disease. Nucl Med Comm (1991) 12:699–707.

Tissingh G, Booij J, Bergmans P et al, Iodine-123-N-ω-fluoropropyl-2β-carbomethoxy-3β-(4-iodophenyl)tropane SPECT in healthy controls and early-stage, drug-naive Parkinson's disease. J Nucl Med (1998) 39:1143–8.

Varma AR, Talbot PR, Snowden JS et al, A ^{99m}Tc-HMPAO single-photon emission computed tomography study of Lewy body disease. J Neurol (1997) 244:349–59.

Varrone A, Marek KL, Jennings D et al, I-123 β-CIT SPECT imaging demonstrates reduced density of striatal dopamine transporters in Parkinson's disease and multiple system atrophy. Mov Disord (2001) 16:1023–32.

Walker Z, Costa DC, Janssen AG et al, Dementia with Lewy bodies: a study of post-synaptic dopaminergic receptors with iodine-123 iodobenzamide single-photon emission tomography. Eur J Nucl Med (1997) 24:609–14.

Walker Z, Costa DC, Walker RWH et al, Differentiation of dementia with Lewy bodies from Alzheimer's disease using a dopaminergic presynaptic ligand. J Neurol Neurosurg Psychiatry (2002a) 73:134–40.

Walker Z, Costa DC, Walker RWH et al, Differentiation of dementia with Lewy bodies from Alzheimer's disease using a dopaminergic presynaptic ligand. J Neurol Neurosurg Psychiatry (2002b) 73:134–40.

chapter 10

Progression of cognitive impairment and duration of illness

Zuzana Walker

Progression of cognitive impairment

Although the illness fluctuates markedly in the short term, patients with dementia with Lewy bodies (DLB) experience a progressive cognitive and functional decline in the long term, which leads to severe dementia and death. Compared with the other aspects of DLB, relatively few studies have specifically focused on the longitudinal course of the illness. One of the first to do so showed that patients with severe DLB had a greater annual rate of decline in verbal fluency than patients with Alzheimer's disease (AD) or patients with vascular dementia (VaD) (Ballard et al, 1996). In addition, the annual mean reduction in Cambridge Cognitive Examination (CAMCOG) score was greater in the DLB group (-27.0 points vs -13.2 points in AD), but this did not reach statistical significance, most probably due to the small numbers of DLB patients ($n=7$). In a much larger autopsy cohort of moderately demented patients (40 DLB patients and 148 AD patients at baseline assessment), the annual decline in Mini-Mental State Examination (MMSE) score was significantly greater for DLB patients (5.8 points per year) than AD patients (4.1 points per year) (Olichney et al, 1998). However significant differences in rate of decline on MMSE score were observed only at 1- and 2-year follow-up but not at 3-year follow-up. The difference became significant again at 4-year follow-up, but by then there were only four patients in the DLB group.

In contrast, more recent studies (Gomez-Isla et al, 1999; Lopez et al, 2000; Ballard et al, 2001; Helmes et al, 2003) did not find significant differences in rate of cognitive decline between DLB and AD. The first of these studies (Gomez-Isla et al, 1999) measured the annual rate of change of the Blessed Dementia Scale and of the Activities of Daily Living (ADL) scale in 53 AD patients and in 8 'mixed' (AD plus Lewy bodies) and 4 'pure' (no or minimal concomitant AD pathology at autopsy) DLB cases. No significant difference was observed between the three groups in the annual rate of decline on the Blessed Dementia Scale, DLB cases had significantly higher rates of decline on the ADL scale than AD cases, but clearly the number of DLB cases was very small. The second study (Lopez et al, 2000) compared the cognitive and functional decline (expressed as the percentage of patients scoring less than 9/30 on an MMSE and more than 12 points on the Blessed Dementia Score for AD) of a large autopsy-confirmed cohort of moderately demented patients with AD+LB ('mixed' DLB) and AD. No significant difference in either functional or cognitive decline was found but patients with 'mixed' DLB had a shorter time to institutionalization. Likewise, the Newcastle group (Ballard et al, 2001), in a study that was much larger than their first study, found no significant difference in the annual rate of decline between DLB and AD patients on MMSE or CAMCOG scores (MMSE: −4.3 vs −4.9; CAMCOG: −11.9 vs −15.0). The most recent study (Helmes et al, 2003) compared the rates of deterioration on the Extended Scale for Dementia (ESD; an extension of the Mattis Dementia Rating Scale with possible scores from 0 to 250) of 15 cases of AD, 7 cases of DLB ('pure' DLB) and 8 cases of 'mixed' DLB. All the cases had autopsy-verified diagnoses. The most severe rate of decline in ESD scores over time was in the 'mixed' DLB group, but nevertheless statistically there was no significant difference between the three dementia groups, perhaps because of the small sample sizes and low statistical power. All groups deteriorated at a rate of approximately 2 ESD points per month. A substantial variability was recorded between individuals in all three groups. In a large Memory Clinic cohort of clinically diagnosed moderately demented patients (mean MMSE score at baseline: DLB 19.2 vs AD 19.0), we observed no significant difference between DLB and AD in annual decline of MMSE and CAM-COG scores at 1, 2, 3 and 4 years (Walker et al, unpublished). Although DLB patients were more impaired at baseline as measured by the Instrumental Activities of Daily Living (IADL) scale, there was no difference in the rate of decline on this scale over the next 4 years.

A small prospective autopsy study (Perry et al, 2003) investigated the longitudinal course of illness and the levels of butyrylcholinesterase in the gray matter of Brodman area 20. In this study of 9 DLB patients, there was a significant association between lower levels of butyrylcholinesterase and a slower rate of cognitive decline as measured by MMSE. Butyrylcholinesterase is one of the two enzymes responsible for the breakdown of acetylcholine in neuronal synapses, and therefore high levels may contribute to the severe cholinergic deficit observed in DLB patients. The study suggested that variation in the butyrylcholinesterase levels might be a factor that influences the rate of progression of illness.

In summary, increasingly the evidence indicates no real difference between DLB and AD in the overall rate of progression of cognitive decline. However, mean values from large studies may conceal disease heterogeneity, and it is recognized for instance that a proportion of DLB patients have a very rapid disease course (Armstrong et al, 1991). Factors that might influence longitudinal course, such as biological markers, symptomatology, gender, age at onset of symptoms and treatment, need to be further investigated.

Age at onset and duration of illness

The position with regard to survival is even less clear than the rate of cognitive decline. The majority of studies are retrospective and based on autopsy series. Consequently, there is the possibility of selection bias. Survival in DLB has been reported to be anything from a few months to 20 years.

In a case series of five 'pure' DLB patients (Lippa et al, 1994), the mean age at onset of illness was 50 years, with a mean duration of illness of 5 years. In another series, 11 cases of diffuse Lewy body disease without neurofibrillary tangles or neuritic senile plaques, the mean age of onset of dementia was 69 years and the duration of illness was 7.7 years (Del Ser et al, 1996). A series of nine 'pure' DLB cases had a mean age at onset of illness of 61.7 years and a mean duration of illness of 8.6 years (Hely et al, 1996). However, a study of 13 'pure' DLB cases with a mean age at onset of 68 years reported a much longer mean duration of illness, namely 10 years (Gomez-Tortosa et al, 1999).

Looking at individual studies of neuropathologically defined cases with mixed pathology (DLB with variable degrees of concomitant AD pathology), the mean age at onset of illness in different cohorts varied between 59 and 79 years and the duration of illness ranged from 1.8 to 9.5 years. The wide ranges of both age at onset and duration of illness highlight the difficulty of drawing conclusions from preselected samples. A meta-analysis (Cercy and Bylsma 1997) of 150 cases reported in the literature derived the same mean survival for 'pure' DLB and 'mixed' DLB (approximately 6 years).

Numerous autopsy studies have compared the duration of illness in DLB and AD, with conflicting results. Some studies (Perry et al, 1990; McKeith et al, 1992, 1994; Olichney et al, 1998; Ballard et al, 1999; Singleton et al, 2002) reported shorter survival in DLB than AD (Table 10.1). However, other studies (Hansen et al, 1990; Klatka et al, 1996; Samuel et al, 1996; Weiner et al, 1996; Papka et al, 1998; Heyman et al, 1999; Del Ser et al, 2001) found no difference in duration of illness between DLB and AD (Table 10.2). In the latest of these studies (Del Ser et al, 2001), the survival was shorter in 'pure' DLB by comparison with 'mixed' DLB (7.7 vs 11 years).

In a study that compared the survival of AD and DLB patients from an unselected cohort of all patients with a clinical diagnosis of dementia referred to a district general hospital over a period of 1 year (Walker et al, 2000) there

Table 10.1 Autopsy studies showing shorter mean duration of illness in DLB than in AD

	DLB		AD		PD	
Study	*Cases*	*Years*	*Cases*	*Years*	*Cases*	*Years*
Perry et al (1990)	18	3.3	46	5.6	12	7.9
McKeith et al (1992)	21	1.8	37	4.8		
McKeith et al (1994)	20	3.1	21	5.5		
Olichney et al (1998)	40	7.7	148	9.3		
Ballard et al (1999)	40	4.3	40	5.6		
Singleton et al (2002)	76	3.5	194	5.3		

Table 10.2 Autopsy studies showing no difference in mean duration of illness between DLB and AD

	DLB		AD	
Study	*Cases*	*Years*	*Cases*	*Years*
Hansen et al (1990)	13	3.0	23	3.5
Klatka et al (1996)	28	9.5	58	9.2
Samuel et al (1996)	14	6.8	12	6.9
Weiner et al (1996)	24	7.5	58	8.5
Papka et al (1998)	18	9.6	21	11.1
Heyman et al (1999)	27	3.8	74	3.6
Del Ser et al (2001)	29	9.7	35	9.6

were no differences between the AD and DLB groups in age of onset (78.1 vs 75.8 years), age at death (84.3 vs 81.7 years) and survival rate. Survival data gathered from a larger cohort of unselected demented patients that have presented to our psychiatric services over a period of 2 years (*n*=183) again showed no significant difference in the survival rates of AD and DLB patients (Figure 10.1) (Walker, unpublished data).

Only one published study has examined the influence of the apolipoprotein E gene on survival rates in patients with DLB (Singleton et al, 2002). In this study, the survival rates were reduced by the presence of the ε4 allele. DLB patients either heterozygous or homozygous for ε4 had significantly higher mortality rates than patients without the ε4 allele.

The conclusion therefore has to be that at present there is no overall convincing evidence regarding age of onset and duration of illness. Only large, prospective, longitudinal studies will be able to determine whether there is no difference between DLB and AD or whether survival really is worse in DLB than in AD. It is possible that disease heterogeneity in DLB is greater than in AD, with some patients surviving a significantly shorter time, while others fare much as AD patients do.

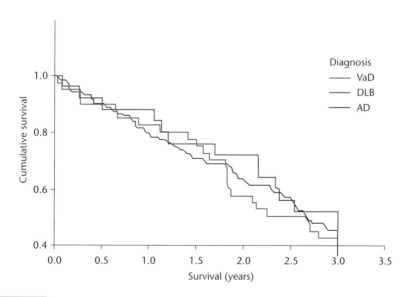

Figure 10.1 *Kaplan–Meier survival curves for AD, DLB and Vascular dementia patients over three years.*

References

Armstrong TP, Hansen LA, Salmon DP et al, Rapidly progressive dementia in a patient with the Lewy body variant of Alzheimer's disease. Neurology (1991) 41:1178–80.

Ballard C, Patel A, Oyebode F, Wilcock G, Cognitive decline in patients with Alzheimer's disease, vascular dementia and senile dementia of Lewy body type. Age Ageing (1996) 25:209–13.

Ballard C, Holmes C, McKeith I et al, Psychiatric morbidity in dementia with Lewy bodies: a prospective clinical and neuropathological comparative study with Alzheimer's disease. Am J Psychiatry (1999) 156:1039–45.

Ballard C, O'Brien J, Morris CM et al, The progression of cognitive impairment in dementia with Lewy bodies, vascular dementia and Alzheimer's disease. Int J Geriatr Psychiatry (2001) 16:499–503.

Cercy SP, Bylsma FW, Lewy bodies and progressive dementia: a critical review and meta-analysis. J Int Neuropsychol Soc (1997) 3:179–94.

Del Ser T, Munoz DG, Hachinski V, Temporal pattern of cognitive decline and incontinence is different in Alzheimer's disease and diffuse Lewy body disease. Neurology (1996) 46:682–6.

Del Ser T, Hachinski V, Merskey H, Munoz DG, Clinical and pathologic features of two groups of patients with dementia with Lewy bodies: effect of coexisting Alzheimer-type lesion load. Alzheimer Dis Assoc Disord (2001) 15:31–44.

Gomez-Isla T, Growdon WB, McNamara M et al, Clinicopathologic correlates in temporal cortex in dementia with Lewy bodies. Neurology (1999) 53:2003–9.

Gomez-Tortosa E, Newell K, Irizarry MC et al, Clinical and quantitative pathologic correlates of dementia with Lewy bodies. Neurology (1999) 53:1284–91.

Hansen L, Salmon D, Galasko D et al, The Lewy body variant of Alzheimer's disease: a clinical and pathologic entity. Neurology (1990) 40:1–8.

Helmes E, Bowler JV, Merskey H et al, Rates of cognitive decline in Alzheimer's disease and dementia with Lewy bodies. Dement Geriatr Cogn Disord (2003) 15:67–71.

Hely MA, Reid WGJ, Halliday GM et al, Diffuse Lewy body disease: clinical features in nine cases without coexistent Alzheimer's disease. J Neurol Neurosurg Psychiatry (1996) 60:531–8.

Heyman A, Fillenbaum GG, Gearing M et al, Comparison of Lewy body variant of Alzheimer's disease with pure Alzheimer's disease: Consortium to Establish a Registry for Alzheimer's Disease, Part XIX. Neurology (1999) 52:1839–44.

Klatka LA, Louis ED, Schiffer RB, Psychiatric features in diffuse Lewy body disease: a clinicopathologic study using Alzheimer's disease and Parkinson's disease comparison groups. Neurology (1996) 47:1148–52.

Lippa CF, Smith TW, Swearer JM, Alzheimer's disease and Lewy body disease: a comparative clinicopathological study. Ann Neurol (1994) 35:81–8.

Lopez OL, Wisniewski S, Hamilton RL et al, Predictors of progression in patients with AD and Lewy bodies. Neurology (2000) 54:1774–9.

McKeith IG, Perry RH, Fairbairn AF et al, Operational criteria for senile dementia of Lewy body type (SDLT). Psychol Med (1992) 22:911–22.

McKeith IG, Fairbairn AF, Bothwell RA et al, An evaluation of the predictive validity and inter-rater reliability of clinical diagnostic criteria for senile dementia of Lewy body type. Neurology (1994) 44:872–7.

Olichney JM. Galasko D, Salmon DP et al, Cognitive decline is faster in Lewy body variant than in Alzheimer's disease. Neurology (1998) 51:351–7.

Papka M, Rubio A, Schiffer RB, Cox C, Lewy body disease: can we diagnose it? J Neuropsychiatry Clin Neurosci (1998) 10:405–12.

Perry E, McKeith I, Ballard C, Butyrylcholinesterase and progression of cognitive deficits in dementia with Lewy bodies. Neurology (2003) 60:1852–3.

Perry RH, Irving D, Blessed G et al, Senile dementia of Lewy body type: a clinically and neuropathologically distinct form of Lewy body dementia in the elderly. J Neurol Sci (1990) 95:119–39.

Samuel W, Galasko D, Masliah E, Hansen L, Neocortical Lewy body counts correlate with dementia in the Lewy body variant of Alzheimer's disease. J Neuropathol Exp Neurol (1996) 55:44–52.

Singleton AB, Wharton A, O'Brien KK et al, Clinical and neuropathological correlates of apolipoprotein E genotype in dementia with Lewy bodies. Dement Geriatr Cogn Disord (2002) 14:167–75.

Walker Z, Allen RL, Shergill S et al, Three years survival in patients with a clinical diagnosis of dementia with Lewy bodies. Int J Geriatr Psychiatry (2000) 15:267–73.

Weiner MF, Risser RC, Cullum CM et al, Alzheimer's disease and its Lewy body variant: a clinical analysis of postmortem verified cases. Am J Psychiatry (1996) 153: 1269–73.

chapter 11

Neuropathology and pathogenesis of dementia with Lewy bodies

Dennis W Dickson

Introduction

Dementia with Lewy bodies (DLB) is a clinical syndrome characterized by mid-to-late life dementia associated with visual hallucinations, parkinsonism and a fluctuating clinical course (McKeith et al, 2004). In this discussion, the term Lewy body disease (LBD) is used to refer to the pathological process associated with neuronal cytoplasmic inclusions first described by Lewy (Dickson, 2002a). As is true for all clinical neurological syndromes, the pathological substrate of DLB is not exclusively a single disease process. For example, parkinsonism, which is the clinical syndrome characterized by bradykinesia, rigidity and resting tremor, has a number of distinct pathological substrates, including LBD, multiple system atrophy (MSA) and progressive supranuclear palsy (PSP) (Dickson, 2002b). These disorders share progressive neuronal loss and gliosis in the dopaminergic neurons of the pars compacta of the substantia nigra, which leads to the striatal dopaminergic deficiencies that cause the extrapyramidal parkinsonian syndrome (Fig. 11.1c). Given that one of the cardinal clinical features of DLB is parkinsonism, it can be predicted that the pathological substrate for this aspect of DLB might be heterogeneous. Indeed, autopsy studies of prospectively diagnosed patients with DLB occasionally have identified neurofibrillary tangle pathology, consistent with PSP, in the substantia nigra rather than Lewy bodies (McKeith et al, 2000).

It should also be noted that a diagnosis of clinically probable DLB is possible in a patient who does not have parkinsonism, if the other criteria

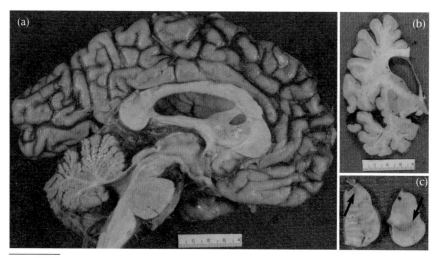

Figure 11.1 *Gross appearance of the brain in a patient with a clinical diagnosis of DLB. (a) The brain shows only mild cortical atrophy. (b) Coronal sections show enlargement of the frontal horn of the lateral ventricle. (c) Sections of the brainstem show depigmentation of the locus ceruleus and substantia nigra (arrows).*

are met – namely, dementia, visual hallucinations and a fluctuating clinical course (McKeith et al, 1996).

Further complicating the clinicopathological correlation of DLB is the fact that dementia with many of the same clinical characteristics occurs during the course of otherwise typical Parkinson's disease (PD) (Emre, 2003). Dementia in PD (PDD) most often occurs late in the disease course. Clinical differences between PDD and DLB are minimal in cross-sectional studies (Aarsland et al, 2004). Clinical differences are more apparent if one considers the temporal aspects of the disease process. Many PD patients never have significant dementia and PDD may follow years later in the course of otherwise typical PD. In contrast, DLB patients may present with significant cognitive and psychiatric impairments long before developing parkinsonism, which is often subtle and sometimes completely absent. The different clinical courses of PDD and DLB remains one of the major unresolved questions about the relationship of these two clinical disorders.

With these caveats in mind, the present discussion describes the neuropathology of DLB. The description is based upon personal experience as well as a review of the literature. With respect to the latter, it must be emphasized that the clinical syndrome of DLB is relatively new. Thus, most of the patients with dementia and LBD have not had antemortem diagnosis of DLB, and often the clinical records do not permit assessment of whether they would have met DLB criteria. The usual reason is lack of documentation of a fluctuating clinical course and extrapyramidal features. The latter are attributed to aging, as it is a commonly held belief that mild parkinsonism, including bradykinesia and gait instability, is a feature of aging, just as some mild degree of cognitive impairment is also often considered a feature of aging. Clearly, with increased interest in identification of the earliest clinical manifestations of dementia as in Alzheimer's disease (AD), this concept has been challenged (Petersen, 2004).

Cardinal histopathological features of DLB

Lewy bodies and Lewy neurites

Lewy bodies (LBs) are hyaline cytoplasmic inclusions within selectively vulnerable neurons (Figure 11.2a and 11.3a). While most LBs are single and spherical, some neurons have multiple or pleomorphic LBs. In some regions of the brain, such as the dorsal motor nucleus of the vagus and the basal nucleus of Meynert, similar inclusions are detected within neuronal

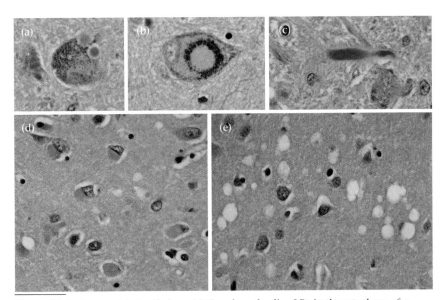

Figure 11.2   *Lewy-related pathology. (a) Two dense hyaline LBs in the cytoplasm of a neuromelanin-containing neuron in the substantia nigra. (b) A less compact pale body within a pigmented neuron. (c) An elongated intraneuritic LB within a neuronal process in the dorsal motor nucleus of the vagus. (d) Multiple neurons in the amygdala have eosinophilic cytoplasmic cortical-type LBs. (e) Microvacuolation of the neuropil in the entorhinal cortex.*

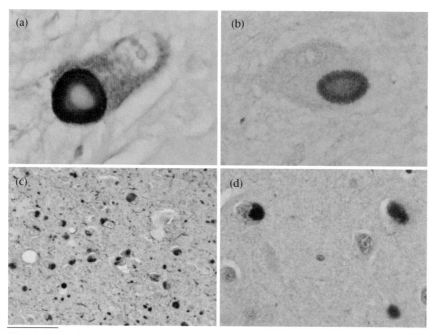

Figure 11.3   *Synuclein immunohistochemistry of an LB (a), a pale body (b) and cortical LBs (c,d).*

processes, and these are often referred to as 'intraneuritic' LBs (Figure 11.2c). Intraneuritic LBs can be detected in routine histopathologic preparations and should be distinguished from Lewy neurites (LNs), which are not visible with routine histopathology.

LNs were first described in the hippocampus (Dickson et al, 1991) (Figure 11.4a), but are also found in other regions of the brain, including the cingulate gyrus, entorhinal cortex (Figure 11.4b), amygdala (Figure 11.4c) and basal ganglia (Figure 11.4d). There is increasing interest in the relationship of neuritic pathology to cognitive impairment in DLB, especially since the number of neurons affected with LBs can be relatively small in some cases.

In addition to the well-circumscribed hyaline inclusions, some neuronal populations develop lesions that are very similar in antigenic properties to LBs, but are poorly circumscribed and easily overlooked in routine histological preparations. These lesions are referred to as pre-Lewy bodies or pale bodies (Figures 11.2b and 11.3b). Pale bodies are most often found in pigmented neurons in the substantia nigra. Similar inclusions within cortical neurons are referred to as cortical LBs (Figures 11.2d and 11.3c,d). They tend to be found

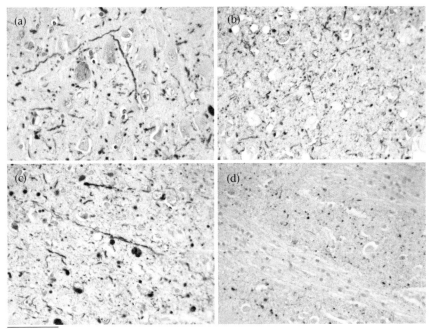

Figure 11.4 *Synuclein immunohistochemistry of LNs in the CA2 region of the hippocampus (a), the superficial cortical layers of the entorhinal cortex (b), the amygdala (c) and the putamen (d). Note the variable mixture of elongated threadlike curvilinear processes and dotlike neurites. The latter are the major type of lesion in the striatum.*

in small nonpyramidal neurons in lower cortical layers, but can also be detected in pyramidal neurons. Occasionally, cortical LBs have a hyaline appearance similar to brainstem LBs.

Ultrastructurally, classical LBs are composed of filamentous and amorphous granular material. The central region of the classical LB contains dense material that lacks discernible detail, while the periphery has radially arranged 10 nm diameter filaments. At the electron-microscopic level, cortical LBs and LNs are also composed of 10 nm filaments, but they lack a dense core and the filaments are haphazardly arranged (Dickson et al, 1991).

Composition of LBs

Biochemical and immunohistochemical methods have indicated that the major structural component of LBs is α-synuclein (Baba et al, 1998). α-synuclein is one of a family of related proteins, including β-synuclein and γ-synuclein (Dickson, 2001). The latter proteins are also expressed in the nervous system, but they do not participate in any appreciable way in LB formation.

α-synuclein is a presynaptic protein that is abnormally distributed to axons and neuronal cell bodies in LBD.

In addition to α-synuclein, immunohistochemical studies have implicated other proteins in LBs (Pollanen et al, 1993). Antibodies to neurofilament label LBs, but each such antibody usually labels only a subset of LBs (Galvin et al, 1997). On the other hand, ubiquitin, a small heat-shock protein involved in energy-dependent protein degradation, is present in most classical and cortical LBs (Kuzuhara et al, 1988). In addition to ubiquitin, several other molecules that play a role in proteasomal protein degradation, including certain chaperone proteins, co-localize with α-synuclein and ubiquitin in LBs (Eriksen et al, 2005).

Tau protein, a microtubule-associated protein that is the major structural component of Alzheimer neurofibrillary tangles, is associated with a subset of LBs (Ishizawa et al, 2003). Indeed, initial biochemical studies of LBs suggested that a major protein constituent of LBs was a 68 kDa protein with cross-reactivity with tau and neurofilament protein (Pollanen et al, 1992). This is of interest given that genetic variants in the gene encoding tau (MAPT) may be a risk factor for Parkinson's disease (Maraganore et al, 2001; Healy et al, 2004).

Distribution of LBs

Based upon initial studies of Parkinson's disease, it was felt that the neurons most vulnerable to LBs were monoaminergic neurons of the substantia nigra, locus ceruleus and dorsal motor nucleus of the vagus, as well as cholinergic neurons in the basal forebrain (Jellinger and Mizuno, 2003). This view has been challenged by immunohistochemical studies with α-synuclein antibodies, which show LBs in other areas not previously suspected, including the cortex and amygdala. Moreover, the earliest type of α-synuclein pathology in vulnerable brain regions appears to be LNs rather than LBs (Braak et al, 2003).

While LBs are rarely detected in the basal ganglia or thalamus, α-synuclein immunohistochemistry often reveals LNs in these areas (Duda et al, 2002). LBs are common in the hypothalamus, especially the posterior and lateral hypothalamus, and in the brainstem reticular formation. The oculomotor nuclear complex is also vulnerable to LBs. In the pons, the dorsal raphe and subpeduncular nuclei are often affected, but neurons of the pontine base are not. LBs have not been described in the cerebellar cortex. In the spinal cord, the neurons of the intermediolateral cell column are most vulnerable. LBs can be found in the autonomic ganglia, including the submucosal ganglia of the lower esophagus and the myenteric plexus of the gastrointestinal tract (Wakabayashi and Takahashi, 1997).

While LBs are increasingly being recognized as affecting cortical neurons, not all cortical neurons are equally vulnerable. The frontal and temporal multimodal association and limbic cortices are most vulnerable, while primary motor and sensory cortices are most resistant. The amygdala is the most vulnerable of the limbic structures (Hamilton, 2000). The cortical areas with the most cortical LBs are the insular cortex and the parahippocampal and cingulate gyri.

LBD can be classified based upon the distribution of LBs (Kosaka et al, 1984). Diffuse Lewy body disease (DLBD) is the pathological diagnosis for cases with LBs widely distributed in the neocortex, while transitional LBD is the term used to describe cases with LBs limited to the limbic lobe. When LBs are minimal in cortical areas, but present in brainstem and forebrain nuclei, the term brainstem-type LBD is used. This staging has been expanded upon by Braak et al (2003), who have added refinements to the brainstem-predominant stage. Table 11.1 summarizes the distribution of LBs in the Kosaka and Braak staging schemes.

Spongiform change

Spongiform change that resembles the fine neuropil microvacuolation that is found in transmissible spongiform encephalopathies, such as Creutzfeldt–Jakob disease, is common in LBD (Hansen et al, 1989) (Figure 11.2e). In transmissible spongiform encephalopathies, spongiform change is widespread, including the cortex, basal ganglia, thalamus and cerebellum, while it is anatomically restricted in LBD. It is most prominent in limbic cortices and the amygdala, but occasionally can be detected in the temporal lobe. Similar changes have been reported in the medial temporal lobe in AD, but recent studies suggest that when marked spongiform change is detected in AD, it is usually accompanied by LBs (Fujino and Dickson, 2003).

Glial lesions

α-synuclein immunoreactive glial lesions are the defining histopathological lesions of MSA (Lantos, 1998), a related synucleinopathy, in which oligodendroglial inclusions parallel the anatomical distribution of neurodegeneration and are associated with demyelination. In contrast, glial lesions are sparse in LBD (Wakabayashi et al, 2000) and are not associated with significant white matter pathology. They appear to be more common in LBD cases with a

Table 11.1   Neuropathological staging of Lewy body disease

Kosaka LBD stage	*Braak PD stage*	*Anatomical distribution of Lewy bodies*
Brainstem-predominant type	1	Medullary tegmentum and the dorsal motor nucleus of the vagus; olfactory bulb
	2	Locus ceruleus, caudal raphe and reticular nucleus of medullary and pontine tegmentum
	3	Substantia nigra and basal forebrain
Transitional (limbic) type	4	Medial temporal (limbic) cortices, including amygdala and CA2 region of the hippocampus
Diffuse cortical type	5	Multimodal association cortices, especially frontal and temporal lobes
	6	Unimodal association cortices and primary cortices

genetic basis (Gwinn-Hardy et al, 2000). As in MSA, glial lesions in LBD are within oligodendroglia, since they are negative for GFAP and positive with markers of pathological oligodendrocytes (Gwinn-Hardy et al, 2000). In some cases of MSA, neuronal inclusions with features similar to LBs are seen (Kato and Nakamura, 1990), but they differ from LBs in their anatomical distribution, being found in the pontine nuclei, inferior olive and putamen – areas that rarely, if ever, have LBs in LBD.

Alzheimer-type pathology

The presence of Alzheimer-type pathology is common in LBD given the advanced age of most patients and the prevalence of Alzheimer pathology with increasing age. In some cases, the density and distribution of Alzheimer-type pathology is consistent with a pathological diagnosis of AD, although clearly this depends upon the pathological criteria used to diagnose AD. The most liberal criteria such as the Khachaturian criteria (Khachaturian et al, 1985) are plaque-based criteria that do not stipulate a particular type of senile plaque and do not require the presence of neurofibrillary tangles. More restrictive criteria include those used by the Consortium to Establish a Registry for Alzheimer's Disease (CERAD), which are based upon neuritic plaques, but also do not require neocortical neurofibrillary tangles (Mirra et al, 1991). The most restrictive criteria, such as those proposed by the Working Group of the National Institutes of Health and the Reagan Institute of the Alzheimer Association (the National Institute of Aging (NIA)–Reagan criteria), require the presence of both neuritic plaques and neurofibrillary tangles (Hyman and Trojanowski, 1997). The NIA–Reagan criteria are summarized in Table 11.2.

Senile plaques

Senile plaques are complex and heterogeneous lesions that are defined by the presence of extracellular deposits of β-amyloid protein, which is derived by proteolytic processing of β-amyloid precursor protein (Dickson, 1997). In some cases, the amyloid deposits are dense, compact spherical lesions (Figure 11.5b,c), while in others they are noncompact, diffuse, irregularly shaped amyloid deposits (Figure 11.5a). Compact amyloid deposits are almost always associated with other cellular elements, such as degenerating neuronal processes ('dystrophic neurites') and reactive glia, including both activated microglia and reactive astrocytes. Diffuse plaques, on the other hand, may not be associated with dystrophic neurites or reactive glia. Plaques with dystrophic neurites are referred to as 'neuritic plaques', and these are also heterogeneous. Some neuritic plaques contain neurites that have abnormal aggregates of tau protein that are similar to those found in neuronal cell bodies in neurofibrillary tangles (Figure 11.5c,e), while other dystrophic neurites

Table 11.2 National Institute of Aging–Reagan Institute criteria for Alzheimer's disease

	Braak neurofibrillary tangle stage			
CERAD[a] senile plaque score	*No NFT*	*I–II*	*III–IV*	*V–VI*
Frequent neuritic plaques	Not AD	Low	Intermediate	High
Moderate neuritic plaques	Not AD	Low	Intermediate	Intermediate
Sparse neuritic plaques	Not AD	Low	Low	Low
No plaques	Not AD	Not AD	Not AD	Not AD

[a]Consortium to Establish a Registry for Alzheimer's Disease.

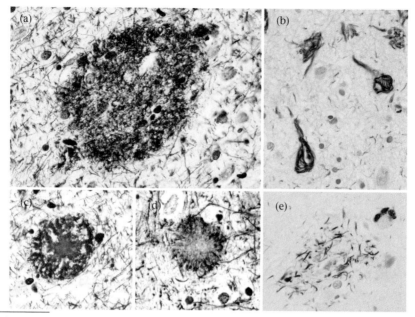

Figure 11.5 *Alzheimer-type pathology in LBD as shown with the Bielschowsky (a,c,d) or the Gallyas (b,e) silver stain. The most prevalent type of senile plaque in LBD is the diffuse amyloid deposit (a). Cored plaques (c,d) show dense amyloid cores either with (d) or without (c) argyrophilic neurites. The neuritic type of plaque (d) is characteristic of concurrent AD. The Gallyas stains show neurofibrillary tangles in the entorhinal cortex (b) and a neuritic plaque (e) in the hippocampus of a case of LBD with concurrent Alzheimer's disease.*

contain membranous organelles and dense bodies, which are immunopositive for ubiquitin and amyloid precursor protein but negative for tau. The latter type of plaque can be detected in nondemented elderly individuals, while the tau-positive neuritic plaque is characteristic of AD. In most cases of DLB, there are many senile plaques, but they do not typically show extensive fibrillar tau pathology-type pathology unless there is concurrent AD (Dickson et al, 1992, 1996).

Amyloid angiopathy

Most patients with AD have amyloid deposits not only in senile plaques, but also within the walls of blood vessels, so called cerebral amyloid angiopathy (CAA). Given that Alzheimer-type pathology is common in LBD, it is not surprising that many cases of LBD also have CAA (Wu et al, 1992). The frequency of CAA in LBD is related to the severity of concurrent Alzheimer-type pathology, which is a function of age and apolipoprotein E genotype (Dickson et al, 1996). Apolipoprotein E is a lipoprotein that may function as a chaperone protein to facilitate amyloid deposition. There are three major genetic variants of apolipoprotein E (ϵ2, ϵ3 and ϵ4), and patients carrying one or two genes with the ϵ4 variant have increased risk of both AD and CAA. The clinical relevance of this observation is that individuals with CAA are more likely to have cerebrovascular pathology, such as microhemorrhages and leukoencephalopathy, which could conceivably contribute to cognitive impairment.

Neurofibrillary tangles

Neurofibrillary tangles are neuronal lesions formed by progressive accumulation of abnormally phosphorylated tau protein within the perikarya and proximal dendrites (Figure 11.5d). The aggregates become filamentous and relatively insoluble as they evolve. In AD, the filaments have a characteristic appearance at the electron-microscopic level and appear to be two filaments helically wound around each other, so-called paired helical filaments. Neurons that are most vulnerable to neurofibrillary tangles in aging and AD have a characteristic distribution with a hierarchical pattern of involvement as the disease progresses. This fact has led to the development of a staging scheme for neurofibrillary degeneration (Braak and Braak, 1991). The initial transentorhinal stage (Braak stages I and II) is characterized by neurofibrillary tangles relatively confined to the medial temporal lobe. Neurons in the hippocampus and temporal lobe are the next most vulnerable in Braak stages III and IV. Higher-order association cortices in frontal, parietal and occipital lobes are affected in stage V, and neurons within primary motor and sensory cortices are affected in stage VI.

While there have been some notable exceptions (Davis et al, 1999; Knopman et al, 2003), in most studies, the majority of individuals with Braak stages III or less have not had significant cognitive impairment (Grober et al, 1999), while patients with Braak stages IV and greater have varying degrees of dementia. The severity of cognitive impairment is a function of both the distribution and density of neurofibrillary pathology (Arriagada et al, 1992).

In patients with a clinical diagnosis of DLB, the severity of AD pathology is usually intermediate or low. Patients in whom severe Alzheimer-type pathology is detected at autopsy have clinical syndromes that are more typical of AD than of DLB. This fact has been incorporated into recent neuropathological criteria for DLB, with the understanding that the likelihood that the patient had a clinical syndrome compatible with DLB is directly related to the severity of LB pathology and inversely related to Alzheimer-type pathology.

When LBs are confined to the brainstem nuclei, most patients are either asymptomatic or have parkinsonism without dementia. Most cases of DLBD have dementia, but the clinical syndrome resembles DLB only if Alzheimer pathology is intermediate or low. Table 11.3 summarizes this scheme.

Clinicopathological correlations

The pathological substrates for the various clinical manifestations of DLB have not been determined with certainty, but given the functional attributes assigned to particular brain regions, it is possible to form working hypotheses as to clinicopathological correlations in LBD.

Dementia

The structural basis for dementia in most neurodegenerative disorders is neuronal and synaptic loss. Synaptic loss has been demonstrated in AD with a variety of complementary methods, including densitometric image analysis, western blot and enzyme-linked immunoassays for synaptic markers, such as synaptophysin. Surprisingly, while decreases in cortical synaptophysin correlate with cognitive decline in AD and in LBD with concurrent AD, they do not correlate in pure LBD (Hansen et al, 1998). Other structural or chemical factors must be important in LBD. Evidence suggests that cortical cholinergic dysfunction may play a critical role in cognitive dysfunction in LBD. Cholinergic deficiencies are profound in LBD and are greater than those found in AD (Dickson et al, 1987). Moreover, there is evidence of loss of cholinergic receptors in LBD, but not in AD (Perry et al, 1990).

Table 11.3 Proposed neuropathological criteria for dementia with Lewy bodies

	Alzheimer-type pathology		
Lewy body-type pathology	*NIA–Reagan low*	*NIA–Reagan intermediate*	*NIA–Reagan high*
Brainstem-predominant	Low	Low	Low
Limbic (transitional)	High	Intermediate	Low
Diffuse neocortical	High	High	Intermediate

While there is evidence of dopaminergic loss in LBD (Langlais et al, 1993), it is unclear what role, if any, loss of dopaminergic innervation of the striatum plays in cognitive impairment. The dopaminergic system most clearly implicated in cognitive dysfunction comprises the dopaminergic neurons in the ventral tegmental region that project to the limbic lobe (the mesolimbic dopaminergic system).

Other possible structural correlates of dementia in DLB include cortical spongiosis and gliosis, as well as LBs and LNs. There are no reported studies correlating the severity of cortical spongiosis with cognitive impairment in LBD. In contrast, there are a number of studies that suggest that the density and distribution of LBs and LNs correlates with cognitive impairment (Lennox et al, 1989; Samuel et al, 1996; Harding and Halliday, 2001). In particular, the density of LNs in the medial temporal lobe structures, such as the amygdala, has been correlated with dementia (Churchyard and Lees, 1997).

Parkinsonism

The best correlate for parkinsonism in DLB is neuronal loss in the pars compacta of the substantia nigra. Dopaminergic deficits have been demonstrated in the striatum, and correlate with the severity of neuronal loss in the substantia nigra and the severity of extrapyramidal signs. There is increasing recognition of the fact that most cases of LBD, especially those with diffuse or transitional type, have neuritic pathology in the striatum. It remains uncertain if this correlates with parkinsonism, but it has been suggested that progressive neuritic degeneration in the striatum may account for progressive loss of responsiveness to levodopa treatment (Apaydin et al, 2002).

Hallucinations and visuospatial disturbance

The pathological substrate of visual hallucinations in DLB has been suggested to be related to medial temporal lobe pathology. In particular, the density of LBs in the amygdala correlates with hallucinations (Harding et al, 2002). Functional imaging studies in DLB consistently demonstrate hypoperfusion of the occipital lobe that is not detected in AD (Albin et al, 1996). Whether this plays a role in the visuospatial disturbances in DLB remains to be determined. The structural basis for occipital hypoperfusion is not clear. A single unconfirmed study suggested that spongiosis in the occipital white matter correlated with occipital hypoperfusion on PET scans (Higuchi et al, 2000). There are almost no LBs and only sparse LNs in the primary visual cortex, but more numerous lesions in the visual association cortices, especially those in the posterior occipitotemporal gyrus.

Fluctuations and sleep disorders

The structural correlates of fluctuating cognition and sleep disorders in DLB have been suggested to be related to pathology in the isodendritic core (Boeve et al, 2004). The isodendritic core refers to the group of neuronal nuclei in the brainstem and basal forebrain that have relatively limited afferents, but widespread efferent projections, especially to the cortex. This core group of nuclei is part of the reticular activating system and includes the locus ceruleus, raphe nuclei and the basal nucleus of Meynert. All of these nuclei are vulnerable to LB pathology. Hypothalamic nuclei also play a role in sleep regulation, and these too are affected in LBD.

Etiology and pathogenesis

Genetic factors

As in most neurodegenerative disorders, the etiology is multifactorial and includes genetic and environmental risk factors. No clear genetic risk factor has been identified in sporadic cases of DLB, but several genes have been implicated in familial PD, and clinical presentations in some kindreds of familial PD (e.g. the Iowa kindred) overlap considerably with DLB (Gwinn-Hardy et al, 2000). The mutation in the Iowa kindred is a triplication of the gene encoding α-synuclein (SCNA) (Singleton et al, 2003). Importantly, polymorphisms in the SNCA promoter that affect expression levels of α-synuclein may also be a risk factor for PD (Chiba-Falek et al, 2003; Farrer et al, 2001). It remains to be determined if SNCA polymorphisms are a risk factor for DLB.

As noted previously, Alzheimer-type pathology is present in most brains of patients clinically diagnosed with DLB. The major genetic risk factor for AD is apolipoprotein E, and ε4 is over-represented in LBD cases with concurrent Alzheimer pathology (Dickson et al, 1996), but not in pure LBD. It may also be a risk factor for DLB independent of its effects on Alzheimer-type pathology (Singleton et al, 2002). The fact that apolipoprotein E is associated with Alzheimer-type and LB pathologies suggests a synergy between amyloid deposition and LBs. Support for this notion comes from transgenic mice expressing both α-synuclein and amyloid precursor protein, which develop more LB-like inclusions than mice expressing only α-synuclein (Masliah et al, 2001).

Variants in the gene encoding tau (*MAPT*), referred to collectively as H1 and H2 haplotypes, have been described, and H1 appears to be a risk factor for several parkinsonian disorders, including PSP and corticobasal degeneration (Baker et al, 1999). Several studies have shown that H1 may also be a risk factor for PD (Maraganore et al, 2001; Healy et al, 2004), but it remains to be determined if this is true for DLB. In a preliminary study of an autopsy cohort of LBD, most of whom were obtained from a dementia brain bank, there was no increased frequency of H1, suggesting the need for a comparable study on cases with antemortem clinical diagnosis of DLB.

Environmental factors

The strongest environmental risk factor for DLB is age. It is clearly a disorder that increases in frequency with age, but the mechanism behind this risk is unknown. In several series, there is also an increased frequency in men, but selection bias has not been completely excluded and it remains a research objective to determine if and how sex-related factors may increase risk for DLB. Environmental toxins have been implicated in PD (Rajput et al, 1986), but there are few or no epidemiological studies of a comparable nature suggesting any environmental risks associated with DLB.

References

Aarsland D, Ballard CG, Halliday G, Are Parkinson's disease with dementia and dementia with Lewy bodies the same entity? J Geriatr Psychiatry Neurol (2004) 17:137–45.

Albin RL, Minoshima S, D'Amato CJ et al, Fluoro-deoxyglucose positron emission tomography in diffuse Lewy body disease. Neurology (1996) 47:462–6.

Apaydin H, Ahlskog JE, Parisi JE et al, Parkinson's disease neuropathology: later-developing dementia and loss of the levodopa response. Arch Neurol (2002) 59:102–12.

Arriagada PV, Growdon JH, Hedley-Whyte ET et al, Neurofibrillary tangles but not senile plaques parallel duration and severity of Alzheimer's disease. Neurology (1992) 42:31–9.

Baba M, Nakajo S, Tu PH, Aggregation of alpha-synuclein in Lewy bodies of sporadic Parkinson's disease and dementia with Lewy bodies. Am J Pathol (1998) 152:879–84.

Baker M, Litvan I, Houlden H et al, Association of an extended haplotype in the *tau* gene with progressive supranuclear palsy. Hum Mol Genet (1999) 8:711–15.

Boeve BF, Silber MH, Ferman TJ, REM sleep behavior disorder in Parkinson's disease and dementia with Lewy bodies. J Geriatr Psychiatry Neurol (2004) 17:146–57.

Braak H, Braak E, Neuropathologic staging of Alzheimer-related changes. Acta Neuropathol (1991) 82:239–59.

Braak H, Del Tredici K, Rüb U et al, Staging of brain pathology related to sporadic Parkinson's disease. Neurobiol Aging (2003) 24:197–211.

Chiba-Falek O, Touchman JE, Mussbaun RL, Functional analysis of intra-allelic variation at NACP–Rep 1 in the alpha-synuclein gene. Human Genet (2003) 113:426–31

Churchyard A, Lees A, The relationship between dementia and direct involvement of the hippocampus and amygdala in Parkinson's disease. Neurology (1997) 49:1570–6.

Davis DG, Schmitt FA, Wekstein DR, Markesbery WR, Alzheimer neuropathologic alterations in aged cognitively normal subjects. J Neuropathol Exp Neurol (1999) 58:376–88.

Dickson DW, Pathogenesis of senile plaques. J Neuropathol Exp Neurol (1997) 56:321–39.

Dickson DW, α-synuclein and the Lewy body disorders. Curr Opin Neurol (2001) 14: 423–32.

Dickson DW, Dementia with Lewy bodies: neuropathology. J Geriat Psychiatry Neurol (2002a) 15:210–16.

Dickson DW, Neuropathology of Parkinsonian disorders. In: Jankovic JJ, Tolosa E, eds, Parkinson's Disease and Movement Disorders (4th edn) (Lippincott Williams & Wilkins: Philadelphia, 2002b) 256–69.

Dickson DW, Davies P, Mayeux R et al, Diffuse Lewy body disease: neuropathological and biochemical studies of six patients. Acta Neuropathol (1987) 75:8–15.

Dickson DW, Ruan D, Crystal H et al, Hippocampal degeneration differentiates diffuse Lewy body disease (DLBD) from Alzheimer's disease: light and electron microscopic immunocytochemistry of CA2-3 neurites specific to DLBD. Neurology (1991) 41:1402–9.

Dickson DW, Wu E, Crystal HA et al, Alzheimer and age-related pathology in diffuse Lewy body disease. In: Boller F, Forcette F, Khachaturian Z, et al, eds, Heterogeneity of Alzheimer's Disease (Springer-Verlag: Berlin, 1992) 168–86.

Dickson DW, Crystal HA, Davies P, Hardy J, Cytoskeletal and Alzheimer type pathology in Lewy body disease. In: Perry RH, McKeith IG, Perry EK, eds, Dementia with Lewy Bodies (Cambridge University Press: Cambridge, 1996) 224–37.

Duda JE, Giasson BI, Mabon ME et al, Novel antibodies to synuclein show abundant striatal pathology in Lewy body diseases. Ann Neurol (2002). 52:205–10.

Emre M, Dementia associated with Parkinson's disease. Lancet Neurol (2003) 2:229–37.

Eriksen JL, Wszolek Z, Petrucelli L, Molecular pathogenesis of Parkinson disease. Arch Neurol (2005) 62:353–7.

Farrer M, Marganore DM, Lockhart P et al, Alpha-synuclein gene haplotypes are associated with Parkinson's disease. Hum Mol Genet (2001) 10:1847–51

Fujino Y, Dickson DW, Spongiosis in Alzheimer's disease not due to concurrent Lewy body disease. J Neuropathol Exp Neurol (2003) 62:553.

Galvin JE, Lee VM, Baba M et al, Monoclonal antibodies to purified cortical Lewy bodies recognize the mid-size neurofilament subunit. Ann Neurol (1997) 42:595–603.

Grober E, Dickson D, Sliwinski MJ et al, Memory and mental status correlates of modified Braak staging. Neurobiol Aging (1999) 20:573–79.

Gwinn-Hardy K, Mehta ND, Farrer M et al, Distinctive neuropathology revealed by α-synuclein antibodies in hereditary Parkinsonism and dementia linked to chromosome 4p. Acta Neuropathol (2000) 99:663–72.

Hamilton RL, Lewy bodies in Alzheimer's disease: a neuropathological review of 145 cases using alpha-synuclein immunohistochemistry. Brain Pathol (2000) 10:378–84.

Hansen LA, Masliah E, Terry RD, Mirra SS, A neuropathological subset of Alzheimer's disease with concomitant Lewy body disease and spongiform change. Acta Neuropathol (1989) 78:194–201

Hansen LA, Daniel SE, Wilcock GK, Love S, Frontal cortical synaptophysin in Lewy body diseases: relation to Alzheimer's disease and dementia. J Neurol Neurosurg Psychiatry (1998) 64:653–6.

Harding AJ, Halliday GM, Cortical Lewy body pathology in the diagnosis of dementia. Acta Neuropathol (2001) 102:355–63.

Harding AJ, Broe GA, Halliday GM, Visual hallucinations in Lewy body disease relate to Lewy bodies in the temporal lobe. Brain (2002) 125:391–403.

Healy DG, Abou-Sleiman PM, Lees AJ et al, Tau gene and Parkinson's disease: a case–control study and meta-analysis. J Neurol Neurosurg Psychiatry (2004) 75:962–5.

Higuchi M, Tashiro M, Arai H et al, Glucose hypometabolism and neuropathological correlates in brains of dementia with Lewy bodies. Exp Neurol (2000) 162:247–56.

Hyman BT, Trojanowski JQ, Consensus recommendations for the postmortem diagnosis of Alzheimer disease from the National Institute on Aging and the Reagan Institute Working Group on diagnostic criteria for the neuropathological assessment of Alzheimer disease. J Neuropathol Exp Neurol (1997) 56: 1095–7.

Ishizawa T, Mattila P, Davies P et al, Colocalization of tau and alpha-synuclein epitopes in Lewy bodies. J Neuropath Exp Neurol (2003) 62:389–97.

Jellinger KA, Mizuno Y, Parkinson's disease. In: Dickson DW, ed, Neurodegeneration: the Molecular Pathology of Dementia and Movement Disorders (ISN Neuropath Press: Basel, 2003) 159–87.

Kato S, Nakamura H, Cytoplasmic argyrophilic inclusions in neurons of pontine nuclei in patients with olivopontocerebellar atrophy: immunohistochemical and ultrastructural studies. Acta Neuropathol (1990) 79:584–94.

Khachaturian ZS, Diagnosis of Alzheimer's disease. Arch Neurol (1985) 42:1097–105.

Knopman DS, Parisi JE, Salviati A et al, Neuropathology of cognitively normal elderly. J Neuropathol Exp Neurol (2003) 62:1087–95.

Kosaka K, Yoshimura M, Ikeda K, Budka H, Diffuse type of Lewy body disease: progressive dementia with abundant cortical Lewy bodies and senile changes of varying degree – a new disease? Clin Neuropathol (1984) 3:185–92.

Kuzuhara S, Mori H, Izumiyama N et al, Lewy bodies are ubiquitinated: a light and electron microscopic immunocytochemical study. Acta Neuropathol (1988) 75:345–53.

Langlais PJ, Thal L, Hansen L et al, Neurotransmitters in basal ganglia and cortex of Alzheimer's disease with and without Lewy bodies. Neurology (1993) 43: 1927–34.

Lantos PL, The definition of multiple system atrophy: a review of recent developments. J Neuropathol Exp Neurol (1998) 57:1099–1111.

Lennox G, Lowe JS, Landon M et al, Diffuse Lewy body disease: correlative neuropathology using anti-ubiquitin immunocytochemistry. J Neurol Neurosurg Psychiatry (1989) 52:1236–47.

Maraganore DM, Hernandez DG, Singleton AB, Case–control study of the extended tau gene haplotype in Parkinson's disease. Ann Neurol (2001) 50:658–61.

McKeith IG, Galasko D, Kosaka K et al, Clinical and pathological diagnosis of dementia with Lewy bodies (DLB): Report of the Consortium on Dementia with Lewy Bodies International Workshop. Neurology (1996) 47:1113–24.

McKeith IG, Ballard CG, Perry RH et al, Prospective validation of consensus criteria for the diagnosis of dementia with Lewy bodies. Neurology (2000) 54:1050–8.

McKeith I, Mintzer J, Aarsland D et al, International Psychogeriatric Association Expert Meeting on DLB. Dementia with Lewy bodies. Lancet Neurol (2004) 3:19–28.

Masliah E, Rockenstein E, Veinbergs I et al, Beta-amyloid peptides enhance alpha-synuclein accumulation and neuronal deficits in a transgenic mouse model linking Alzheimer's disease and Parkinson's disease. Proc Natl Acad Sci USA (2001) 98:12245–50.

Mirra SS, Heyman A, McKeel D et al, The Consortium to Establish a Registry for Alzheimer's Disease (CERAD). Part II. Standardization of the neuropathologic assessment of Alzheimer's disease. Neurology (1991) 41:479–86.

Perry EK, Smith CJ, Court JA, Perry RH, Cholinergic nicotinic and muscarinic receptors in dementia of Alzheimer, Parkinson and Lewy body types. J Neural Transm Park Dis Dement Sect (1990) 2:149–58.

Petersen R, Mild cognitive impairment as a diagnostic entity. J Intern Med (2004) 256:183–94

Pollanen MS, Bergeron C, Weyer L, Detergent insoluble cortical Lewy body fibrils share epitopes with neurofilament and tau. J Neurochem (1992) 58:1953–6

Pollanen MS, Dickson DW, Bergeron C, Pathology and biology of the Lewy body. J Neuropathol Exp Neurol (1993) 52:183–91.

Rajput AH, Uitti RJ, Stern W, Laverty W, Early onset Parkinson's disease in Saskatchewan – environmental considerations for etiology. Can J Neurol Sci (1986) 13:312–6.

Samuel W, Galasko D, Masliah E, Hansen LA, Neocortical Lewy body counts correlate with dementia in the Lewy body variant of Alzheimer's disease. J Neuropathol Exp Neurol (1996) 55:44–52.

Singleton AB, Wharton A, O'Brien KK et al, Clinical and neuropathological correlates of apolipoprotein E genotype in dementia with Lewy bodies. Dement Geriatr Cogn Disord (2002) 14:167–75.

Singleton AB, Farrer M, Johnson J et al, Alpha-synuclein locus triplication causes Parkinson's disease. Science (2003) 302:841.

Wakabayashi K, Takahashi H, Neuropathology of autonomic nervous system in Parkinson's disease. Eur Neurol (1997) 38(Suppl 2):2–7.

Wakabayashi K, Hayashi S, Yoshimoto M et al, NACP/alpha-synuclein-positive filamentous inclusions in astrocytes and oligodendrocytes of Parkinson's disease brains. Acta Neuropathol (2000) 99:14–20.

Wu E, Lipton RD, Dickson DW, Amyloid angiopathy in diffuse Lewy body disease. Neurology (1992) 42, 2131–2135.

chapter 12

Neurochemical pathology of dementia with Lewy bodies

Paul T Francis, Elaine K Perry, Margaret A Piggott and John E Duda

Introduction

It is now some 30 years since the beginning of intensive efforts to understand the neurotransmitter biochemistry of dementia as exemplified by Alzheimer's disease (AD), and such studies have led to the development of rational treatment strategies that are continuing to benefit patients (Francis et al, 1999). However, as studies became more sophisticated and clinicians rediscovered an interest in dementia because of the potential for symptomatic treatment, it has become clear that there are several different neurodegenerative conditions that give rise to dementia syndromes and that each has a distinct neurochemical pathology (Francis et al, 1999; Duda, 2004). This has important treatment implications, since what works for one patient may not work for another or (at the extreme) may make matters worse. It is therefore clear that a detailed understanding of neurotransmitter function in each condition is not merely academic but can lead to rational drug design and treatment strategies appropriate for that group of patients. Dementia with Lewy bodies (DLB) has clinicopathological features that overlap with either AD or Parkinson's disease (PD), as well as features that help to distinguish it, such as fluctuations in cognitive impairment and a higher prevalence of visual hallucinations. On this basis, it would be expected that the neurochemistry would have some similarities with both disorders.

Cholinergic neurotransmission

The status of the cholinergic system in DLB is summarized in Table 12.1. One notable feature of DLB is the more profound loss of cholinergic neurons and choline acetyltransferase (ChAT) activity compared with AD. Not only are neocortical presynaptic cholinergic activities reduced to a greater extent than in AD, but there are additional losses in DLB, but not AD, in the basal ganglia, including the striatum, and in the pedunculopontine pathway that projects to such areas as the thalamus. It is interesting to note that ChAT deficits are greater in some regions of the temporal cortex of DLB patients with visual hallucinations compared with those without. In particular, the greatest differences were seen in areas of the temporal cortex involved with visual recognition (Broadmann's area 36) compared with the parietal cortex, which is involved with the representation of visual objects in space and interpreting visual input into appropriate motor activity (Ballard et al, 2000a). In this study, many of the DLB patients experiencing visual hallucinations were being treated with levodopa, which is known to induce visual hallucinations in some patients with DLB or PD with dementia (PDD). An imbalance in cholinergic and dopaminergic activity may exacerbate or precipitate hallucinations in these patients. It has been suggested that the striatal cholinergic deficiency may contribute to the lesser degree of extrapyramidal symptoms seen in DLB compared with PD, in which striatal cholinergic activity is normal. However, this has not yet been supported by clinical–pathological correlations, and it is likely that less extensive substantia nigra neuronal loss is also responsible. The loss of thalamic cholinergic activity, which occurs particularly in the reticular formation, is likely to reflect degeneration of pedunculopontine neurons, which no doubt occurs in DLB as in PD. Whether this relates to attentional dysfunction and/or disturbances in consciousness, which are more extensive in DLB compared with AD, remains to be established.

In two studies, M_1 receptors were preserved or upregulated in the temporal cortex in DLB compared with AD, but appeared to be reduced in the hippocampus in both DLB and AD (Shiozaki et al, 1999, 2001; Ballard et al, 2000b). Furthermore, there is some evidence of uncoupling of M_1 receptors from the intracellular cascade in AD. Preservation of M_1 receptor number and function in the temporal cortex in DLB may partially explain why patients with DLB have a particularly beneficial response to cholinergic agents, such as acetylcholinesterase inhibitors (AChEI) (McKeith et al, 2000).

Table 12.1 Cholinergic activities in dementia with Lewy bodies (DLB) compared with Alzheimer's disease (AD) and Parkinson's disease (PD)[a]

	DLB	AD	PD
ChAT			
Cerebral cortex	↓↓	↓	↓[b]
Hippocampus	↓	↓↓	↓
Striatum	↓	↓	→
Thalamus	↓	→/↓	→[h]
AChE			
Cerebral cortex	↓↓[c]	↓	↓
BuChE			
Cerebral cortex	→	↓	→[b]
VAChT			
Cerebral cortex		↓	↓[b,c]
Muscarinic receptors			
M_1			
Cerebral cortex	↑	→	↑[b,c]
Striatum	↓	↑	→
M_2			
Cerebral cortex	↑	↓	
Striatum	↑/→	→	
M_4			
Cerebral cortex	↑	↓	
Striatum	→	↓	
Nicotinic receptors			
αBT binding (α_7):			
Cerebral cortex	→/↓	→	
Thalamus	↓	↓	
High-affinity agonist site (α_4/β_2):			
Cerebral cortex	↓	↓	↓
Striatum	↓	→/↓	↓↓
Thalamus	→/↓	→/↓	→

ChAT, choline acetyltransferase; AChE, acetylcholinesterase; BuChE, butyrylcholinesterase; VAChT, vesicular acetylcholine transporter; αBT, α-bungarotoxin.

[a] Summary of neurochemical findings, modified and updated from McKeith et al (2001).

[b] Reduced or more extensive in PD+ dementia.

[c] Alteration reported using PET or SPECT neuroimaging.

Nicotine binding is significantly reduced in the substantia nigra in both PD and DLB (Perry et al, 1995); however, neuronal loss accounts for much of the nicotinic receptor loss in PD, but not in DLB. PD and DLB patients had neuronal losses of 70% and 40%, respectively, while nicotine binding was reduced by 70% in both diseases. This suggests that, as in other parts of the brain, loss of cholinergic function in the substantia nigra precedes the degeneration and loss of neurons in DLB.

High-affinity nicotinic receptor loss has also been investigated in the temporal cortex in DLB and AD (Perry et al, 1995; Martin-Ruiz et al, 2000). In AD, the loss of nicotinic receptors in the temporal cortex parallels the loss of ChAT and AChE; however, in DLB, the nicotinic receptor loss was not as great as that in AD, despite the greater reduction of ChAT in patients with DLB compared with AD. Interestingly, the area of highest Lewy body (LB) density in the parahippocampal gyrus did not correlate with the greatest nicotinic receptor loss in DLB; nicotinic receptor levels were actually higher in this region in DLB. However, both AD and DLB had significant receptor loss in the dentate granular area, which may be significant in terms of memory loss in these patients. AD patients also have reduced projections from the entorhinal cortex to the dentate granular area, which may account for the greater severity of memory deficits in AD patients compared with DLB patients.

Nicotinic receptor changes in the cortex include a loss of the high-affinity agonist-binding site (reflecting the $\alpha_4\beta_2$ subtype), but no consistently reported change in the α_7 subunit or α-bungarotoxin binding site. In the thalamus, in contrast, there is little change in nicotine binding, but a highly significant reduction in α-bungarotoxin binding in the reticular nucleus. Similar nicotinic receptor abnormalities occur in AD and, as far as has been investigated, in PD. In the striatum, there is a greater loss of nicotine binding in PD than in DLB (Perry et al, 2000), in keeping with the more extensive reduction in basal ganglia dopaminergic projections, but no loss in neuroleptic-free AD patients.

Nicotinic receptors of the α_7 subtype were reduced in DLB compared with AD or controls (Wonnacott, 1997). This could have significance for DLB, since α_7 nicotinic receptors are thought to play a role in the release of the transmitter glutamate. Deficiencies in α_7 nicotinic receptors may also affect hallucinations in patients with DLB. In a study of DLB patients who either did or did not experience hallucinations, only those who experienced hallucinations had a deficiency in α_7 nicotinic receptors in the temporal cortex in areas associated with encoding complex recognition (Brodmann's areas 20 and 36)

(Court et al, 2001). There were no significant differences in high-affinity nicotinic receptors for DLB patients who experienced hallucinations compared with those who did not. However, this study and another (Martin-Ruiz et al, 2000) showed that there were significant differences in high-affinity nicotinic receptor levels between DLB and age-matched controls. In contrast, high-affinity nicotinic receptor binding in the temporal cortex (Brodmann's areas 20 and 36) did differentiate DLB patients with or without disturbances of consciousness, with a relative preservation in patients experiencing them (Ballard et al, 2002c).

Dopaminergic neurotransmission

For DLB and PD, neuronal losses in the substantia nigra from the medial to the lateral region appear to correspond to neuropsychiatric and motor symptoms, respectively. In DLB and idiopathic PD, neuronal loss in this region is correlated with the presence of Lewy pathology. However, in PD, neuronal loss is more asymmetrical than in DLB, leaving the medial region of the substantia nigra less affected in patients with PD (Ransmayr et al, 2001). This appears to be reflected in the levels of the dopamine transporter determined using single-photon emission computed tomography (SPECT), which is differentially affected in DLB compared with AD, and while there are some subtle differences between DLB and PD, further work is required for their use in differential diagnosis (O'Brien et al, 2004;Walker et al, 2004). Differences between DLB and PD in dopaminergic activities (summarized in Table 12.2) are of particular importance due to the differences in the response to levodopa (McKeith et al, 1996) and neuroleptics in DLB and PD patients (Ballard et al, 1998). Some patients with DLB have a poor response to levodopa treatment and can have a severe reaction to treatment with neuroleptics. This suggests that there may be neuropathological differences between PD and DLB with respect to dopamine. Piggott et al (1999) determined that dopamine D_2 receptor levels were significantly reduced (17%) in the caudal putamen in DLB patients compared with controls and patients with PD. In patients with PD, there were increases in D_2 receptors in all coronal sections, especially in the rostral putamen (an increase of 71%). In addition, increases in the amount of neuritic pathology in the striatum have been demonstrated in DLB and concomitant AD/DLB compared with PD (Duda et al, 2002). These differences may begin to explain the poor response of some DLB patients to levodopa and do provide a foundation for studying the severe reactions of many DLB patients to neuroleptics. Furthermore, D_2 receptors represent an important diagnostic tool to distinguish DLB from AD (Walker et al, 1997).

Other neurotransmitter systems

Changes in serotonergic neurotransmission in AD include neuron loss and neurofibrillary tangle formation in the raphe nucleus and receptor changes in

Table 12.2 Dopaminergic activities in dementia with Lewy bodies (DLB) compared with Alzheimer's disease (AD) and Parkinson's disease (PD)[a]

	DLB	AD	PD
DA			
Striatum	↓	→	↓↓
Cortex		→	↓↓
HVA			
Striatum	↓	↓→	↓↓
Cortex	↓		
Tyrosine hydroxylase			
Striatum			↓↓
Cerebral cortex		→	
Dopa decarboxylase			
Striatum			↓→
DAT			
Striatum	↓	→	↓↓
Dopaminergic receptors			
D_1			
Striatum	→	→	↑
Cerebral cortex	??	→	
D_2			
Striatum	↓	→	↑
Cerebral cortex	↓	→	↑
Thalamus	↓/→	→	↑

DA, dopamine; HVA, homovanillic acid; Dopa, 3,4-dihydroxy-L-phenylalamine; DAT, dopamine transporter.
[a]Summary of neurochemical findings, modified and updated from McKeith et al (2001).

the neocortex. Recent work indicates a loss of serotonin reuptake sites in the temporal cortex in AD associated with depression, but with preservation of serotonergic function in the frontal cortex, as indicated by the ratio of 5-hydroxyindoleacetic acid (5-HIAA) to serotonin (Chen et al, 1996). In DLB, Lewy bodies occur in the dorsal raphe nucleus, and marked reductions in serotonin levels have been reported in the striatum, neocortex and frontal cortex. In contrast, DLB patients with major depression had a relative higher binding to the serotonin transporter reuptake sites in the parietal cortex, compared with those without depression. However, while no control data were reported in this study (Ballard et al, 2002a) both groups had lower mean values than control (EK Perry, unpublished observations). In PD, the association between serotonergic dysfunction and depression is clearer, with a number of studies identifying reduced 5-HIAA in the cerebrospinal fluid (Mayeux et al, 1988; Kuhn et al, 1996).

Only two studies have been published to date examining the glutamatergic system: they reported no change in the expression of a glutamate transporter protein in a small number of DLB cases (Scott et al, 2002) and reduced glutamate receptor immunoreactivity in the hippocampus and entorhinal cortex of patients with the Lewy body variant of AD (Thorns et al, 1997). Clearly, further studies are required to determine the possible role of glutamatergic neurons in DLB using a range of markers (Francis, 2003).

Conclusions and future directions

Considerable progress has been made over the last two decades in the investigation of the neurochemical pathology of AD and PD, and this has led to the development of new treatments and the refinement of existing therapies. Although much less is known about neurotransmission changes in DLB, an understanding is emerging of the reasons why some drugs developed for AD work better in DLB patients while those for PD work less well (or indeed may be harmful) in DLB. Likewise, correlative studies have begun to determine the neurochemical basis of particular symptoms associated with the condition, which may help with more fundamental aspects of neuroscience research. It is hoped that future studies will lead to the development of drugs that are particularly suitable in DLB, to the benefit of patients and carers, and to the identification of novel diagnostic markers and ligands suitable for imaging.

References

Ballard C, Grace J, McKeith I, Holmes C, Neuroleptic sensitivity in dementia with Lewy bodies and Alzheimer's disease. Lancet (1998) 351:1032–3.

Ballard C, Johnson M, Piggott M et al, A positive association between 5HT re-uptake binding sites and depression in dementia with Lewy bodies. J Affect Disord (2002a) 69:219–23.

Ballard C, Piggott M, Johnson M et al, Delusions associated with elevated muscarinic binding in dementia with Lewy bodies. Ann Neurol (2002b) 48:868–76.

Ballard CG, Court JA, Piggott M et al, Disturbances of consciousness in dementia with Lewy bodies associated with alteration in nicotinic receptor binding in the temporal cortex. Conscious Cogn (2002c) 11:461–74.

Chen CPL-H, Alder JT, Bowen DM et al, Presynaptic serotonergic markers in community-acquired cases of Alzheimer's disease: correlation with depression and neuroleptic medication. J Neurochem (1996) 66:1592–8.

Court J, Martin-Ruiz C, Piggott M et al, Nicotinic receptor abnormalities in Alzheimer's disease. Biol Psychiatry (2001) 49:175–84.

Duda JE, Pathology and neurotransmitter abnormalities of dementia with Lewy bodies. Dement Geriatr Cogn Disord (2004) 17(Suppl 1):3–14.

Duda JE, Giasson BI, Mabon ME et al, Novel antibodies to synuclein show abundant striatal pathology in Lewy body diseases. Ann Neurol (2002) 52:205–10.

Francis PT, Glutamatergic systems in Alzheimer's disease. Int J Geriatr Psychiatry (2003) 18:S15–21.

Francis PT, Palmer AM, Snape M, Wilcock GK, The cholinergic hypothesis of Alzheimer's disease: a review of progress. J Neurol Neurosurg Psychiatry (1999) 66:137–47.

Kuhn W, Muller T, Gerlach M et al, Depression in Parkinson's disease: biogenic amines in CSF of 'de novo' patients. J Neural Transm (1996) 103:1441–5.

McKeith IG, Galasko D, Kosaka K et al, Consensus guidelines for the clinical and pathological diagnosis of dementia with Lewy bodies (DLB) – Report of the Consortium on DBL International Workshop. Neurology (1996) 47:1113–24.

McKeith IG, Grace JB, Walker Z et al, Rivastigmine in the treatment of dementia with Lewy bodies: preliminary findings from an open trial. Int J Geriatr Psychiatry (2000) 15:387–92.

McKeith IG, Burn D, O'Brien J et al, Dementia with Lewy bodies. In: Davis KL et al, eds, Neuropsychopharmacology: The Fifth Generation of Progress (Lippincott, Williams & Wilkins: Baltimore, 2001) 1301–16.

Martin-Ruiz C, Court J, Lee M et al, Nicotinic receptors in dementia of Alzheimer, Lewy body and vascular types. Acta Neurol Scand Suppl (2000) 176:34–41.

Mayeux R, Stern Y, Sano M et al, The relationship of serotonin to depression in Parkinson's disease. Mov Disord (1998) 3:237–44.

O'Brien, J. T., Colloby, S., Fenwick, J et al, Dopamine transporter loss visualized with FP-CIT SPECT in the differential diagnosis of dementia with Lewy bodies. Arch Neurol (2004) 6:919–25.

Perry EK, Morris CM, Court JA et al, Alteration in nicotine binding sites in Parkinson's disease, Lewy body dementia and Alzheimer's: possible index of early neuropathology. Neuroscience (1995) 64:385–95.

Perry E, Martin-Ruiz C, Lee M et al, Nicotinic receptor subtypes in human brain ageing, Alzheimer and Lewy body diseases. Eur J Pharmacol (2000) 393:215–22.

Piggott MA, Marshall EF, Thomas N et al, Dopaminergic activities in the human striatum: rostrocaudal gradients of uptake sites and of D1 and D2 but not of D3 receptor binding or dopamine. Neuroscience (1999) 90:433–45.

Ransmayr G, Seppi K, Donnemiller, E et al, Striatal dopamine transporter function in dementia with Lewy bodies and Parkinson's disease. Eur J Nucl Med (2001) 28:1523–8.

Scott HL, Pow DV, Tannenberg AE, Dodd PR, Aberrant expression of the glutamate transporter excitatory amino acid transporter 1 (EAAT1) in Alzheimer's disease. J Neurosci (2002) 22:RC206.

Shiozaki K, Iseki E, Uchiyama H et al, Alterations of muscarinic acetylcholine receptor subtypes in diffuse Lewy body disease: relation to Alzheimer's disease. J Neurol Neurosurg Psychiatry (1999) 67:209–13.

Shiozaki K, Iseki E, Hino H, Kosaka K, Distribution of m1 muscarinic acetylcholine receptors in the hippocampus of patients with Alzheimer's disease and dementia with Lewy bodies – an immunohistochemical study. J Neurol Sci (2001) 193:23–8.

Thorns V, Mallory M, Hansen L, Masliah E, Alterations in glutamate receptor 2/3 sub-units and amyloid precursor protein expression during the course of Alzheimer's disease and Lewy body variant. Acta Neuropathol (Berl) (1997) 94:539–48.

Walker Z, Costa DC, Janssen AG et al, Dementia with Lewy bodies: a study of post-synaptic dopaminergic receptors with iodine-123 iodobenzamide single-photon emission tomography. Eur J Nucl Med (1997) 24:609–14.

Walker Z, Costa DC, Walker RW et al, Striatal dopamine transporter in dementia with Lewy bodies and Parkinson disease: a comparison. Neurol (2004) 62:1568–72.

Wonnacott S, Presynaptic nicotinic ACh receptors. Trends Neurosci (1997) 20:92–8.

chapter 13

Nosological confusion regarding the boundaries of dementia with Lewy bodies

John Hardy

Defining the clinical and pathological boundaries of the diagnosis of dementia with Lewy bodies (DLB) with respect to both Parkinson's disease (PD) and Alzheimer's disease (AD) has been an intractable problem. Here, I argue that this intractability probably reflects the underlying biology of the disease processes.

DLB was first recognized as a rare pathological entity (Kosaka et al, 1984), but with the increasing use of, first, ubiquitin staining (Lennox et al, 1989a,b) and then α-synuclein staining (Spillantini et al, 1989), it was gradually realized by many groups that cortical Lewy bodies were also frequent findings in dementia cases with plaque pathology (Hansen et al, 1989; Lennox et al, 1989a,b; Perry et al, 1990) and in PD, especially in cases where the latter had progressed to involve cognitive problems (Gibbs et al, 1987). Thus, the diagnosis of DLB grew in the area between AD and PD (McKeith et al, 1996). The diagnosis is useful because it seems that the cognitive symptoms in individuals with DLB respond particularly well to cholinergic therapy (Pakrasi et al, 2003), in a fashion rather reminiscent to dopamine therapy in PD (Hornykiewicz, 2002). In general, there is a cluster of clinical features that predict the findings of Lewy bodies in the cortex (McKeith et al, 1996): it is a troubled diagnosis, however, because the overlaps on the one hand with AD and on the other hand with PD are clearly arbitrary and difficult to define (Hansen, 1997). Here I argue from a genetic perspective that these difficulties in diagnosis are inevitable. I adduce three primary pieces of evidence: first, the occurrence of Lewy bodies in genetically defined cases of AD; second, the potentiation of α-synuclein pathology in synuclein transgenic animals by *APP* transgenes; and third, by analogy with the work linking Aβ with tau and tangles in both humans and transgenic animals.

While the occurrence of Lewy bodies in 'typical' AD is widespread, in such cases it is not possible to be certain that their occurrence is not coincidental and reflecting two separate pathogenic processes (Hansen and Samuel, 1997). However, the occurrence of Lewy bodies in cases of AD with *APP* mutations (Hardy, 1994; Lantos et al, 1994), with presenilin mutations or with Down syndrome (Lippa et al, 1998, 1999) is revealing because these individuals get the disease very early, at an age at which incidental Lewy bodies are a rare event, and also, in these individuals, it is clear that the Lewy bodies are downstream of the primary pathogenic insult, which relates to Aβ42 production and deposition (Hardy, 1994). Thus it is clear that Lewy body formation can be initiated, in humans, by Aβ42.

However, the occurrence of mutations in α-synuclein in hereditary Lewy body diseases – both those manifesting as PD and those manifesting as dementia – shows that Lewy body formation can also be initiated by mutations in the *a-synuclein* gene (Polymeropoulos et al, 1997). In fact, most (possibly all) mutations can manifest as either a dementing illness or a movement disorder (Muenter et al, 1998, Kruger et al, 2001, Zarranz et al, 2004). The fact that this statement holds true in those families who have multiplications of the *a-synuclein* locus shows that genetic variability in α-synuclein expression is a key variable in determining whether Lewy body disease occurs (Farrer et al, 2001; Singleton et al, 2003).

So far, it has not proved possible to model Lewy body formation in transgenic mice: however, mice overexpressing the *a-synuclein* gene develop an α-synuclein pathology, and crossing these mice with amyloid transgenic mice potentiates this pathology (Masliah et al, 2000, 2001).

There is a similar literature for tau and tangles as for α-synuclein and Lewy bodies: tangle formation is clearly downstream of Aβ42 in AD (Hardy et al, 1998), but mutations in tau can lead directly to tangle formation (Hutton et al, 1998) – and tangle formation is potentiated, especially in the cortex, in transgenic mice by overproduction of Aβ42 (Lewis et al, 2000, 2001). For tau, this has led to the proposal that the pathogenic mechanism is as illustrated in Figure 13.1: clearly, it is equally logical to propose a similar scheme for α-synuclein (Figure 13.2) (Hardy et al, 1998).

Application of the logical hierarchy implicit in this scheme suggests the following:

- There will be those individuals who, probably in part because of their expression levels of α-synuclein, will be predisposed to get Lewy body disease. Analysis of the families so far described suggests that this may manifest primarily as either a movement disorder or as a dementia.

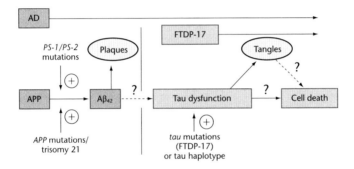

Figure 13.1 *Relationship between amyloid and tau in Alzheimer's disease and frontotemoral dementia with parkinsonism linked to chromosome 17 (FTDP-17).*

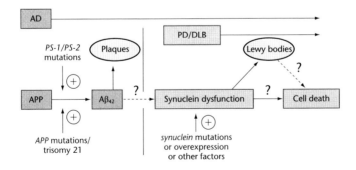

Figure 13.2 *Relationship between amyloid and α-synuclein in Alzheimer's disease and the Lewy body diseases.*

- In those older individuals, and especially in those who have an apolipoprotein ε4 allele, in addition to a high α-synuclein expression, the consequent Aβ pathology will drive Lewy body formation, especially in cortical areas. In this regard, it is of interest that DLB has shown an ε4 association (Hardy et al, 1994; Lippa et al, 1994), whereas PD shows a weak association with the E2 allele (Maraganore et al, 2000) – presumably because this latter allele is 'protective' against the amyloid deposition of AD (Chartier Harlin et al, 1994). Thus, the probable reason why the apolipoprotein ε2 allele is weakly associated with PD is because of its indirect 'protective' effect against Aβ deposition and cortical pathology.

This scheme allows only three variables: α-synuclein expression, apolipoprotein E genotype and age, with high α-synuclein expression predisposing to Lewy body disease in general and the precise nature of the resultant phenotype being influenced by the other variables, with high age and an ε4 allele predisposing to a cortical/dementing phenotype and low age and an ε2 allele predisposing to a movement disorder phenotype. Clearly, this is a gross oversimplification, and it must remain likely that the tau/tangle phenotype is an alternative to the α-synuclein/Lewy body phenotype and that this will also influence the precise nature of the phenotype.

However, of the three variables, α-synuclein expression levels will presumably be a nearly continuous variable, age is a continuous variable, and although apolipoprotein E genotype is a discrete variable, there are six possible genotypes: in such circumstances, dissecting the precise edges of the phenotypic spectra is likely to always be a forlorn task (Hansen, 1997). In these overlap syndromes, strict differential diagnoses are impossible, and it is more fruitful to appreciate the diseases as interacting pathological processes (Hardy and Gwinn-Hardy, 1999).

References

Chartier-Harlin MC, Parfitt M, Legrain S et al, Apolipoprotein E, ε4 allele as a major risk factor for sporadic early and late-onset forms of Alzheimer's disease: analysis of the 19q13.2 chromosomal region. Hum Mol Genet (1994) 3:569–74.

Farrer M, Maraganore DM, Lockhart P et al, α-synuclein gene haplotypes are associated with Parkinson's disease. Hum Mol Genet (2001) 10:1847–51.

Gibbs WR, Esiri MM, Lees AJ, Clinical and pathological features of diffuse cortical Lewy body disease (Lewy body dementia). Brain (1987) 110:1131–53.

Hansen LA. The Lewy body variant of Alzheimer disease. J Neural Transm Suppl (1997) 51:83–93.

Hansen LA, Masliah E, Terry RD, Mirra SS, A neuropathological subset of Alzheimer's disease with concomitant Lewy body disease and spongiform change. Acta Neuropathol (Berl) (1989) 78:194–201.

Hansen LA, Samuel W, Criteria for Alzheimer's disease and the nosology of dementia with Lewy bodies. Neurology (1997) 48:126–32.

Hardy J, Lewy bodies in Alzheimer's disease in which the primary lesion is a mutation in the amyloid precursor protein. Neurosci Lett (1994) 180:290–2.

Hardy J, Gwinn-Hardy K, Neurodegenerative disease: a different view of diagnosis. Mol Med Today (1999) 5:514–7.

Hardy J, Crook R, Prihar G et al, Senile dementia of the Lewy body type has an apolipoprotein E ε4 allele frequency intermediate between controls and Alzheimer's disease. Neurosci Lett (1994) 182:1–3.

Hardy J, Duff K, Gwinn-Hardy K et al, Genetic dissection of Alzheimer's disease and related dementias: amyloid and its relationship to tau. Nat Neurosci (1998) 1:95–9.

Hornykiewicz O, Dopamine miracle: from brain homogenate to dopamine replacement. Mov Disord (2002) 17:501–8

Hutton M, Lendon CL, Rizzu P et al, Association of missense and 5′-splice-site mutations in tau with the inherited dementia FTDP-17. Nature (1998) 393:702–5.

Kosaka K, Yoshimura M, Ikeda K, Budka H, Diffuse type of Lewy body disease: progressive dementia with abundant cortical Lewy bodies and senile changes of varying degree – a new disease? Clin Neuropathol (1984) 3:185–92.

Kruger R, Kuhn W, Leenders KL et al, Familial parkinsonism with synuclein pathology: clinical and PET studies of A30P mutation carriers. Neurology (2001) 56:1355–62.

Lantos PL, Ovenstone IM, Johnson J et al, Lewy bodies in the brain of two members of a family with the 717 (Val to Ile) mutation of the amyloid precursor protein gene. Neurosci Lett (1994) 172:77–9.

Lennox G, Lowe J, Morrell K et al, Anti-ubiquitin immunocytochemistry is more sensitive than conventional techniques in the detection of diffuse Lewy body disease. J Neurol Neurosurg Psychiatry (1989a) 52:67–71.

Lennox G, Lowe J, Landon M et al, Diffuse Lewy body disease: correlative neuropathology using anti-ubiquitin immunocytochemistry. J Neurol Neurosurg Psychiatry (1989b) 52:1236–47.

Lewis J, McGowan E, Rockwood J et al, Neurofibrillary tangles, amyotrophy and progressive motor disturbance in mice expressing mutant (P301L) tau protein. Nat Genet (2000) 25:402–5.

Lewis J, Dickson DW, Lin WL et al, Enhanced neurofibrillary degeneration in transgenic mice expressing mutant tau and APP. Science (2001) 293:1487–91.

Lippa CF, Smith TW, Saunders AM et al, Apolipoprotein E genotype and Lewy body disease. Neurology (1994) 45:97–103.

Lippa CF, Fujiwara H, Mann DM et al, Lewy bodies contain altered alpha-synuclein in brains of many familial Alzheimer's disease patients with mutations in presenilin and amyloid precursor protein genes. Am J Pathol (1998) 153:1365–70

Lippa CF, Schmidt ML, Lee VM, Trojanowski JQ, Antibodies to alpha-synuclein detect Lewy bodies in many Down's syndrome brains with Alzheimer's disease. Ann Neurol (1999) 45:353–7.

McKeith IG, Galasko D, Kosaka K et al, Consensus guidelines for the clinical and pathologic diagnosis of dementia with Lewy bodies (DLB): Report of the Consortium on DLB International Workshop. Neurology (1996) 47:1113–24.

Maraganore DM, Farrer MJ, Hardy JA et al, Case–control study of debrisoquine 4-hydroxylase, N-acetyltransferase 2, and apolipoprotein E gene polymorphisms in Parkinson's disease. Mov Disord (2000) 15:714–19

Masliah E, Rockenstein E, Veinbergs I et al, Dopaminergic loss and inclusion body formation in alpha-synuclein mice: implications for neurodegenerative disorders. Science (2000) 287:1265–9.

Masliah E, Rockenstein E, Veinbergs I et al, β-amyloid peptides enhance α-synuclein accumulation and neuronal deficits in a transgenic mouse model linking Alzheimer's disease and Parkinson's disease. Proc Natl Acad Sci USA (2001) 98:12245–50.

Muenter MD, Forno LS, Hornykiewicz O et al, Hereditary form of parkinsonism's dementia. Ann Neurol (1998) 43:768–81.

Pakrasi S, Mukaetova-Ladinska EB, McKeith IG, O'Brien JT, Clinical predictors of response to acetyl cholinesterase inhibitors: experience from routine clinical use in Newcastle. Int J Geriatr Psychiatry (2003) 18:879–86.

Perry RH, Irving D, Blessed G et al, Senile dementia of Lewy body type. A clinically and neuropathologically distinct form of Lewy body dementia in the elderly. J Neurol Sci (1990) 95:119–39.

Polymeropoulos MH, Lavedan C, Leroy E et al, Mutation in the alpha-synuclein gene identified in families with Parkinson's disease. Science (1997) 276:2045–7.

Singleton A, Farrer M, Johnson J et al, α-synuclein locus triplication causes Parkinson's disease. Science (2003) 302:841.

Spillantini MG, Crowther RA, Jakes R et al, α-synuclein in filamentous inclusions of Lewy bodies from Parkinson's disease and dementia with Lewy bodies. Proc Natl Acad Sci USA (1998) 95:6469–73.

Zarranz JJ, Alegre J, Gomez-Esteban et al, The new mutation, E46K, of alpha-synuclein causes Parkinson and Lewy body dementia. Ann Neurol (2004) 55:164–73.

chapter 14

Pharmacological treatment of dementia with Lewy bodies

Ian G McKeith and Serge Gauthier

Introduction

The pharmacological management of dementia with Lewy bodies (DLB) can be one of the most challenging issues facing neurologists, psychiatrists, geriatricians, primary care physicians and others caring for older people. (McKeith et al, 1995; Burn and McKeith, 2003) On the one hand, there lies the risk of severe, sometimes fatal, neuroleptic sensitivity reactions (McKeith et al, 1992); on the other hand, there are the potentially gratifying positive effects of cholinesterase inhibitors (ChEI) (Aarsland et al, 2004). Polypharmacy is the norm, with multiple pharmacological treatment targets including motor parkinsonism, cognitive failure, psychiatric symptoms and autonomic dysfunction. Since at the time of writing, little category A (randomized, placebo-controlled, trial-based) evidence is available, most prescribing for DLB is 'off-licence', outside of recognized treatment guidelines. This chapter reflects the authors' personal experience and practice of managing DLB patients, citing the evidence that is available in an increasing number of case reports and from controlled and (more typically) uncontrolled trials. Since the literature suggests that pharmacological responses are similar in both DLB and Parkinson's disease (PD) with dementia (PDD), reference will be made to both clinical situations, assuming that the same general principles apply to each.

General considerations

When dealing with the management of DLB or PDD patients, it is helpful first to draw up a problem list of cognitive, psychiatric and motor disabilities and to then ask the patient and carer to identify the symptoms that they find most disabling or distressing and that carry highest priority for treatment (Barber et al, 2001). There may be discrepant views about this, which have to be resolved; for example, a carer may complain that his or her sleep is being disrupted by the patient's nocturnal restlessness, whereas the patient is more preoccupied with motor slowness through the day. The clinician should explain, before any drugs are prescribed, that treatment gains in target symptoms may be associated with worsening of symptoms in other domains. The specific risks of neuroleptic sensitivity reactions should be mentioned in all cases, and it is prudent to mark patient case notes and records with an alert to reduce possibility of inadvertent neuroleptic prescribing, particularly in primary care or emergency room settings.

Nonpharmacological strategies for cognitive symptoms, including explanation, education, reassurance, orientation and memory prompts, attentional cues, and targeted behavioral interventions, are dealt with in Chapter 15 and will not be discussed here. They are an integral part of the management of DLB and pharmacological treatment is most successful when prescribed as part of a comprehensive management approach. Similarly, if a patient with DLB has become acutely confused and psychotic, then intercurrent infection and subdural hematoma, in particular, should be actively excluded (McKeith et al, 1996). It cannot always be assumed that worsening of symptoms is simply part of the natural fluctuating history of DLB. Non-essential medications capable of causing confusion such as cimetidine and oxybutinin should be discontinued.

Specific medications

Antiparkinsonian agents

There are two situations commonly faced by the clinician prescribing antiparkinsonian agents to DLB patients. The same general principles can be applied to both. The first scenario is the need to initiate treatment for motor symptoms – typically bradykinesia and rigidity, and less commonly tremor. The second is when considering whether to reduce or withdraw an antiparkinsonian drug regime that is suspected of aggravating confusion and psychotic symptoms.

There is general agreement that if antiparkinsonian drugs are prescribed, the clinician should aim for the lowest acceptable dose of levodopa monotherapy (Burn and McKeith, 2003). Although the effectiveness of levodopa on motor symptoms in DLB has not been established, it is probably less than in uncomplicated PD, possibly due to additional intrinsic striatal pathology and dysfunction (Duda et al, 2002). Other antiparkinsonians, including anticholinergics, amantadine, selegiline, catechol-O-methyl transferase (COMT) inhibitors and dopamine agonists, should generally be avoided and if already being prescribed may be slowly withdrawn in that order. Patients and carers will usually indicate when they feel that the lower acceptable limit of antiparkinsonian treatment has been reached. It is not uncommon to find that confusional and psychotic symptoms are not significantly ameliorated by dose reductions in antiparkinsonians, nor is motor disability substantially aggravated. This suggests that nondopaminergic mechanisms may be playing a major role in symptom formation.

Cholinesterase inhibitors

There is converging and consistent evidence that cholinesterase inhibitor (ChEI) drugs are effective and relatively safe in the treatment of neuropsychiatric and cognitive symptoms in DLB and PDD, but the number of patients studied is relatively small and larger trials are still needed (Aarsland et al, 2004). Apathy, anxiety, impaired attention, hallucinations, delusions, sleep disturbance, and cognitive changes are the most frequently cited treatment-responsive symptoms in DLB patients treated with ChEIs (Kaufer et al, 1998; McKeith et al, 2000b; Maclean et al, 2001; Reading et al, 2001). Improvements are generally reported as greater than those achieved in AD (Samuel et al, 2000; Aarsland, 2002).

Hutchinson and Fazzini (1996) were the first to report the benefits of tacrine in an open-label trial with seven PDD patients of mean age 74 years. Although tacrine is now not generally available because of problems with hepatotoxicity, reference to the original study remains informative. The mean duration of PD before the onset of dementia was 7.6 years. In all cases, the use of tacrine was associated with a 'greatly reduced' frequency of visual hallucinations (VH). Furthermore, both Mini-Mental State Examination (MMSE) scores and full-scale Unified Parkinson's Disease Rating Scale (UPDRS) scores improved significantly after treatment, the latter being particularly impressive (mean score before treatment 79.3, mean score after treatment 29.6; $p < 0.0001$). Despite the shortcomings of the study design, this work suggested that not only could a ChEI improve neuropsychiatric features of PDD, but, contrary to theoretical predictions and previous beliefs, this improvement might not occur at the expense of worsening motor features (in fact, the converse seemed to be the case).

The ChEI generally available at present are rivastigmine, donepezil and galantamine, all three preventing the inactivation of acetylcholine after its release from the neuron. Recent studies have suggested that, in addition to acetylcholinesterase, butyrylcholinesterase also plays an important role in cholinergic transmission (O'Brien et al, 2003). Of the available ChEIs, rivastigmine is a dual inhibitor of acetylcholinesterase and butyrylcholinesterase, while donepezil and galantamine are acetylcholinesterase-selective. Galantamine, the most recently licensed ChEI, is additionally an allosteric modulator of nicotinic receptors. At the time of writing, there are very few published data about its effects in Lewy body disease (Aarsland et al, 2003b; Edwards et al, 2004), but its effects seem broadly similar to the other two drugs.

A multicenter, randomized placebo-controlled study assessed the effect of rivastigmine (mean dose 7 mg/day) in DLB patients over 20 weeks, followed by a 3-week withdrawal period (McKeith et al, 2000a). One hundred and twenty patients with a clinical diagnosis of probable DLB, and an MMSE score greater than 10, were treated with up to 12 mg/day of rivastigmine or placebo. A four-item subscore of the Neuropsychiatric Inventory (NPI) comprising delusions, hallucinations, apathy and depression was used as the primary efficacy criterion (Del Ser et al, 2000). Approximately twice as many patients on rivastigmine (63.4%) than on placebo (30.0%) showed at least a 30% improvement from baseline on their NPI-4 scores ($p = 0.001$), with psychotic features resolving almost completely in over half of the treated patients. These symptoms rapidly re-emerged during a 3-week washout period. Nonsignificant improvements were also seen at 20 weeks in MMSE score and clinical global change-plus rating, in favor of the rivastigmine-treated group. Parkinsonian signs did not worsen on treatment, although an emergent tremor was noted in four rivastigmine-treated patients. Predominant adverse effects were cholinergic in nature, and the frequency of nausea (37%), vomiting (25%), anorexia (19%) and somnolence (9%) was significantly higher in the rivastigmine-treated patients. Most adverse events were rated as either mild or moderate, however, and only 7 of 59 patients receiving the ChEI withdrew for this reason (not significantly different from the placebo group).

The presence, rather than absence, of VH in DLB predicted a good response to rivastigmine, as evidenced by improved attention measures (Wesnes et al, 2002; McKeith et al, 2004b). In autopsy studies, DLB cases with VH have lower levels of cortical choline acetyltransferase, particularly in temporoparietal regions, compared with DLB patients without VH (Perry et al, 1990). This may allow greater clinical improvements to occur, with cholinergic replacement therapy having a more marked effect upon a lower neurochemical baseline. Cognitive reaction time (calculated by subtracting simple from choice reaction times) was not improved by rivastigmine. Such variability in the responsiveness of different cognitive parameters to ChEIs may give an insight into their neurochemical basis. Thus, it may be postulated that failure to improve choice reaction time by cholinomimetic therapy is because this is also dopaminergically mediated, perhaps via loss of mesocortical dopaminergic projections.

ChEIs are generally well tolerated in DLB, dosage being in the usual Alzheimer's disease (AD) range and with dropout rates (10–31%) and gastrointestinal side-effects similar to those found in AD. Hypersalivation, rhinorrhoea and lacrimation may also occur in approximately 15% of DLB and PDD patients treated with donepezil (Thomas et al, in press), and postural hypotension, falls and syncope are possibly increased. An early report of worsening of parkinsonism in two of nine patients treated with donepezil has not been replicated in other studies, which have consistently demonstrated either no change or improvement in motor function during ChEI therapy (Shea et al, 1998). Abrupt withdrawal of ChEIs is associated with rapid return of neuropsychiatric symptoms and cognitive decline in DLB and PDD (Minett et al, 2003). Although reinstatement of treatment may reverse such deterioration, it is recommended that DLB patients who are assessed as responding to ChEI be maintained on long-term treatment. A follow-up study of DLB patients receiving rivastigmine (Grace et al, 2001) found MMSE and NPI scores to be stable over the first 12 months of treatment, then to gradually worsen, although not significantly so even 2 years after baseline. Motor UPDRS scores tended to improve, probably because some antiparkinsonian treatment was initiated. Attempts at switching from one ChEI to another were associated with clinically significant withdrawal effects (Bhanji and Gauthier, 2003) and this treatment strategy is not recommended.

Typical and atypical antipsychotics

D_2 receptor antagonists, particularly traditional neuroleptic agents, can provoke severe neuroleptic sensitivity reactions in up to 50% of DLB patients, with a two- or threefold increased mortality (McKeith et al, 1992; Grace et al, 1998; Aarsland et al, 2003a). These reactions are generally acute or subacute, becoming evident within the first few doses or after an increase from a previously tolerated dose. The pre-existence or severity of spontaneous parkinsonism does not appear to be a reliable guide to the probability of neuroleptic sensitivity occurring. If acute deterioration occurs in a confused elderly patient following neuroleptic administration, DLB should always be considered as part of the differential diagnosis. Newer atypical antipsychotics used at low dose may be safer in this regard, but since sensitivity reactions have been documented with most, they should all be used with caution. Risperidone and olanzapine have recently been associated with two- to threefold increased stroke risk in patients with dementia, and therefore their use in DLB cannot be advocated. There is limited evidence available about the use of quetiapine, which does appear to have a lower incidence of parkinsonian side-effects and which is reported as effective in nondemented PD. Clozapine is also useful in treating PD psychosis, but its antimuscarinic properties may increase confusion in DLB patients (Burke et al, 1998).

If DLB or PDD patients exhibit psychotic symptoms or behavioral disturbances that are not responsive to other treatment strategies and that are intolerably distressing or pose a threat to themselves or other people, it may not be possible to avoid a trial of a low-dose neuroleptic. Very low doses should be administered under close supervision, with frequent reassessment for potential side-effects. The drug should be withdrawn immediately if there is a suspicion of deterioration, particularly with increasing parkinsonian features, diminishing alertness or reduced intake of food and fluid. Injectable and slow-release preparations should never be used in DLB. Preliminary experience suggests that ChEIs may safely be used in combination.

Other pharmacological agents

Other non-neuroleptic medications may have a role to play in the management of DLB, including the use of low-dose clonazepam (0.5–1 mg) for sleep disturbance with the characteristics of REM sleep behavior disorder (Boeve et al, 2001). Disturbed sleep with thrashing limb movements, vocalizations and vivid dreams may precede DLB as an early manifestation, and may persist, sometimes in attenuated form. Daytime drowsiness and unsteadiness may occur. The frequent occurrence of EEG abnormalities in DLB with transient temporal slow waves has prompted the use of carbamazepine and sodium valproate, but no systematic reports of efficacy or side-effects are available. The

5-HT$_3$ antagonist ondansetron was reported as having antipsychotic effects in hallucinated PD patients, but this has not been independently replicated and the high doses required make the cost prohibitive for routine practice (Harrison and McKeith, 1995). Up to 30% of DLB patients have significant depressive symptoms, although these can be hard to assess because of coexistent cognitive dysfunction and parkinsonism. A trial of antidepressant medication is warranted for persistent or severe depressive states. Conventional tricyclics with anticholinergic side-effects should be avoided, and one of the newer classes of agents should be used. No trial data exist in this population.

Trial designs and regulatory issues

Regulatory issues

There are no treatments currently licensed for DLB (McKeith et al, 2004a). As a consequence, all prescribing to this group of patients is essentially 'off-licence'. This situation has always been the norm in dementia care, but the recent licensing of drugs for treating AD has paradoxically highlighted the lack of recommended treatments for other dementia types, including DLB. In addition to the medicolegal and liability issues that this can pose for prescribers, healthcare providers may be reluctant to reimburse drug costs for DLB patients receiving for example, ChEIs.

Regulatory authorities seem to be prepared to accept DLB as an indication for regulatory approval on condition that (a) its existence is widely accepted by the field of experts, (b) it can be operationally defined by reliable and valid criteria and (c) outcomes for studies use validated and standardized outcome measures. The US Food and Drug Administration (FDA) has considered DLB as an indication, and has initially suggested that there be dual primary outcomes – namely global and a specified measure of cognition. Large-scale randomized placebo-controlled trials need to be presented to the regulators, but at the time of writing none are in progress.

Trial designs and outcome measures

Few DLB treatment trials have been reported, partly because it is still a relatively 'new' disorder, and partly because of restricted expertise in clinical diagnosis. The current approach is to address DLB and PDD studies separately, but the close relationship of these disorders and the logistics of recruitment may provide the opportunity for both patient populations to enter into a single clinical trial with a harmonized set of entry criteria. Post hoc subanalysis might be used to examine for differential responses. Cognitive outcome measures from AD clinical trials, which are predominantly memory-based, need not necessarily be used in DLB studies, and more appropriate instruments should be considered. The acceptability of a primary behavioral outcome measure in DLB clinical trials has not yet been clarified. Potential confounding factors for global and functional scales in DLB include the additional disabilities arising from motor disability and for all outcome measures, the inherent fluctuations of the untreated illness. Specific measures of attention and cognitive fluctuation, which are both part of the clinical profile of DLB/PDD, have been shown to be sensitive to response to treatment intervention. Other key domains of executive functioning, visual perception and memory systems must also be measured. The most important neuropsychiatric target symptoms include visual hallucinations, delusions, delusional misidentification, apathy, anxiety and depression. The desired behavioral outcomes might be reductions in both the intensity and frequency of these key behavioral symptoms. Functional and global assessments will be influenced by the presence of parkinsonism. Scales measuring extrapyramidal motor function can be modified to account for the confounding effects of cognitive impairment on motor performance (Ballard et al, 1997).

In view of the limited number of randomized controlled trials in either DLB or PDD, it is considered that the use of placebos is still ethical, noting, however, that ChEIs are already in widespread use in some countries.

Conclusions

ChEIs offer the greatest hope for symptomatic improvement in both psychotic and cognitive features of DLB and seem to offer these benefits without significant compromise of motor function. Ongoing multicenter, double-blind, placebo-controlled studies will hopefully clarify these issues, while long-term studies are required to assess the duration of benefit. Neuroleptics may need to be used sparingly, particularly when other pharmacological and nonpharmacological approaches fail to prevent severe distress or injurious behavior to self or others. Clinicians should be vigilant for severe sensitivity reactions. Clonazepam may have a particular role to play in the management of sleep disorders, but the role of other sedatives and anticonvulsants is unproven. New generation antidepressants may be helpful for persistent depressive symptoms. Disease-modifying treatments are urgently required. Clinical trial data suggest that ChEIs may potentially slow disease progression in AD, and similar effects could be anticipated in DLB. Better understanding of the pathobiological processing of synuclein proteins could ultimately lead to the development of novel therapeutic interventions for DLB.

References

Aarsland D, Donepezil for cognitive impairment in Parkinson's disease: a randomised controlled study. J Neurol Neurosurg Psychiatry (2002) 73:354.

Aarsland D, Ballard C, Larsen JP et al, Marked neuroleptic sensitivity in dementia with Lewy bodies and Parkinson's disease. Nord J Psychiatry (2003a) 57:94.

Aarsland D, Hutchinson M, Larsen JP, Cognitive, psychiatric and motor response to galantamine in Parkinson's disease with dementia. Int J Geriatr Psychiatry (2003b) 18:937–41.

Aarsland D, Mosimann UP, McKeith IG, Role of cholinesterase inhibitors in Parkinson's disease and dementia with Lewy bodies. J Geriatr Psychiatry Neurol (2004) 17:164–71.

Ballard C, McKeith I, Burn D et al, The UPDRS scale as a means of identifying extra-pyramidal signs in patients suffering from dementia with Lewy bodies. Acta Neurol Scand (1997) 96: 366–71.

Barber R, Panikkar A, McKeith IG, Dementia with Lewy bodies: diagnosis and management. Int J Geriatr Psychiatry (2001) 16:S12–18.

Bhanji NH, Gauthier S, Dementia with Lewy bodies: preliminary observations on switching cholinesterase inhibitors. Int Psychogeriatrics (2003) 15(Suppl 2):179.

Boeve B, Silber M, Ferman T et al, Association of REM sleep behavior disorder and neurodegenerative disease may reflect an underlying synucleinopathy. Mov Disord (2001) 16:622–30.

Burke WJ, Pfeiffer RF, McComb RD, Neuroleptic sensitivity to clozapine in dementia with Lewy bodies. J Neuropsychiatry Clin Neurosci (1998) 10:227–9.

Burn DJ, McKeith IG, Current treatment of dementia with Lewy bodies and dementia associated with Parkinson's disease. Mov Disord (2003) 18:S72–9.

Del Ser T, McKeith I, Anand R et al, Dementia with Lewy bodies: findings from an international multicentre study. Int J Geriatr Psychiatry (2000) 15:1034–45.

Duda JE, Giasson BI, Mabon ME et al, Novel antibodies to synuclein show abundant striatal pathology in Lewy body diseases. Ann Neurol (2002) 52:205–10.

Edwards KR Hersey L, Wray L et al, Efficacy and safety of galantamine in patients with dementia with Lewy bodies: a 12–week interim analysis. Dement Geriatr Cogn Disord (2004) 17(S1):40–8.

Grace J, Ballard C, McKeith IG, Neuroleptic sensitivity in dementia with Lewy bodies (DLB) and Alzheimer's disease (AD). In: Proceedings of 5th International Geneva/Springfield Symposium on Advances in Alzheimer Therapy (1998) 144.

Grace J, Daniel S, Stevens T et al, Long-term use of rivastigmine in patients with dementia with Lewy bodies: an open-label trial. Int Psychogeriatrics (2001) 13:199–205.

Harrison RH, McKeith IG, Senile dementia of Lewy body type – a review of clinical and pathological features: implications for treatment. Int J Geriatr Psychiatry (1995) 10:919–26.

Hutchinson M, Fazzini E, Cholinesterase inhibitors in Parkinson's disease. J Neurol Neurosurg Psychiatry (1996) 61:324–5.

Kaufer DI, Catt KE, Lopez OL, DeKosky ST, Dementia with Lewy bodies: response of delirium-like features to donepezil. Neurology (1998) 51:1512.

McKeith I, Fairbairn A, Perry R et al, Neuroleptic sensitivity in patients with senile dementia of Lewy body type. BMJ (1992) 305:673–8.

McKeith IG, Galasko D, Wilcock GK, Byrne EJ, Lewy body dementia – diagnosis and treatment. Br J Psychiatry (1995) 167:709–17.

McKeith IG, Galasko D, Kosaka K et al, Consensus guidelines for the clinical and patho-logic diagnosis of dementia with Lewy bodies (DLB): report of the Consortium on DLB International Workshop. Neurology (1996) 47:1113–24.

McKeith I, Del-Ser T, Spano PF et al, Efficacy of rivastigmine in dementia with Lewy bodies: a randomised, double-blind, placebo-controlled international study. Lancet (2000a) 356:2031–6.

McKeith IG, Grace JB, Walker Z et al, Rivastigmine in the treatment of dementia with Lewy bodies: Preliminary findings from an open trial. Int J Geriatr Psychiatry (2000b) 15:387–92.

McKeith I, Mintzer J, Aarsland D et al, Dementia with Lewy bodies. Lancet Neurol (2004a) 3:19–28.

McKeith IG, Wesnes KA, Perry E, Ferrara R. Hallucinations predict attentional improve-ments with rivastigmine in dementia with Lewy bodies. Dement Geriatr Cogn Disord (2004b)18:94–100.

Maclean LE, Collins CC, Byrne EJ, Dementia with Lewy bodies treated with rivastigmine: effects on cognition, neuropsychiatric symptoms, and sleep. Int Psychogeriatr (2001) 13:277–88.

Minett TSC, Thomas A, Wilkinson LM et al, What happens when donepezil is suddenly withdrawn? An open label trial in dementia with Lewy bodies and Parkinson's disease with dementia. Int J Geriatr Psychiatry (2003) 18:988–93.

O'Brien KK, Saxby BK, Ballard CG et al, Regulation of attention and response to therapy in dementia by butyrylcholinesterase. Pharmacogenetics (2003) 13:231–9.

Perry EK, Marshall E, Kerwin J et al, Evidence of a monoaminergic-cholinergic imbal-ance related to visual hallucinations in Lewy body dementia. J Neurochem (1990) 55:1454–6.

Reading PJ, Luce AK, McKeith IG, Rivastigmine in the treatment of parkinsonian psychosis and cognitive impairment. Mov Disord (2001) 16:1171–4.

Samuel W, Caligiuri M, Galakso D et al, Better cognitive and psychopathologic response to donepezil in patients prospectively diagnosed as dementia with Lewy bodies: a preliminary study. Int J Geriatr Psychiatry (2000) 15:794–802.

Shea C, MacKnight C, Rockwood K, Donepezil for treatment of dementia with Lewy bodies: a case series of nine patients. Int Psychogeriatr (1998) 10:229–38.

Thomas AJ, Burn DJ, Rowan E et al, Efficacy of donepezil in Parkinson's disease with dementia and dementia with Lewy bodies. Int J Geriatr Psychiatry (2005) in press.

Wesnes KA, McKeith IG, Ferrara R et al, Effects of rivastigmine on cognitive function in dementia with Lewy bodies: a randomised placebo-controlled international study using the Cognitive Drug Research computerised assessment system. Dement Geriatr Cogn Disord (2002) 13:183–92.

chapter 15

Nonpharmacological approaches to the care of dementia with Lewy bodies

Jiska Cohen-Mansfield

Introduction

Nonpharmacological approaches to the care of people with dementia include a range of theoretical orientations and methodologies. Unlike pharmacological approaches, where the focus of treatment is on the diseased individual, nonpharmacological interventions focus treatment on the interactions between a person and the environment. While specific goals of treatment can also differ between the two approaches, both can be used to improve function or decrease behavioral problems. Nonpharmacological interventions have been used specifically to enhance cognition, affect and Activities of Daily Living (ADL) performance, to reinforce a positive sense of self, and to reduce agitation/behavioral problems and psychotic symptoms. Other targets have included decreasing the burden on caregivers or promoting independence. When examining which of these goals is worthwhile for a specific person in a specific situation, the importance of overarching goals, such as maximizing quality of life, needs to be examined. Before embarking on any treatment, the decision maker(s) need to clarify answers to such questions as: Who needs to be treated? Whose problem is being treated? Whose reality is being considered? Whose needs and preferences take precedence? Answers to these questions will determine the ultimate goal, which will then dictate the specific nonpharmacological method(s) to be used.

In contrast to pharmacological approaches that try to treat problems through interventions directed at the patient, the nonpharmacological approach views the treatment in a systems context, in which the 'problem' is caused by a failure in the interaction between patient, caregiver, environment and the current system. The system can include the finances of care/reimbursement, the regulatory system, or the institution's administration, management and care style, and other policies. The caregiver can be a formal caregiver, such as a nursing assistant, or an informal caregiver, such as a relative, who has a specific style and knowledge base regarding care. The environment refers to the physical environment in which care is provided, and includes attributes such as safety, privacy, homelike qualities, etc. In addition, another environmental attribute is the availability of resources for the patient or caregiver. Examples include the presence of an enclosed, safe outdoor area, the availability of stimuli for the patient to manipulate, the availability of large, soft towels for bathing, or the provision of hearing aids for a hearing-impaired person.

In targeting the system, caregiver or environment for intervention, the nonpharmacological approach imparts a greater significance to the patient's point of view. First, understanding this point of view forms an important stage in the determination of treatment. Second, patients' habits or preferences are given precedence over those of the environment, thereby making the social and physical environment the target of change. Under such a scenario, it is the institution that may need to change meal times, for example, rather than expect residents to get up in time for a meal that fits the institutional schedule. Similarly, if a patient has a hallucination that does not cause discomfort or harm to himself or others, this would then be accepted as the reality for that patient, and changing the hallucination would not be considered a treatment goal.

The areas of life in which interventions are needed can be divided into those whose decline is associated with the dementia process, including loss of memory, loss of ability to perform activities of daily living, and manifestation of behavioral problems or agitation. There are also specific areas that are unique to dementia with Lewy bodies (DLB), including fluctuations in cognition, fluctuations in communication, rigidity, and an increased incidence of hallucinations and delusions.

Before describing nonpharmacological approaches to each of these challenges, we need to acknowledge that no information has been found in the literature about nonpharmacological treatment of DLB. This chapter will therefore be based largely on extrapolation from other work in dementia that deals with nonpharmacological treatments.

Table 15.1 demonstrates the breadth of treatments that can be used for disruptive behaviors in dementia by listing specific interventions, sorted by general approaches and goals, into a 'nonpharmacological toolkit'. An overview of the theoretical approaches underlying nonpharmacological interventions and the specific treatments involved is available in Cohen-Mansfield (2004) and Kasl-Godley and Gatz (2000). Even within the more thoroughly investigated arena of nonpharmacological interventions in dementia in general (in contrast to DLB specifically), most of these interventions have shown promise but have not yet been proven conclusively to be efficacious (for a review of interventions for behavioral problems, see Cohen-Mansfield, 2001; Opie et al, 1999). Furthermore, the parameters of efficacy themselves have not yet been clarified. The main question should not be whether a treatment is helpful in dementia, but for whom is the intervention helpful, i.e., for what specific problem and within which context would an intervention be helpful. It becomes crucial to know the characteristics of the person, such as cognitive, functional, sensory and other characteristics that would make the patient likely to benefit from any specific treatment.

Basics of nonpharmacological interventions: caregiver education, communication training and a favorable practice style

While the hallmark of dementia is cognitive decline, DLB is associated in particular with fluctuating levels of cognitive and communicative ability. The most important nonpharmacological intervention at this point is the provision of information about the manifestations of dementia in general, and about the unique features of DLB in particular. This will enhance the caregiver's understanding of the disease, so that when symptoms such as rigidity or fluctuations in cognition occur, they are not attributed to the patient's resistance, malicious intent or indifference. Furthermore, a caregiver who is knowledgeable about the manifestations of DLB is likely to become less alarmed and helpless than a caregiver who is confronting new symptoms with no preparation. Thus, the educated caregiver is likely to experience less burden and to react to new symptoms more appropriately than one with no prior awareness of the disease process. Ongoing caregiver support that offers

Table 15.1 The nonpharmacological tool kit: examples of types of interventions

Cognitive	Self-affirming	Functional	Social	Behavioral	Sensory	Structured activities	Environmental
Memory books	Reminiscence therapy	Enhanced communication	Pet therapy	Differential reinforcement	Therapeutic touch	Activity programs	Cues/signs to room, toilet
			Simulated			Exercise/walking	
Spaced retrieval	Validation therapy	Use of prompts: physical and/or verbal	presence therapy	Stimulus control	Massage	Outdoor walks	Homelike environment
					Music		
Cognitive remediation	Self-identity activities	Equipment/ Technology	Family videotapes		Aroma-therapy	Reinforcing activities	Optimize light/noise; reduce glare
Reality orientation	Use of objects that were meaningful in the past	Environmental intervention: e.g. cues, enhanced lighting	One-on-one interaction		Snoozelen	Arts/crafts	Provide access to secure walking area
Cognitive tasks (e.g. sorting) and games		Staffing and staff training	Small-group interactions and games		Providing hearing aids or glasses	Meaningful roles	Camouflage exits
Signs to improve orientation			Dolls				Alarm systems

Note: This is not a comprehensive list, but a list that provides examples of the types of available interventions. Note that some interventions may belong to several categories. For example, massage can be considered a sensory stimulation intervention, but can also be used for providing social contact, especially in late stages of dementia. Similarly, camouflaging exits is also a stimulus control intervention. All the interventions could potentially be useful for decreasing problem behaviors under the appropriate circumstances. © Cohen-Mansfield, 2003.

continuous opportunities to seek advice has been shown to help caregivers and postpone the institutionalization of persons with dementia (Mittleman et al, 1993).

A second nonpharmacological intervention that needs to be universally implemented is communication training. With advanced dementia, the patient's ability to communicate declines, yet that communication ability is crucial for maintaining quality of life and for understanding the patient's perspective. Communication techniques can help in this regard. Caregivers need to learn to observe, listen, talk and ask questions, and offer alternatives in ways that will maximize the patient's ability to receive and transmit information. Communication training for caregivers of persons with dementia includes elements pertaining to the environmental aspects of communication, the content of communication, the phrasing of communication, and the understanding of nonverbal or confused verbal communication. Examples of environmental aspects involve approaching slowly so as not to frighten the person with dementia, getting to the person's eye level and making eye contact. In terms of content, it is often useful to address only aspects of communication that can be understood by the patient – such that if a person has lost his or her sense of time, asking about a preferred time would be useless. Also, phrasing sentences in a short and clear way, and asking questions in a simple (preferably yes/no) format can be helpful. Finally, paying attention to the words uttered by the person with dementia, even if the sentence does not make sense, is crucial, because the intent of the message may be embedded in those words. Most essential is not to ignore, discount or negate the verbalizations of the patient, but rather to accept these and try to work to improve the situation from that person's perspective.

To maximize the effects of any nonpharmacological intervention, the intervener, therapist or caregiver needs to approach caregiving with a style that is conducive to understanding the patient's perspective and maximizing his or her quality of life. This requires, in addition to observation and communication skills, respect for the patient as a person, empathy, willingness to enhance patient autonomy, flexibility in addressing both care and environmental issues, and compassion towards the patient.

Behavioral problems/agitation

A large number of the interventions enumerated in Table 15.1 have been used in studies to decrease behavioral problems or agitation in persons with dementia (Cohen-Mansfield, 2001). The interventions are based on several different conceptualizations of the etiology of behavioral problems. For example, behavioral theory posits that inappropriate behavior may be reinforced by consequences such as attention. Treatment in this case would therefore involve altering contingencies so that attention is provided when the behavioral problem is not manifested, rather than having it follow an occurrence of the problem behavior. Theories that focus on the low stress threshold of persons with dementia advocate the development of low-stimulation environments. The unmet needs theory holds that there is a mismatch between the person's needs based on his or her physical and psychological condition, lifelong habits, preferences, and identity, and the way in which the current physical and psychological environment addresses these needs. The TREA (Treatment Routes for Exploring Agitation) approach involves a series of steps to clarify what the unmet need is, and to choose a treatment that addresses the need in a way that takes cognitive, sensory, functional and psychological attributes of the individual into account. (A more detailed description of the different theoretical approaches and the TREA interventions can be found in Cohen-Mansfield (2000a,b).) The needs underlying agitated behaviors are correlated with their manifestations. Specifically, verbal/vocal agitation (e.g. screaming or repeated requests for help) is more likely to be related to physical pain, discomfort, loneliness and depressed affect. Alternately, physical nonaggressive or restless agitation (e.g. wandering or inappropriately handling objects) is often related to a need for activity and stimulation, while aggressive behaviors tend to occur most often during ADL, and are associated with the person with dementia trying to avoid discomfort or with invasion of the patient's personal space by another person. The wide variety of treatment options illustrated in Table 15.1 allows for the choice of an intervention that addresses the unmet need and also matches the sensory, cognitive and personal characteristics of the patient.

We have had the opportunity to study two persons with DLB who participated in our large study of nonpharmacological interventions for behavioral problems in dementia (Cohen-Mansfield et al, in review). The first, Mrs A, is a 74-year-old woman who smiles occasionally and speaks so softly that it is very difficult to hear her. She had a Mini-Mental State Examination (MMSE) score of 5. She was identified as agitated by the nursing staff because of grabbing things when there was nothing there, handling things inappropriately and pulling on a lap restraint. Systematic observations, which were obtained using the Agitation Behavior Mapping Instrument (Cohen-Mansfield et al,

1989), showed that her physical agitation occurred mostly in the activity room, when the radio or television was on and she was not involved in any activities. Based on the type of agitated behaviors that she displayed and the context in which they occurred, we hypothesized that Mrs A was suffering from insufficient stimulation for her cognitive level. In order to select an intervention, we checked that her hearing and vision were adequate and assessed her sense of identity and preferences with a self-identity question-naire (Cohen-Mansfield et al, 2000) administered to a relative. Results of the self-identity questionnaire revealed that Mrs A had been a homemaker and took care of her children, and that the relationship with her children was the most important one in her life. Her selflessness and sacrifice were personal attributes of which she was the most proud. Based on her love of family and taking care of others, we offered her a baby doll and family pictures as inter-ventions. We also tried to accommodate her restless behaviors by providing more acceptable stimuli to handle, namely, an activity apron and a soft toy. Her responses to the different treatments were varied. She loved the baby doll, kissing it and caressing its hair while holding and talking to it. She often did not want to return the doll. In contrast, she looked at the family pictures only briefly. She responded well to the two stimuli that were introduced to accom-modate her agitated behavior. She showed interest in the activity apron and handled the different objects attached to it, and she had a very dramatic response to the soft toy. A research assistant approached her at a time when she was agitated – in this case she was pulling on her lap restraint and sweat-ing. When given a soft toy caterpillar, she squeezed it, and a few minutes later she was totally calm and relaxed. While providing the interventions, the research assistants noticed that her hands were often very cold. For this rea-son, we provided her with a warm water bag to hold, and she enjoyed this as well. Mrs A was responsive to the interventions, with observations showing that she paid attention to the stimuli provided and had a positive attitude towards these. Her restless behaviors decreased dramatically during the interventions, in the absence of any changes in her medications.

In reviewing the interventions for Mrs. A, several points should be highlighted.

- *Use of physical restraints.* Mrs A was restrained, and physical restraints have been shown to be associated with agitation (Werner et al, 1989). Therefore, whenever an agitated person is restrained, the removal of restraints needs to be the first line of intervention. This intervention is sometimes met with staff and institutional resistance. In this case, for example, one of the research assistants spoke with the staff about removal of the restraint, but was told that Mrs A would fall out of her chair if it were removed, and refused to remove it.

- *The need for multiple interventions.* Several different interventions need to be tried in order to find the most appropriate intervention for any given person, as some may not work for various reasons. For instance, Mrs A may not have remembered the family as seen in the pictures provided, or the pictures may not have provided sufficiently engaging stimulation – perhaps because just looking at pictures is a mostly passive activity. For some people, it is possible to use the pictures as part of preparing an album, or to start a discussion about family members, either of which is a more engaging activity. Additionally, given that restless agitation can continue for a significant amount of time, having multiple interventions is helpful to caregivers. For this reason, those providing or instructing about nonpharmacological interventions need to become familiar with most of the techniques exemplified in Table 15.1 as well as other nonpharmacological interventions.
- *Using dolls as interventions.* The use of dolls has been a controversial intervention because it is sometimes considered to be infantilizing the older person. Despite this reservation, we have found that from the older person's (mostly woman's) perspective, a doll can provide an activity that is meaningful beyond that of most other stimuli. The doll can be both an object to love (and possibly to feel loved by), especially in the nursing home environment when there is little other love available, and it provides a meaningful activity in that the resident can provide care for it. Obviously, other meaningful activities can be tried (e.g. cooking, setting a table or folding towels) that may be more age-appropriate. It is difficult to estimate the responsiveness to such activities without an actual trial, but generally these seem to require more advanced cognition and dexterity than loving a doll.
- *Cost.* Finally, most of the interventions provided in this example cost little in terms of materials or staff time.

The second person, Mr B, is an 86-year old man with a diagnosis of DLB and a MMSE score of 10, who was described by the nursing staff as being agitated. He presented with physical agitation, including aimless wandering, inappropriate disrobing or dressing, pacing (in his wheelchair), and wanting to get out of the chair or out of the lap belt. In addition, Mr B would ask for help continuously, often to go to the bathroom when it was not in fact necessary (according to the nursing staff). Like Mrs A, he seemed to lack appropriate stimulation, but had a higher level of cognitive ability and a different personal background. Mr B had held a high administrative role in a company, he enjoyed the outdoors, fishing and boating, and his relationship with his wife was the most important relationship throughout his life. During the treatment period, the lap belt was changed to a 'fall sensor', consisting of a thin cord that clipped to the back of his shirt and was attached to an alarm box on the back of his wheelchair. While this device did not hinder him, an alarm would go off if it were to be dislodged. Interventions that engaged him included pictures of a vacation in Yellowstone National Park that he enjoyed looking at, talking about his outdoor experiences, and a Hawaii travel video with which he got so engaged that he watched it intently without any signs of restlessness. He talked about his trip to Hawaii, and about how he had enjoyed the scenery and the water.

Three aspects of the interventions seemed to be important for Mr B. The first was the ability to move freely, which was accommodated by the removal of the lap restraint in favor of the fall sensor. The second was the connection with his past identity, which was addressed with the stimuli related to outdoor leisure. Finally, he had a need to be engaged interpersonally, which was manifested by his interest in playing card games repeatedly with a research assistant, and in discussing the outdoor leisure stimuli. In contrast to Mrs A, stimuli that only addressed the ability to manipulate objects, such as a stress ball or woodworking equipment, did not hold his attention to the same extent.

These two cases underscore the importance of understanding both the needs and the personal attributes of the resident when tailoring interventions for inappropriate behaviors.

Psychotic symptoms: hallucinations and delusions

When addressing psychotic symptoms, the clinician first needs to ask several questions: Do these symptoms present real psychosis? What are the consequences of the symptoms to the patient and to caregivers? What are possible reasons for the symptoms? Each of these queries is briefly reviewed in the following.

Do these symptoms present real psychosis?

Smith (2000) describes an elderly nursing home resident referred for acute psychotic symptoms, in which she complained that people in the ceiling were talking to her. During a visit to this resident's room, the physician noticed the frequent announcements through the loudspeaker system and realized that, because of her hearing difficulties, she misinterpreted announcements to 'Hall C' as announcements to 'Elsie' – her name. Once the intercom system was turned off in her room, those delusions ceased. Similarly, Tune (2003) describes a resident who developed delusions that Monica Lewinsky was bothering her, which disappeared when the TV was turned off. These are examples of misinterpretations of real stimuli that are caused by a combination of sensory and cognitive deficits. Stimuli reflected in mirrors and windows often lead to such misinterpretations. An unanticipated approach of a person, such as a staff member coming into the room to provide assistance with an ADL, can also provoke fear and, consequently, lead to the resident misinterpreting the identity or the motives of the person. Nonpharmacological treatment in these cases is straightforward, and involves clarifying the stimulus that is being misinterpreted as well as the reason for misinterpretation, and then changing the stimulus or the manner in which the stimulus emerges.

What are the consequences of the symptoms to the patient and to caregivers?

It is not unusual for persons with dementia to have hallucinations that seem to be pleasing to them. Some people talk with seemingly familiar but currently non-existent persons for long periods of time. These examples illustrate the importance of clarifying the overarching goal of care. Most often, if this is to enhance the quality of life of the person with dementia, other possible goals, such as helping the person perceive reality, become of secondary importance or lose their importance altogether. Consequently, if the person seems to enjoy his or her hallucinations and does not suffer any ill effects from these, a possible course may be to explain this situation to caregivers in a manner that will make the practice acceptable to them.

What are possible reasons for the symptoms?

Hallucinations have been shown repeatedly to correlate with visual problems (Cohen-Mansfield et al, 1998; Holroyd, 1998; Chapman et al, 1999; Forsell, 2000), and may be linked to sensory deprivation (Zubek et al, 1961; Holroyd and Sheldon-Keller, 1996). Therefore, medical examination and treatment of eye disease should be considered the first line of intervention. Alternative sensory stimulation, such as music, massage and aromatherapy, could also be tried. As mentioned above, many delusions are misinterpretations of actual events or stimuli in the environment. Delusions need to be analyzed with that in mind. For example, the nursing home resident who complains repeatedly that objects are stolen may either be describing a true reality (as theft is not uncommon in nursing homes) or forgetting where she has placed her personal belongings and interpreting her inability to find them as a confabulation of theft. A number of potential solutions can be offered for residents, including marking personal belongings in clear ways so that they are easily identifiable, attaching a finder (see http://www.keyringer.com/) device to a personal belonging, or purchasing multiple inexpensive copies of personal articles so that they can easily be replaced when necessary. Delusions can also result from a delirium associated with acute medical conditions that should be addressed. A more detailed analysis of a nonpharmacological approach to psychotic symptoms can be found in Cohen-Mansfield (2003).

Activities of daily living

The ability to perform ADL deteriorates in all forms of dementia. This poses a major burden to patients and their caregivers. Nonpharmacological interventions include communication training on approaching a person, requesting permission to perform an ADL task, announcing the task before starting it, responding to complaints and verbal abuse, engaging the person in the task or in conversation during the task, calming a person, etc. Both verbal and physical prompts are essential components of helping a person engage in ADL. A verbal prompt may involve asking the person to engage in the next subtask of an activity. A physical prompt may include modeling the activity, starting the activity for the person, or providing a trigger, such as spreading the clothes on the bed to remind the person to dress (Namazi and Johnson, 1992). For further discussion of nonpharmacological approaches to ADL, see Beck et al. (1997). Environmental interventions are also crucial for optimizing performance of ADL, in that they adjust the surroundings, including physical access, temperature, color, furniture or wall design, to facilitate the activity for both patient and caregiver.

ADL are very private activities that are normally conducted by each person for him or herself. Providing this care for another adult requires a high degree of respect and attention to the comfort of the other person. The methodology for providing ADL with dignity is yet to be definitively established, but some gains have been made. Procedures for bathing, for example, based on work by Sloane et al (1995), are presented in a video (Barrick et al, 2003). Technological innovations may also help with some ADL, such as the use of wash-and-dry toilets for toileting (Cohen-Mansfield and Biddison, in press), the use of various nonrinse products for bathing (see http://www.bathingwithoutabattle.unc.edu/main_page.html), or improved equipment to warm the bathroom to avoid patients being cold before or after bathing. Finally, in order to optimize nonpharmacological interventions in general, and ADL care in particular, it is also crucial to pay attention to the demands on the caregiver. Some tasks require more than one caregiver, while others require technology or modifications in environmental design to spare caregivers from discomfort or injuries, which are extremely common (Cohen-Mansfield et al, 1996).

Cognitive decline and fluctuations

The extent to which cognitive interventions (see Table 15.1 for examples) may be helpful is unknown, but, generally, in the early stages of the disease, maintaining lifelong habits that have been overlearned through long-term practice can be beneficial. Similarly, employing reminders, such as lists or alarms, can be useful. If the person forgets to use the list or to attend to the alarms, then spaced retrieval (Camp et al, 2002), in which small amounts of information are rehearsed consistently with a growing time lag between rehearsals, can be utilized to help the person employ the memory aids. In later stages of dementia, memory books (Bourgeois et al, 2001) can assist with communication. Technology, such as the use of electronic memory aids or environmental sensors (Cohen-Mansfield et al., in press; and see http://rehab-www.eng.cam.ac.uk/cwuaat/02/20.pdf) are expected to play increasingly greater roles in the future as prostheses for cognitive losses.

Understanding the role of nonpharmacological interventions for persons with DLB is obviously in its infancy. Data are needed concerning the prevalence of different types of caregiving challenges that require intervention, and the extent to which these differ from those in other types of dementia. Research needs to examine the etiologies of these problems and the efficacy of different nonpharmacological approaches for improving care and enhancing quality of life. Findings of this research would then need to be translated into practice, and investigations into how best to train or mentor caregivers in employing these interventions would be required. Finally, cost analyses and investigation of reimbursement structures for nonpharmacological interventions are needed.

References

Barrick AL, Rader J, Sloane P, Bathing without a battle. Video designed by Eo Studios (University of North Carolina at Chapel Hill, 2003).

Beck CK, Heacock P, Mercer SO et al, Improving dressing behavior in cognitively impaired nursing home residents. Nurs Res (1997) 46:126–32.

Bourgeois M, Dijkstra K, Burgio L et al, Memory aids as an augmentative and alternative communication strategy for nursing home residents with dementia. Augment Altern Commun (2001) 17:196–210.

Camp CJ, Cohen-Mansfield J, Capezuti EA, Use of nonpharmacologic interventions among nursing home residents with dementia. Psychiatric Serv (2002) 53: 1397–1401.

Chapman FM, Dickinson J, McKeith I, Ballard C, Association among visual hallucinations, visual acuity, and specific eye pathologies in Alzheimer's disease: Treatment implications. Am J Psychiatry (1999) 156:1983–5.

Cohen-Mansfield J, Theoretical frameworks for behavioral problems in dementia. Alzheimer's Care Q (2000a) 1:8–21.

Cohen-Mansfield J, Nonpharmacological management of behavioral problems in persons with dementia: The TREA model. Alzheimer's Care Q (2000b) 1:22–34.

Cohen-Mansfield J, Nonpharmacologic interventions for psychotic symptoms in dementia. J Geriatr Psychiatry Neurol (2003) 16:219–24.

Cohen-Mansfield J, Cognitive and behavioral interventions for persons with dementia. In: Encyclopedia of Applied Psychology Vol 1., Elsevier Inc.; 2004; 377–85.

Cohen-Mansfield J, Biddison J, The potential of 'wash and dry' toilets to improve in toileting care in elderly nursing home residents. Gerontologist (in press).

Cohen-Mansfield J, Werner P, Marx M, An observational study of agitation in agitated nursing home residents. Intern Psychogeriatr (1989) 1:153–65.

Cohen-Mansfield J, Culpepper J, Carter P, Back injuries to nursing staff in long term care facilities. AAOHN (1996) 44:9–17.

Cohen-Mansfield J, Taylor L, Werner P, Delusions and hallucinations in an adult day care population: a longitudinal study. Am J Geriatr Psychiatry (1998) 6:104–21.

Cohen-Mansfield J, Golander H, Arnheim G, Self-identity in older persons suffering from dementia: preliminary results. Soc Sci Med (2000) 51:381–94.

Cohen-Mansfield J, Creedon MA, Kilpatrick MJ, Malone TB, Electronic memory aids for community dwelling elderly persons: attitudes, preferences, and potential utilization J Appl Gerontol (2005) 24: 3–20.

Cohen-Mansfield J, Libin A, Marx MS, The efficacy of non-pharmacological treatment of agitation using a systematic individualized approach (Treatment Routes for Exploring Agitation – TREA) (in review).

Forsell Y, Predictors for depression, anxiety and psychotic symptoms in a very elderly population: data from a 3-year follow-up study. Soc Psychiatry Psychiatr Epidemiol (2001) 35:259–63.

Holroyd S, Hallucinations and delusions in Alzheimer's disease. In Vellas BJ, Fitten J, Frisconi G, eds, Research and Practice in Alzheimer's Disease: Intervention in Gerontology (Serdi Publishing: Paris, 1998) 213–22.

Holroyd S, Sheldon-Keller A, A study of visual hallucinations in Alzheimer's disease. Am J Geriatr Psychiatry (1996) 3:198–205.

Kasl-Godley J, Gatz M, Psychosocial interventions for individuals with dementia: an integration of theory, therapy, and a clinical understanding of dementia. Clin Psychol Rev (2000) 20:755–82.

Mittelman M, Ferris S, Steinberg G et al, An intervention that delays institutionalization of Alzheimer's disease patients: treatment of spouse-caregivers. Gerontologist (1993) 33:730–40.

Namazi KH, Johnson BD, Dressing independently: a closet modification model for Alzheimer's disease patients. Am J Alzheimer's Care Rel Disord Res (1992) 7:22–8.

Opie J, Rosewarne R, O'Connor D, The efficacy of psychosocial approaches to behaviour disorders in dementia: a systematic literature review. Aust NZ J Psychiatry (1999) 33:789–99.

Sloane P, Rader J, Barrick A et al, Bathing persons with dementia. Gerontologist (1995) 35:672–8.

Smith DA, Elsie's hallucination. Ann Long-Term Care (2000) 8:68.

Tune L, Dementia management: regulations, rules, and research. J Am Med Directors' Assoc (2003) July/August, Supplement: H13–16.

Werner P, Cohen-Mansfield J, Braun J, Marx MS, Physical restraints and agitation in nursing home residents. J Am Geriatr Soc (1989) 37:1122–6.

Zubek JP, Pushkar D, Sansom W, Gowing J, Perceptual changes after prolonged sensory isolation (darkness and silence). Can J Psychol (1961) 15:83–100.

chapter 16

Dementia with Lewy bodies – a carer's view

Meg Wilkes

Introduction

This is a brief account of my experience of caring for my husband who has dementia with Lewy bodies (DLB).

I will give thumbnail sketches, describe the effects of his illness and give personal examples from the 'core conditions'. Although personal and written, in global terms, from the privileged position of a comfortable home in the UK, some of the experiences will be familiar to other carers.

A frequent cry from carers is 'no-one can understand how it is unless they've been there'. It must be equally true for those we care for. None of us has the full picture. I am sure that understanding and knowledge will grow if professional and informal carers are more honest with each other, more courageous, trusting each other's expertise.

DLB is a horrible illness. Anything we can do to be more effective will be worth the effort.

Then

In our student days, I fell in love with a lively, clever, creative, athletic, thoughtful, deeply spiritual, charming young man who had vision and great skills in communicating. He graduated from the University of Cambridge with a science degree, went on to ordination as a priest in the Church of England, and later became recognized as one of the Church's authorities in the field of education, holding nationally influential and responsible posts. We married in our 20s and had two children, trying hard to combine family care with a demanding working life.

Now

We are in our early 70s. My husband is in a nursing home in a Special Unit for Elderly Mentally Infirm patients, living as best he can with DLB. He has to be fed, washed, dressed and helped from bed to wheelchair. He sits slumped, like a puppet without strings. He is doubly incontinent. He is unable to read or write or to control the radio, TV or phone. He sleeps a lot and often keeps his eyes closed when he is awake. His speech is mostly incoherent and so quiet that few people can hear him. His attention span can be measured in seconds and rarely lasts a whole sentence. He seems unable to distinguish between his dreams, his waking thoughts and what is happening around him. My heart aches to see him like this.

When I arrive, he greets me briefly, often with a smile, though sometimes he doesn't know me. He usually has something to tell me. Recurring themes are meetings he thinks he is chairing, train journeys, visits to Ireland to meet the IRA . . . once, it was that one of us was dead but he didn't know which. Among the most heartbreaking was when he greeted me in tears of joy after hearing a programme about stem cell research, declaring that he was cured. His news said, he turns his head away for the rest of the time I am with him. I long for some sign of affection, some reassurance that I am still special to him. Mostly, I have to be content that I am the one he takes for granted.

When visitors come, he usually responds for a few minutes, especially if they have connections with his work; at other times, he will resist or reject their approaches. His lifelong conversational skills can mask his lack of understanding. His habitual response, 'yes', means, ' yes', 'no' or, more often, 'I know that you have said something and I'm trying to fathom its meaning'. His descriptions of imaginary events can sound plausible.

Often, he is having auditory or visual hallucinations, unable to recognize or focus on objects in front of him, perhaps talking to our son or daughter, who are many miles away. He seems not to notice the unusual behavior of his fellow patients, though he is disturbed and easily distracted by noises, shouting out in response to someone else's conversation in the corridor. Now and then, he astonishes people by a sudden burst of energy and determination, getting up quickly and walking. This usually ends in a fall. I have come to associate these times with talk of trains and journeys, which symbolize escape for him.

There are fleeting, infrequent times when his thoughts are clearer. He might remark on events, perhaps asking after people we know or commenting on his care.

I am with him for several hours every other day, witnessing the relentless progress of the disease. I rejoice that he has excellent care and I grieve for the husband I knew.

Early signs

A few stumbles, a slight blurring of speech. My husband was stooped, slow, acting like an old man, though not yet 60. At home, he became increasingly tired and dull, with a grim expression; unresponsive, rarely making eye contact, seldom laughing, seldom talking, except about his work. He avoided making decisions, rarely initiated things. He had a disturbingly bad short-term memory and 'holes' in his concentration when he was apparently unable to grasp the meaning of things. He would repeat phrases back but not respond, no longer following the normal rules of conversation; hearing, but only with his ears. He did things by rote, often inappropriately. Once, he burst into tears after trying for half an hour to work out how to wire a three-pin plug.

At times, my husband followed me round like a puppy, as if needing my reassurance. He had strange, distorted ideas about our relationship, our hopes and our life together. It was all so unbelievable that I wrote down some of the things he was saying and checked with him that he meant them. I came across the scrap of paper recently and recognized signs of now-familiar delusion and paranoia. At the time, I was bewildered and distressed. We became caricatures of ourselves; my husband is a walk-away man, I am a talk-it-through person. What had once been a happy mix was painful exaggeration. We were becoming strangers. We kept up our public image, but home was a cheerless place.

I tried to share my worries but it was always the same – people dismissed them with 'explanations', hinted that I had unreasonable expectations. I questioned my perceptions. I questioned my worth as a wife.

When my husband's illness was diagnosed as atypical Parkinson's, he was afraid that he would be written off by friends and colleagues, so we kept it a secret for a couple of years. The medication helped him physically. When he did share his news, people judged his condition by their knowledge of Parkinson's and assumed that he was little affected, particularly as he showed none of the expected tremor.

At work, colleagues' apparent expectations put an enormous strain on him. It all became such an effort for him that he shrank his world to what he saw as the essentials. He tried so hard. In many ways, he succeeded. He pushed himself to the limit. He was probably unable to realize the demands he was making. It was a relief when he decided to take early retirement. It would have been a bitter blow for him to have continued until he was asked to stand down. It was a difficult and painful decision for him, as his work brought him into contact with interesting and stimulating people. It was his life, not just a job. He was scarcely aware of his declining ability and planned to write another book in his retirement. The book was never written.

How symptoms developed

Our diaries for the years following my husband's retirement show me that we continued to pursue our interests and play our part in the many activities of our friendly little town, that our youngest grandchild was born, that we went away for holidays, spent time with family and friends, planted some trees, went to the theater, to the swimming pool, to the dentist, that the dog and cats were wormed, that we changed the car . . . it all seems so normal, put like that.

Perhaps it even looked reasonably normal from the outside. It was far from normal.

My husband's Parkinson's symptoms were increasing. He managed to keep going, but every activity involved a supreme effort, and some habitual ones were now beyond him.

More disabling, though less obvious to other people, was his progressive mental impairment. He was unable to deal with builders, letters, tax forms and bills, to think ahead, to hold a normal conversation. We would talk in zigzags, as his responses were only vaguely near the target.

He still helped local clergy by taking familiar services for them, but read his old sermons.

There was one seemingly trivial change – whenever he went food shopping, he used only paper money, coming back with a purse overflowing with coins. It took me a long time to discover the reason. My assumption was that it was forgetfulness or his impaired dexterity (or, on a bad day, just to annoy!). None of those. It was because he couldn't work out the change. That shocked me and filled me with foreboding. I linked it with logic and reason. Loss of memory and loss of reasoning power are both devastating, the one perhaps ultimately due to the other, but for me the latter is the deeper wound. I experience it as a profound loss in my life's partner, one that has been difficult to acknowledge. Those years ago, before I knew what was to come, it was comparatively easy to accept that I had to write lists for him, even for two purchases. It had begun to seem quite normal until old friends came to stay and laughed when I did the same for them.

A few years into his illness, as well as avoiding eye contact, he told me he didn't like me touching him. Even holding hands as we walked or accidental contact indoors was unpleasant for him. I must just watch him if he fell, not try to help him up. He told me all this in a light, matter-of-fact way as though it was a trifling matter. It persisted for years, except for an occasional time when he denied it all and said I must be mentally ill to say such things. There were times when I felt the need of some comfort and asked him if he would give me a hug. He couldn't. I found it acutely painful. To me, touching is a way of expressing love. It felt like a punishment, banishment, an over-harsh reaction to my shortcomings.

My husband seemed to be cocooned, careless about his clothes, indifferent to his appearance, unaware of the impact he had on other people. That led to some surprises, for example reaching across a restaurant table to take food from a stranger's plate. Once, when we were having tea out, he went in search of the gents. Half an hour later, he returned, holding out his smeared and smelly hands for all to see. He had got lost, soiled himself on the way and had not washed in the toilet because there was someone else there. To him, coming back to the café seemed the right choice

At night, he would use the receptacles by the bed, then empty them onto the carpet. Sometimes he headed for the bathroom but ended up trying to get through the window.

Other difficulties, little things in themselves, but a taste of something bigger: he couldn't sort the cutlery into the drawer or papers into the filing cabinet, fold his clothes, measure a suitcase or tie a functional knot. He spent a whole morning trying to saw a piece of plywood to fit the catflap hole. He kept changing the dimensions of both, so never achieved his goal.

I had to be sure to pick up the post before him, or important letters would be taken to the study and lost or torn up and put in the dustbin. The answerphone baffled him and messages left with him were forgotten.

'Helping' me to get ready for our last holiday, he emptied his suitcase and repacked it with nothing but seven vests and some underpants.

Regularly, he turned the central heating off because he couldn't work out the function of the room thermostat. He cancelled or made duplicate appointments at Outpatients, turned the washing machine off mid-program whenever he went past it, wrote illegible reminder lists, addressed empty envelopes, cut buttons off his shirts when he couldn't undo them, had difficulty turning his clothes the right way out, trying to push the fabric instead of pulling . . . on and on.

He did some potentially dangerous things – shattered a glass dish by using it on the gas cooker, turned on an electric fire too near to furniture, took my medication. I couldn't relax for a moment.

He walked out of hospital in a snowstorm, without a coat, the day after he was sent for investigations following collapse and was missing for five hours.

At home, he would set off to do something, apparently forget before he got there, forget that he had forgotten, and later assure me that the job was done. The worst example of this was his once regular chore of keeping the rainwater drain from the roof free of debris; a tricky job he insisted on doing himself. Very soon after it was 'done', we had a heavy downpour in the middle of the night. Ceilings on the top floor collapsed, the water poured down the stairwell. As I clambered about on the flooded roof in nightie and wellies and my husband rested calmly in bed, I realized that in many ways I was now on my own. I raged to the night sky but resolved to survive. It was a dramatic moment, now a strengthening memory when things get hard. He did remember that he had 'forgotten' to do the job. I think it is more likely that he couldn't bring himself to admit that it was beyond him. Poor, dear, once vigorous and talented man. My deep and shameful regret is that he shared so few of his fears with me. Male friends have told me that he would have seen it as a matter of pride, of not wanting to worry me, wanting to go on being the supportive husband he wished to be. I shall never know.

The hidden element of DLB

From the beginning, the main difficulties in other people's recognition of his illness were:

1. Some of the changes were different only in degree and frequency, not in kind, from normal ones – poor memory, increasingly bad driving, weariness, 'absent-mindedness', fixed ideas.
2. Superficially, he retained his public self while losing his grasp on day-to-day living. He could seem all right during a short conversation, particularly to people who had not known him before he was ill. He was living a life of contrasts, as though inhabiting two worlds. 'On stage', he could, for

example, discuss current affairs with sufficient skill to seem his normal self to all but the most focused listener, while, behind the scenes, he was exhibiting bizarre behavior. It was different from fluctuating confusion, more like entirely different areas of consciousness. There was an element of the surreal about it.

For years, professional and lay people alike normalized his mental state and disregarded or rejected my attempts to alert them to the changes. Several times, they even told me that if what I was saying was true, I was the cause of it. It seemed as though my descriptions of his changing behavior were taken by clinicians as nothing more than criticism of their charming patient.

Core features and supportive symptoms

My husband's hallucinations are vivid, long-lasting and bizarre, sometimes disturbing, sometimes pulsating or oscillating, always detailed and clear. Examples are dead babies lined up on a bed, printed words on clean paper, bollards walking to and fro, pineapples swelling and shrinking, the center of a town in a field of sheep, a station at the bottom of the garden. I have not known him to recognize them as unreal.

At other times, he fails to see what is there, though his eyesight is good. He has peered behind me, looking for me, telling me that I am 'behind you somewhere', looked at photos or the TV and failed to make sense of the images. Optical illusions are taken at face value.

He has frequent delusions, some short-lived, some lasting for a year or more. Those about his work almost invariably involve praise for his contribution – poignant, seen in relation to his 'real' feelings of uselessness. He has told me that the care staff are killing him and I am in collusion with them. A friend found him in tears in church when I was away one weekend. He told her that I had died in the night. (The same friend who tried to persuade me to have more time off!). He was convinced for months that our son had AIDS.

A delusion about an imaginary letter lasted longer. He searched for it diligently, crawling on all fours round the edges of our sitting room, checking the cellar, accusing me of hiding it. He told a friend that he was going to get a builder in to remove the skirting boards in case it had slipped behind them.

Only once has he told me that he realized he had been deluded. He added that he was glad that I was still talking sense, because his world was all confused. That reinforced my belief that it is wrong to pretend to see or believe his fantasies. If I did that, what secure base could he rely on? It would be a bit like his piece of wood and the catflap. No constant.

He has told me that he goes along with people when they change the subject, to 'keep them sweet', but it frustrates him and leaves the delusion intact. I think that the best approach, which I don't always manage, is to explain that I am not experiencing the same things but to respond to his descriptions. Some seem to be metaphors. The obvious ones are his talk of prisons and journeys. One was about coins jangling in a mower, which turned out to be his way of expressing his lack of control over his life. That, sadly, is all too real. Some, only the two of us can understand.

My husband broke his hip a few years ago. That is a whole story in itself. It was pinned very satisfactorily but I think that the effects of the anesthetic never really cleared. He has frequent falls, some due to his poor balance, some from misjudging the distance to a chair, some due to his postural hypotension.

Transient loss of consciousness was a frequent problem at home. He would crumple to a heap after stepping out of the car, rising from a chair, walking up stairs or getting out of bed in the night. Neither reminders nor pleadings would stop him making sudden moves. I had noticed his uneven pulse rate, which may also have been a contributory factor. He was eventually given medication to control it.

Syncope was rare until a few months ago. He had two short episodes at home and another at the General Practitioner's surgery. The Nursing Home has reported several longer ones.

There are other changes:

- sudden severe sweats, unrelated to exercise or ambient temperature
- a craving for sugar and a voracious appetite, though loss of weight
- occasional increase in overnight urine output – up to 4 liters
- changed sleep patterns – thrashing about with arms and legs, talking and walking in his sleep; falling asleep suddenly during the day, often in the middle of a meal
- a lack of awareness of the position of his body

When he was still driving, he would slow down sometimes to 20 mph or less in an unrestricted zone on a clear road, without realizing it. At nearly every road junction, he tells me that I am going the wrong way. He has lost his sense of direction and his ability to read a map.

In recent years, my husband has needed a wheelchair. Until he became too ill, it gave us the freedom to go out and about together, but lifting the chair and small (but heavy) electric motor in and out of the car, helping my husband in and out of the car, in and out of the chair and attending to his needs was very hard work for me. Lack of public awareness added to the difficulties – cars are parked across ramps, drivers are impatient at road crossings, pedestrians expect wheelchair users to take avoiding action, swing doors crash into chair or carer. Some public toilets for disabled people are ill equipped and too small for a wheelchair user who needs help. Even inadequate ones are few and far between and often occupied by an able-bodied person. We used the chair in staid and sensible ways, but also struggled along rough footpaths, up hills to viewpoints and had picnics in the rain like 'normal' ramblers. It was worth all the effort, giving us some precious happy times together.

Medication

My husband has medication for his physical symptoms. We found that the best regime was to divide his tablets into appropriate doses six times a day. I was able to fine-tune them for him, cutting back when he showed signs of overdose, keeping him sufficiently mobile for what he wanted to do without affecting his mental condition too much. I am sad that a detailed response to his needs for medication is not possible in residential care.

At home, when he had been more active than usual, he would need an additional small dose of Sinemet (carbidopa/levodopa) to get him into the house or up to bed, as though the exercise 'used up' the drug more quickly. The experts have told me that theoretically this is not so. From daily observation for 12 years, it does seem to be.

Neuroleptics for DLB patients are of particular significance, but I am concerned about the criteria for the use of 'calming' drugs for patients with all types of dementia in care homes.

Gratitude

I am grateful to the editors of this book for including a contribution from a carer. I shall always be deeply grateful to our wonderful children and their families, to patient and supportive friends and to the life-enhancing therapists and clinicians whose help and expertise have allowed for my husband's individual needs, who have valued him, listened with imagination and worked with flexibility; who have not needed to be all-powerful and all-knowing.

I feel less warmth towards those who have offered unworkable textbook solutions to problems and directed their frustration towards me, telling me that I must be grateful and 'make an effort'. Wife/carers, by definition, will be near exhaustion, oversensitive and anxious. We already know that we are inadequate for our task. I know that we can be difficult and challenging, but it is a thin and fragile protection of our true feelings of anguished helplessness. We respond well to gentleness!

Guilt

I feel an unreal, illogical guilt that I was not able to keep my husband well for his children and grandchildren. I begin to understand the phrase 'survivor's guilt'. My husband is locked in a diseased body. Now he is also locked in a building, and I sent him there. Each time I drive away, I feel I need forgiveness, although I know I had to do it. It is not real guilt, I did my best, but it is hard to shake it off.

I feel real guilt for the times that I have expressed my anger and been impatient, unkind, resentful and critical. I have even secretly wished my husband dead when everything has seemed too painful, too demanding, overwhelming. I would like to be able to claim a purely unselfish reason, that he would be free of a life that looks so burdensome. If I am truthful, it would be to ease my own pain. I feel so lonely when I am with him. His body is there but the essence of our life together has gone. There is unfinished business between us, so many things to say, but no way to share them. I hope he knows I love him.

Suggestions and thoughts about clinic visits

- Your work for your patients implies your sorrow that they are having to cope with this disease. I think it would mean a lot to them to hear you tell them so.
- Be kind to yourself! It is not your fault that your patient's health is deteriorating. Your patients and their carers do know, deep down, that you are only human. A carer who is sure that you have their loved one's welfare at heart can tolerate not knowing all the answers. I have squeezed some fun out of consultations over the years from observing clinicians' different

versions of the 'argument weak, speak louder' ploy. 'I don't know' is more reassuring and equally effective.

- Make full use of carers in your assessments. Create an atmosphere where a carer's contribution is acceptable and given credence. You will need the information they can give you. Ask them the right questions, while remembering that it is a painful experience for them to be there, watching their loved one struggle. Also, they will be well aware of the pressures and will not want to 'waste the busy doctor's time'.

- Ask carers to describe in some detail what they had to do that day to present the patient on time, looking clean and tidy. That will produce a lot of otherwise untapped information, though the carer might be reluctant to say some of it in the patient's presence. They will want to preserve his dignity. If you suspect this, see them on their own. The rules about confidentiality are for the benefit of patients. They must not be used to their detriment.

- Reassure carers that they are not being disloyal by being honest. They are the only people present who will be able to judge the patient from the baseline of their healthy state. There is room for very significant deterioration while still keeping within the 'normal' limits.

- There is enormous power lurking in a clinic visit. In terms of time, it is a drop in the ocean of the patient's life, but the ripples of its influence can last his lifetime. The carer's information can minimize the inevitably distorted impression of the patient's condition.

- Before writing notes during a consultation, check that your interpretation of what was said is shared by the patient and carer. 'Facts' and opinions once recorded will become the accepted truth.

- Check for accuracy the notes from the previous consultation or from a third party, realizing that a patient with memory loss is not a good source of factual information and that a deluded patient can sound entirely plausible. At each link in the chain, errors can be introduced or amplified.

- Resist the temptation to tailor your assessment of the patient's needs for support and help to fit into what you know is available. There will always be a shortfall, and whole areas of need may not have been considered at all in traditional arrangements. Even within tight budgets, improvements can be made. Your patients need your help to bring about changes.

- Check that instructions have reached the appropriate place and been activated.

These suggestions may seem to be asking for more clinic time. I think that they would actually save time in the long run, reduce unnecessary waste of precious resources and certainly relieve some of the pressure on carers.

Please be aware

There seems to be a worryingly high proportion of wife/carers who feel the need to take prescribed drugs to cope with their days and nights. There is an urgent need for effective support and a forum for their voices to be heard.

Disabled people have lives to live. Please, overworked social worker/therapist, don't send a message saying that you will be coming next day but leaving neither name nor contact number. Imagine a scene: Do we go for our long-anticipated and carefully planned outing and risk my husband being put on the bottom of the list because he 'didn't keep the appointment'? Do we leave a note on the doorstep and risk being burgled? Perhaps I should leave my husband alone and therefore in danger, while I dash round with a key and try to persuade a neighbor to be in our house most of the day to explain our absence? Or do we abandon our plans? Too many avoidable stresses can nearly overwhelm an exhausted carer. A thoughtful 'would it be convenient?' can make all the difference.

That dreaded phrase, 'I know exactly how you feel', brings up feelings of isolation in me. These kind people who want to make it all better for us often go on to tell me their justification for their claim – perhaps that they have spent an hour with a 98-year-old second cousin who is getting a bit forgetful! (I know I am exaggerating.) Finding the kindness behind the words takes precious energy.

When a wife/carer asks for help, she probably needs it. Almost certainly, she has already tried all the obvious things before troubling anyone else. I still laugh about one of the times my husband collapsed on the front doorstep. I did all the right things but couldn't get him up. Our neighbors were out. There was nobody in sight. I phoned our GP's surgery for advice and spoke to an unknown locum, explaining the situation. 'Get him into bed', he said. If I couldn't find anyone to help me, what should I do? 'You could always phone us', came the reply. Presumably, to be told to get him into bed!

Residential care

A frequent response to my husband's move to residential care was 'You must be so relieved that he is being well (do they mean 'better'?) cared for'. I am hugely relieved that there was a vacancy, as I could not have managed caring on my own for much longer. But relief is only part of it. It is a profound and heartrending change; the most difficult decision I have ever had to make. It was the end of our life together.

Suddenly there is no privacy. We are lucky that he has a single room, but the staff have to come in and out with laundry, tablets, cups of tea. Their sudden arrival can feel like an intrusion. That room is our home now. No longer our 'castle'.

My husband has lost all the comforting familiar things that we have shared for so long. The things I like to be busy with are elsewhere.

There are innumerable changes that seem to rob me of my wifehood. My husband is in strangers' hands. They are making decisions on his behalf and I am on the sidelines. I see the subtle changes but can no longer adjust his drugs for him. He has difficulty in communicating and I see him being misunderstood. His gentle politeness can give the impression that all is well. The carers in the home can't know. They have not been with him for 48 years, as I have.

Very little is said about sex and residential care. Photographs in brochures show smiling elderly people holding hands, the wooden arms of their chairs between them. Partners who have shared their bed for over half their lifetime may or may not have been 'having sex' but may still crave the comfort of closeness, the feeling of their skin against their partner's. A 'Do Not Disturb' notice is as difficult to use as it would be to hang a notice on the gate at home, telling all passers-by that they and their partner are having a special time together. We have lost the possibility of a natural comforting closeness.

It is certainly easier, though not always better, to be a carer with no emotional involvement, but this truism can spill over into another dimension, that of avoiding the expression of emotions at all costs. A passive patient sitting quietly is not necessarily a contented one; they may be just enduring. They are vulnerable and dependent. There can be fear behind their compliance.

It is tempting to dismiss patients' bizarre utterances as meaningless, easy to make a thoughtless, patronizing response. We must surely find a way to relieve their palpable frustration as they try to communicate from their confused worlds. I dream of a time when there will be skilled and unhurried listeners for them.

Conclusions

DLB is a whole-person disease. It is heartening to hear of all the work being done towards understanding it and lessening its devastating effect.

This is written at a time when an effective treatment is on the horizon. In future, it may be even more important to recognize DLB in its early stages. That can only happen with input from all those involved.

Correct diagnosis is vital for the best treatment. Carers are a rich source of immensely valuable and otherwise unobtainable information. If this is left untapped, knowledge of the patient's state of health will be the poorer, diagnosis possibly delayed and an opportunity lost to learn of the patient's personhood.

On all counts, pooling our knowledge makes good sense. It is the least we can do for those suffering from this horrible illness.

Post script

My husband has died, aged 73. Neuropathological autopsy examinations revealed that he had been suffering from 'pure' Lewy body disease, i.e. without other significant pathologies.

chapter 17

Dementia in Parkinson's disease

Dag Aarsland

Introduction

Parkinson's disease (PD) is a common neurodegenerative disorder affecting about 1.5% of people aged 65 or older (de Rijk et al, 1997). PD is defined pathologically as cell loss in the pigmented dopaminergic cells of the pars compacta, of the substantia nigra and synuclein pathology (Lewy neurites and Lewy bodies) in the surviving cells. In addition, cholinergic forebrain nuclei and other brainstem nuclei, including the serotonergic raphe nuclei and the noradrenergic locus ceruleus, are usually affected. From these brainstem changes, the topographical progression subsequently involves the anteromedial temporal mesocortex, including the transentorhinal region, and reaches into adjoining high-order sensory association areas and important limbic structures such as amygdala and hippocampus (Braak et al, 2003; Jellinger, 2003). In addition, amyloid plaques and even neurofibrillary tangles are found in most patients at autopsy ((Mattila et al, 1999; Jellinger et al, 2002). The cardinal clinical features of PD are resting tremor, bradykinesia, rigidity and postural abnormalities (Gelb et al, 1999). However, due to the wide distribution of neurodegeneration, it is not surprising that a wide range of nonmotor symptoms also occur, including neuropsychiatric symptoms and autonomic dysfunction.

The treatment of the motor symptoms of PD involves dopamine replacement therapy with levodopa and dopamine agonists (Lees, 2002). The monoamine oxidase inhibitor selegiline, with a potential neuroprotective effect, may slow disease progression. The use of anticholinergic agents has declined drastically due to concerns relating to their risk of cognitive impairment and delirium, particularly in the elderly. Deep cerebral stimulation with implantation of electrodes can be very helpful for selected patients. A wide range of behavioral side-effects can occur during drug and surgical treatments (Burn and Troster, 2004).

During the last decade, a considerable literature has shown that cognitive impairment is common even in early PD, and that, as the disease progresses, a substantial proportion of patients develop dementia (Emre, 2003). In addition, other neuropsychiatric symptoms, such as visual hallucinations, depression and apathy, are also common (Aarsland et al, 1999). It is thus increasingly recognized that PD is a neuropsychiatric disorder and not merely a movement disorder. Independent of the motor symptoms, cognitive impairment in patients with PD affects quality of life, contributes to caregiver distress and increased risk of nursing home placement, and is associated with more psychiatric symptoms such as depression and hallucinations, higher mortality and functional disability, and higher risk for drug toxicity. This chapter will discuss the epidemiology, pathophysiological mechanism, clinical presentation, relationship to DLB and management of dementia in patients with PD.

Cognitive impairment in early PD

Cognitive impairment is present even at the earliest stages of PD. In a series of 91 PD patients with a mean duration of PD of less than 2 years, impairment on a range of neuropsychological tests was found (Reid et al, 1996), and in a community-based study, more than 50% of the nondemented PD subjects had some form of cognitive impairment (Janvin et al, 2003b). The cognitive profile in early PD varies. Executive impairment, including working memory and attention shift, is the earliest cognitive manifestation in PD, but visuospatial dysfunctions, and even memory, may also be impaired in some patients (Dubois and Pillon, 1997). In a study of 42 PD patients with mild cognitive impairment (MCI), 20% exhibited predominantly memory deficits and 30% a dominant executive impairment, and 50% had a more global cognitive impairment (Janvin et al, 2003b). In the only community-based study of cognitive impairment in early PD to date, 36% of the PD patients had evidence of cognitive impairment. Cognitive subgroups were identified, as 30% of the cognitively impaired subjects had a frontostriatal-type deficit, whereas 21% had a temporal lobe-type deficit (Foltynie et al, 2004). With advancing PD, there is an increase in the severity and broadening of cognitive impairment, with superimposition of deficits typically associated with cortical dementia upon the early executive deficits (Reid et al, 1996), and thus the cognitive profile is intermediate between Alzheimer's disease (AD) and a classical subcortical dementia such as progressive supranuclear palsy (Aarsland et al, 2003c). Again, within the PDD group, there are different profiles, with some patients showing a memory-dominant pattern, others an executive pattern, and finally a more globally impaired group (Figure 17.1). It might be argued that the memory impairment in PDD is secondary to executive dysfunction. However, in a detailed study of memory and executive functioning in nondemented PD patients, Weintraub (2004) found that two-thirds of PD patients with mild memory impairment showed a subcortical memory profile, while the remaining one-third showed a limbic–cortical pattern, i.e. impaired free recall and recognition.

Few prospective studies of mild cognitive impairment (MCI) in PD exist. The annual decline on the Mini-Mental State Examination (MMSE) in PD is 1 point, but with wide interindividual variations (Aarsland et al, 2004c). Mild executive and memory impairments are predictors of subsequent dementia in PD, independent of age and stage of PD (Levy et al, 2002a). We reassessed 29 nondemented PD patients with MCI (5 with amnestic, 13 with single non-memory and 11 with multiple-domain MCI) after 4 years, and found that 62% had developed dementia (Janvin et al, 2004), which is consistent with the conversion rate to dementia in non-PD MCI patients (Petersen et al, 2001). The proportion that progressed to dementia did not differ between the three different MCI groups, but was higher than among cognitively intact patients (23%) ($p<0.05$) (Janvin et al, 2004).

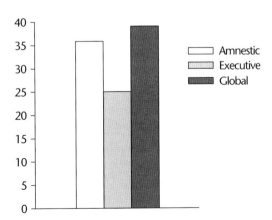

Figure 17.1 *Percentage of Parkinson's disease patients with dementia with different cognitive profiles (Janvin et al, 2003a).*

Epidemiology of dementia in PD

Wide variations in prevalence estimates of dementia in PD have been reported, based on differences in the selection and number of patients studied, diagnostic criteria for PD, assessment of cognition, and diagnostic criteria for dementia. Information on the frequency of PDD is largely available from two sources: studies assessing prevalence of dementia subtypes and studies of dementia in PD samples. Studies of the prevalence of different types of dementia indicate that 3–4% of dementia patients have PDD (Table 17.1). However, such studies usually do not use standardized diagnostic criteria for PD or assessment of parkinsonism. The exception is the Cardiovascular Health Cognition Study, where 21 of 707 (3.0%) dementia patients were classified as having PD (Lopez et al, 2003), and the Honolulu–Asia Aging Study, where PD was the only diagnosis of 7 of 226 (3.1%) patients with dementia, although PD and other conditions were diagnosed in an additional 6 (2.7%) of cases (White et al, 1996).

Large community-based studies using standardized cognitive assessment and DSM-IIIR criteria for dementia show that 23% to 41% of patients with PD have dementia (Levy and Marder, 2003) (Table 17.2). Thus, taken together, the results from community-based studies of dementia and of PD suggest that the prevalence of PDD in subjects aged 65 or older is 0.3–0.5%. Since dementia is associated with increased mortality in PD (Levy et al, 2002d), prevalence studies underestimate the true frequency of dementia in PD, and longitudinal studies are thus required to accurately describe the frequency of dementia in PD.

Few studies of the incidence of dementia in PD populations exist. Estimates vary from 42.6 (Hughes et al, 2000) to 112.5 (Marder et al, 1995) per 1000 patient-years. In the two community-based studies, the incidence was 95.3 (Aarsland et al, 2001a) and 112.5 (Marder et al, 1995), indicating that about 10% of PD patients develop dementia per year, and the risk for developing dementia in PD is six times higher than in non-PD subjects (Aarsland et al, 2001a). Although little is known regarding the lifetime risk of developing dementia in patients with a diagnosis of PD, the available evidence suggests that the risk is high. Only one study to date has prospectively followed de novo PD patients to assess the frequency of dementia. After 5 years, a cumulative prevalence of dementia of 36% could be estimated from the data presented (Reid et al, 1996). We performed an 8-year prospective study of a community-based sample of 224 PD patients with a mean duration of disease

Table 17.1 Proportion of Parkinson's disease (PD) in community-based studies of dementia

Study	Age group	Dementia cases	Dementia case-finding method	Standardized assessment and diagnosis of PD	Dementia criteria	Prevalence of dementia (%)	Proportion of dementia with PD (%)
White et al (1996)	71–93	226	Stratified random sample	Criteria specified	DSM-IIIR	9.3	3.1 (5.8[a])
Lopez et al (2003)	≥65	707	Total population screened	Standardized assessment	DSM-IV	19.6[b]	3.0
Stevens et al (2002)	≥65	107	Stratified random sample	None	DSM-IV	9.9	2
Ott et al (1995)	≥55	474	Total population screened	None	DSM-IIIR	6.3	6.3
Group (1994)	≥65	1125	Stratified random sample	None	?	8	2.4

DSM, Diagnostic and Statistical Manual.
[a]Including PD plus other cause.
[b]Cumulative prevalence.

Table 17.2 Point-prevalence of dementia in community-based studies of Parkinson's disease (PD)

Study	PD cases	Method of case identification[a]	PD criteria	Dementia criteria	Standardized cognitive assessment	Prevalence of dementia (%)	Estimated population prevalence (per 100 000)
Aarsland et al (1996)	245	(1)	Larsen et al (1994)	DSM-IIIR	MMSE	27.7	30
Marttila and Rinne (1976)	444	(1)	Hoehn and Yahr (1967)	Celesia and Wanamaker (1972)	No	28.8	35
Marder et al (1995)	279	(1)	Hughes et al (1992)	DSM-IIIR	Neuro-psychological test battery	37.3	–
Mayeux et al (1992)	179	(1) + announcements	2 of 4 cardinal features	DSM-IIIR	Neuro-psychological test battery	41.3	41
Tison et al (1995)	60	(2)	UK Brain Bank Criteria (Hughes et al, 1992)	DSM-III	Neuro-psychological test battery	17.6	–

DSM, Diagnostic and Statistical Manual; MMSE, Mini-Mental State Examination.

[a](1) All PD cases known to the health system in a defined geographical area.

(2) Questionnaire administered to a stratified random sample aged ≥65.

of 9 years at baseline. Of these, 122 subjects received a diagnosis of dementia at baseline or at subsequent evaluations. After controlling for attrition due to death, the 8-year cumulative prevalence of dementia was calculated to 78% (Aarsland et al, 2003a). Thus, it is clear that a substantial proportion of patients with PD develop dementia, which is usually diagnosed for the first time more than 10 years after the diagnosis of PD (Hughes et al, 2000; Aarsland et al, 2003a).

Risk factors for dementia in PD

Several factors have been reported to be associated with dementia in PD, including male sex, low education, depression, hallucinations, age, age at onset, mild cognitive impairment, family history of dementia and genetic factors (Emre, 2003). However, prospective studies that use multivariate statistical approach indicate that age, advanced parkinsonism and MCI are predictors of dementia in PD (Hughes et al, 2000; Levy et al, 2002b; Aarsland et al, 2003a). With regard to parkinsonian symptoms, rigidity and symptoms mediated mainly by nondopaminergic systems, such as speech, gait and postural disorders, are particularly related to subsequent development of dementia, whereas patients with a tremor-dominant pattern have a lower risk (Levy et al, 2000). Although some studies suggest that patients with late onset of PD have a higher risk of dementia, the evidence suggests that it is age, and not age at onset, that is associated with incident dementia in PD (Hughes et al, 2000; Levy et al, 2002b; Aarsland et al, 2003a). The relationship with age and severity of parkinsonism seems to be related to their combined effect rather than separate effects (Levy et al, 2002b).

Although PD was long thought not to be a genetic disorder, over the past few years, several genes for the disorder have been cloned, including *a-synuclein* and *parkin*, both of which are involved in the ubiquitin-dependent protein degradation pathway (Gwinn-Hardy, 2002). The relationship of these genes to dementia is not clear, but there are mutation carriers both with PD and with PDD (Muenter et al, 1998). Several studies have explored the effect of apolipoprotein E (ApoE) polymorphism, a risk factor for AD, on the risk for PD and dementia, with conflicting results. Increased risk of PD and, in particular, PDD, in carriers of the ApoE ε2 allele has been reported (Harhangi et al, 2000), while another study reported an association between the ApoE ε4 allele and Alzheimer pathology in PD patients

(Mattila et al, 2000). Most studies, however, have failed to find an association between ApoE polymorphism and dementia in PD.

Diagnosis of dementia in PD

There are no generally accepted clinical criteria for the dementia in PD, and when applying DSM-IV (1994), it can be difficult to decide whether cognitive impairment adds to the social and occupational impairment caused by the motor symptoms of the disease. A careful history emphasizing the onset, course, profile and chronology of motor, cognitive and psychiatric symptoms is crucial. Cognitive rating scales should be used, taking into account the disabilities due to motor symptoms. Screening tests that assess executive dysfunction should be employed, such as the Dementia Rating Scale (Mattis, 1976) or CAMCOG, the cognitive section of CAMDEX (Roth et al, 1986). Neuropsychological assessment is useful in the diagnosis of mildly affected cases. Although visuospatial, attentional and executive dysfunction is typical, the cognitive profile varies with stage of disease and between patients, and thus the finding of cognitive impairment per se is of greater importance than the pattern of neuropsychological deficits in the diagnosis of PDD. Particular care should be taken to distinguish between dementia and confusional states due to drug toxicity.

Mechanisms underlying cognitive impairment in PD

The etiology of cognitive impairment in PD is not yet clear. The heterogeneous cognitive deficits in PD probably reflect differing forms of neuropathological involvement. The executive impairment in early PD is related to the dopaminergic deficits, caused by disruption of nigrostriatal circuitry with altered outflow of the caudate nuclei to the frontal cortex via the thalamus (Rinne et al, 2000; Lewis et al, 2003) or by diminished dopamine activity in the frontal projections consequent to degeneration of mesocortical projections (Mattay et al, 2002), or by both. This is supported by the worsening of executive functioning, but not memory, after withdrawal of levodopa (Lange et al, 1995). The effects of nondopaminergic lesions on the cognitive impairments in PD is not known, but the cortical noradrenergic system has been linked to extradimensional shift performance, whereas visual memory may be dependent on acetylcholine (Robbins et al, 2003)

The broadening of cognitive impairment suggests that cortical regions are becoming involved in later disease stages, a notion supported by functional and structural imaging studies. In a study using single-photon emission computed tomography (SPECT), nondemented but cognitively impaired PD patients with decrements in multiple spheres of cognition had diminished temporal perfusion relative to controls. A differential pattern of relationships between cortical perfusion and cognitive functions was observed, with temporal and parietal perfusion showing relationships to global cognitive impairment, while dorsolateral frontal perfusion was related to executive impairment (Jagust et al, 1992). A positron emission tomography (PET) study revealed that nondemented PD patients had widespread cortical glucose hypometabolism, involving mainly frontal but also left temporal and parietal regions, compared with a more marked and global reduction, including severe bilateral temporoparietal defects, in PDD patients (Peppard et al, 1992). In studies using structural magnetic resonance imaging (MRI), annual brain volume loss correlated with cognitive decline (Hu et al, 2001). Reduced hippocampal volumes in PD patients have been shown, and in PDD patients, hippocampal volumes were even smaller than in AD patients (Laakso et al, 1996). Hippocampal atrophy is associated with memory impairment in PD, in contrast with prefrontal atrophy, which is more related to attentional impairment (Bruck et al, 2004). In a recent study using voxel-based morphometry, frontal and temporal cortical loss was found in PDD compared with normal controls, and these changes were indistinguishable from those in patients with DLB (Burton et al, 2004). However, cortical atrophy is mild compared with other dementia syndromes.

Different pathologies may contribute to the cortical changes observed in patients with PDD, including synuclein degeneration, amyloid plaques and cerebrovascular pathology. The heterogeneous cognitive profile of dementia in PD, with features of both subcortical and cortical dementia (see above), suggests that the relative severity and impact of the various neuropathological and neurochemical changes differs among patients with PDD. An association between cortical Lewy bodies (LBs) with dementia in PD has been found in some studies (Hurtig et al, 2000), but not all (Colosimo et al, 2003), suggesting that LBs are not the only pathology contributing to dementia in PD. There is evidence that Alzheimer-like changes contribute to dementia in PD (Jellinger et al, 2002). Finally, vascular changes may also contribute, although the contribution of vascular factors to dementia in PD seems to be modest (Levy et al, 2002c; Haugarvoll et al, 2004).

Much interest has focused on the relationship between cholinergic deficits and dementia in PDD. Selective loss of cells in the cholinergic nucleus basalis of Meynert and cortical cholinergic losses of similar degrees as in AD have been reported, and these changes are more pronounced in PDD patients compared with non-demented patients (Whitehouse et al, 1983; Perry et al, 1993; Kuhl et al, 1996; Tiraboschi et al, 2000). Interestingly, cholinergic deficits also occur in the frontal and temporoparietal cortex, as well as the hippocampus (Bohnen et al, 2003) and thalamus (Ziabreva et al, 2004) and cholinergic neuronal loss has also been reported in the pedunculopontine nucleus (Jellinger, 1988), with potential relevance for key clinical symptoms such as REM sleep abnormalities (Boeve et al, 2003) and fluctuating attention. Nicotinic receptor reductions have been reported in neocortex, striatum and thalamus in PD (Aubert et al, 1992; Perry et al, 1993; Reid et al, 2000; Pimlott et al, 2004), whereas, in contrast to the finding in AD, muscarinic receptors seem to be upregulated in PD (Perry et al, 1993). These receptor changes have potential therapeutic relevance (see below).

What is the relationship between PDD and DLB?

There is considerable overlap in the clinical, neurochemical and pathological features found in DLB and PDD. Both have parkinsonism, similar cognitive deficits, similar patterns of atrophy, similar amounts of LB pathology, and similar substantial cholinergic and dopaminergic deficits, which appear amenable to similar treatments The available evidence suggests that the heterogeneity within the two syndromes (i.e. PD with or without dementia; DLB with or without parkinsonism) may be more crucial than the differences between them (Aarsland et al, 2004a). However, the severity of executive dysfunction (Downes et al, 1998; Aarsland et al, 2003c) and in particular the frequency of psychiatric symptoms (Aarsland et al, 2001b), are significantly greater in DLB than in PDD. Subtle neurochemical and pathological differences are likely to underlie these differences. Executive dysfunction may relate to the loss of the hippocampal projection to the frontal lobe in DLB but not in PD (Harding et al, 2002b), and both increased cholinergic deficits and LB pathology in the temporal cortex strongly relate to the increased frequency of psychiatric features in DLB but not in PDD (Ballard et al, 2000; Harding et al, 2002a).

The most obvious difference is the earlier onset of dementia in DLB than in PDD. The explanation for this relationship may be the presence of substantial cortical Aβ deposition in DLB but not in PDD (Harding and Halliday, 2001;

Aarsland et al, 2004a). Thus, DLB is similar to AD in that it has two major pathologies – cortical Aβ and LBs in DLB versus cortical Aβ and neurofibrillary tangles in AD – whereas PDD has mainly the LB pathology and a late (slower) onset of dementia.

There are four possible models that could be used to classify DLB and PDD:

1. They could be considered as distinct conditions.
2. They could be considered as part of a spectrum of dementia related to cortical LB disease.
3. DLB with parkinsonism and PDD could be considered as a distinct condition, but separate from DLB without parkinsonism and PD without dementia.
4. They could be considered as part of a spectrum of LB and AD pathology.

The commonality of the presenting symptoms, treatment response and many neuropathological/neurochemical substrates would seem to best support a spectrum model, although the additional cortical Aβ deposition in DLB suggests important differences underlying dementia at onset.

Treatment of cognitive impairment in PD

There are several pharmacological agents available to treat the various motor and psychiatric manifestations of PD, all of which have the potential to improve one symptom domain at the expense of exacerbating another. However, no pharmacological agents have been approved for the treatment of cognitive impairment in PD. The only evidence-based treatment for neuropsychiatric symptoms in PD is the use of clozapine for hallucinations (Goetz, 2002). Nonspecific measures such as reviewing and removing drugs that may cause worsening of cognition (e.g. anticholinergic agents) and treating comorbid medical conditions must be considered in PD patients with cognitive impairment. Informing the patient and family about the risk of progressive worsening of cognitive functioning in addition to motor symptoms is also important.

Levodopa treatment may improve some and impair other cognitive functions (see above), but probably has no effect on dementia. Other drugs frequently prescribed for PD patients may potentially improve cognition. In a placebo-controlled trial, neither selegiline nor vitamin E had a significant effect on cognitive functioning in nondemented PD patients (Kieburtz et al,

1994). An observational study suggested that postmenopausal estrogen use was protective for the development of dementia within the setting of PD (Marder et al, 1998), but controlled studies supporting this promising result have not been performed.

The cholinergic loss in PDD, the increase in muscarinic receptor binding and the relatively fewer neocortical neurodegenerative changes suggest that cholinergic drugs may be particularly useful in PDD. This hypothesis received support from an early study showing remarkable improvements of cognition, hallucinations and even parkinsonism during treatment with tacrine (Hutchinson and Fazzini, 1996). Subsequent uncontrolled case series have shown improvement of cognition and visual hallucinations in PDD during treatment with the more recently developed cholinesterase inhibitors rivastigmine (Reading et al, 2001) and galantamine (Aarsland et al, 2003b), although the improvements were less dramatic than those reported with tacrine. These promising results were supported by two small placebo-controlled trials showing some cognitive improvement after treatment with donepezil (Aarsland et al, 2002; Leroi et al, 2004). In a recent review of cholinesterase inhibitors in PD, we identified 14 studies with a total of 144 patients (details from the most important studies are found in Table 17.3). Across studies, the mean Mini-Mental State Examination (MMSE) score improved from 20 to 22, and improvement of hallucinations was reported in 92% of patients who had this symptom at baseline (Aarsland et al, 2004b). The improvement of neuro-psychiatric symptoms on rivastigmine in a large randomized trial with DLB patients (McKeith et al, 2000) also supports the usefulness of cholinesterase inhibitors for PDD. Worsening of motor symptoms occurred in some patients with PD, although most patients tolerated the drug well without increasing parkinsonism. These promising results were confirmed in a recent large-scale trial showing significant improvement of cognition, activities of daily living and psychiatric symptoms in patients with PDD after treatment with rivastigmine (Emre et al, 2004).

The currently available cholinergic drugs differ in their pharmacodynamic profiles. It is not known at present whether these differences, such as the additional effect on butyrylcholinetransferase (rivastigmine) and the modulating effect on nicotinic receptors (galantamine) have therapeutic relevance in the treatment of PDD. However, there is evidence that temporal cortex butyrylcholine esterase is associated with cognitive decline in DLB (Perry et al, 2003), and nicotine appears to have a beneficial effect on arousal, attention and processing speed, and may even improve motor symptoms in PD

Table 17.3 Summary of studies with cholinesterase inhibitors in patients with Parkinson's disease (PD)

Study	Drug	N	Drop-out	Age (years)	Hoehn and Yahr score	Duration of PD (years)	Study design	Treatment duration (weeks)	Baseline MMSE score	Outcome			
										Parkinsonism	VH	Cognition	Mean MMSE change
Hutchinson and Fazzini (1996)	Tacrine	7	0	74	4.4	8	Open	8	17	+	+	+	7.1[a]
Fabbrini et al (2002)	Donepezil	8	0	74	ND	8	Open	8	25.2	−(n=2)	+	0	0.3
Minett et al (2003)	Donepezil	15	4	ND	ND	ND	Open, treat/ withdraw/ treat	20/6/12	18	0	+	+	3.8[a]/ −4.4/5.4
Aarsland et al (2002)	Donepezil	14	2	71	2.4	11	RCT crossover	10+10	20.8	0	ND	+	2.1 (0.3 on (placebo)[a]
Leroi et al (2004)	Donepezil	16	5/7	66	2.5	11	RCT	18	26	0	0	+	−0.7
Reading et al (2001)	Rivastigmine	15	3	71	ND	12	Open/ washout	14/3	20	0	+	+	5.0[a]/−4.2
Giladi et al (2003)	Rivastigmine	28	8	75	3.1	7	Open/ washout	26+8	19.5	0	ND	+	1.4/−1.2
Aarsland et al (2003b)	Galantamine	16	3	76	3.6	13	Open	8	17.7	+(n=6) −(n=4)	+	+	2.3[a]

N, number of patients included; MMSE, Mini-Mental State Examination; VH, visual hallucinations; ND, no data; RCT, randomized controlled trial.
[a]Statistically significant.

(Rusted et al, 2000), suggesting that the cholinesterase inhibitors may differ in their clinical effects in PDD. However, comparative clinical trials are necessary to corroborate these hypotheses.

Conclusions

Cognitive impairment and dementia are very common in patients with PD, with important clinical consequences for patients and their caregivers. Clinicians need to focus on these and other neuropsychiatric symptoms in addition to the motor symptoms in order to provide optimal care for these patients. The underlying etiology and the clinical presentation of cognitive impairment in PD are highly variable, and the nosological classification of PDD and its relationship to other dementias, in particular DLB, is not yet clarified. The complex clinical presentation in these frail and elderly individuals poses considerable challenges for their clinical management. Recent evidence suggests that cholinergic agents are useful for patients with PD and dementia, although further large-scale, randomized clinical trials are needed.

References

Aarsland D, Tandberg E, Larsen JP, Cummings JL, Frequency of dementia in Parkinson disease. Arch Neurol (1996) 53:538–42.

Aarsland D, Larsen JP, Lim NG et al, Range of neuropsychiatric disturbances in patients with Parkinson's disease. J Neurol Neurosurg Psychiatry (1999) 67:492–6.

Aarsland D, Andersen K, Larsen JP et al, Risk of dementia in Parkinson's disease: A community-based, prospective study. Neurology (2001a) 56:730–6.

Aarsland D, Ballard C, Larsen JP, McKeith I, A comparative study of psychiatric symptoms in dementia with Lewy bodies and Parkinson's disease with and without dementia. Int J Geriatr Psychiatry (2001b) 16:528–36.

Aarsland D, Laake K, Larsen JP, Janvin C, Donepezil for cognitive impairment in Parkinson's disease: a randomised controlled study. J Neurol Neurosurg Psychiatry (2002) 72:708–12.

Aarsland D, Andersen K, Larsen JP et al, Prevalence and characteristics of dementia in Parkinson disease: an 8-year prospective study. Arch Neurol (2003a) 60:387–92.

Aarsland D, Hutchinson M, Larsen JP, Cognitive, psychiatric, and motor response to galantamine in Parkinson's disease with dementia. Int J Geriatr Psychiatry (2003b) 18:937–41.

Aarsland D, Litvan I, Salmon D et al, Performance on the dementia rating scale in Parkinson's disease with dementia and dementia with Lewy bodies: comparison with progressive supranuclear palsy and Alzheimer's disease. J Neurol Neurosurg Psychiatry (2003c) 74:1215–20.

Aarsland D, Ballard CG, Halliday G, Are Parkinson's disease with dementia and dementia with Lewy bodies the same entity? J Geriatr Psychiatry Neurol (2004a) 17:137–45.

Aarsland D, Mosimann UP, McKeith IG, Role of cholinesterase inhibitors in Parkinson's disease dementia and dementia with Lewy bodies. J Geriatr Psychiatry Neurol (2004b) 17:164–71.

Aarsland D, Anderson K, Larsen JP et al, The rate of cognitive decline in Parkinson disease. Arch Neurol (2004c) 61:1906–11.

Aubert I, Araujo DM, Cecyre D et al, Comparative alterations of nicotinic and muscarinic binding sites in Alzheimer's and Parkinson's diseases. J Neurochem (1992) 58:529–41.

Ballard C, Piggott M, Johnson M et al, Delusions associated with elevated muscarinic binding in dementia with Lewy bodies. Ann Neurol (2000) 48:868–76.

Boeve BF, Silber MH, Parisi JE et al, Synucleinopathy pathology and REM sleep behavior disorder plus dementia or parkinsonism. Neurology (2003) 61:40–5.

Bohnen NI, Kaufer DI, Ivanco LS et al, Cortical cholinergic function is more severely affected in Parkinsonian dementia than in Alzheimer disease: an in vivo positron emission tomographic study. Arch Neurol (2003) 60:1745–8.

Braak H, Del Tredici K, Rub U et al, Staging of brain pathology related to sporadic Parkinson's disease. Neurobiol Aging (2003) 24:197–211.

Bruck A, Kurki T, Kaasinen V et al, Hippocampal and prefrontal atrophy in patients with early non-demented Parkinson's disease is related to cognitive impairment. J Neurol Neurosurg Psychiatry (2004) 75:1467–9.

Burn DJ, Troster AI Neuropsychiatric complications of medical and surgical therapies for Parkinson's disease. J Geriatr Psychiatry Neurol (2004) 17:172–80.

Burton EJ, McKeith IG, Burn DJ, Williams ED, OBrien JT, Cerebral atrophy in Parkinson's disease with and without dementia: a comparison with Alzheimer's disease, dementia with Lewy bodies and controls. Brain (2004) 127:791–800.

Celesia GG, Wanamaker WM, Psychiatric disturbances in Parkinson's disease. Dis Nerv Syst (1972) 33:577–83.

Colosimo C, Hughes AJ, Kilford L, Lees AJ, Lewy body cortical involvement may not always predict dementia in Parkinson's disease. J Neurol Neurosurg Psychiatry (2003) 74:852–6.

de Rijk MC, Tzourio C, Breteler MM et al, Prevalence of parkinsonism and Parkinson's disease in Europe: the EUROPARKINSON Collaborative Study. European Community Concerted Action on the Epidemiology of Parkinson's disease. J Neurol Neurosurg Psychiatry (1997) 62:10–15.

Downes JJ, Priestley NM, Doran M et al, Intellectual, mnemonic, and frontal functions in Lewy bodies: A comparison with early and advanced Parkinson's disease. Behav Neurol (1998) 11:173–83.

DSM-IV, Diagnostic and Statistical Manual of Mental Disorders (DSM IV). Fourth Edition. Revised. (American Psychiatric Association: Washington, DC, 1994).

Dubois B, Pillon B, Cognitive deficits in Parkinson's disease. J Neurol (1997) 244:2–8.

Emre M, Dementia associated with Parkinson's disease. Lancet Neurol (2003) 2:229–37.

Emre M, Aarsland D, Albanese A et al, Rivastigmine for dementia associated with Parkinson's disease. N Engl J Med (2004) 351(24):2509–18.

Fabbrini G, Barbanti P, Aurilia C et al, Donepezil in the treatment of hallucinations and delusions in Parkinson's disease. Neurol Sci (2002) 23:41–3.

Foltynie T, Brayne CE, Robbins TW, Barker RA, The cognitive ability of an incident cohort of Parkinson's patients in the UK. The CamPaIGN study. Brain (2004) 127:550–60.

Gelb DJ, Oliver E, Gilman S, Diagnostic criteria for Parkinson disease. Arch Neurol (1999) 56:33–9.

Giladi N, Shabtai H, Gurevich T et al, Rivastigmine (Exelon) for dementia in patients with Parkinson's disease. Acta Neurol Scand (2003) 108:368–73.

Goetz CG, Koller WC, Poewe W et al, Management of Parkinson's disease: An evidence-based review. Mov Disord (2002) 17(Suppl 4):112–27.

Group CSoHaAW, Canadian study of health and aging: Study methods and prevalence of dementia. CMAJ (1994) 150:899–913.

Gwinn-Hardy K, Genetics of parkinsonism. Mov Disord (2002) 17:645–56.

Harding AJ, Halliday GM, Cortical Lewy body pathology in the diagnosis of dementia. Acta Neuropathol (Berl) (2001) 102:355–63.

Harding AJ, Broe GA, Halliday GM, Visual hallucinations in Lewy body disease relate to Lewy bodies in the temporal lobe. Brain (2002a) 125:391–403.

Harding AJ, Lakay B, Halliday GM, Selective hippocampal neuron loss in dementia with Lewy bodies. Ann Neurol (2002b) 51:125–8.

Harhangi BS, de Rijk MC, van Duijn CM et al, APOE and the risk of PD with or without dementia in a population-based study. Neurology (2000) 54:1272–6.

Haugarvoll K, Aarsland D, Larsen JP, In: Proceedings of 8th International Congress of Parkinson's Disease and Movement Disorders, Rome, Italy (2004).

Hoehn M, Yahr M, Parkinsonism: Onset, progression and mortality. Neurology (1967) 17:427–42.

Hu MT, White SJ, Chaudhuri KR et al, Correlating rates of cerebral atrophy in Parkinson's disease with measures of cognitive decline. J Neural Transm (2001) 108:571–80.

Hughes AJ, Daniel SE, Kilford L, Lees AJ, Accuracy of clinical diagnosis of idiopathic Parkinson's disease: a clinico-pathological study of 100 cases. J Neurol Neurosurg Psychiatry (1992) 55:181–4.

Hughes TA, Ross HF, Musa S et al, A 10-year study of the incidence of and factors predicting dementia in Parkinson's disease. Neurology (2000) 54:1596–602.

Hurtig HI, Trojanowski JQ, Galvin J et al, Alpha-synuclein cortical lewy bodies are markers for dementia. Neurology (2000) 54:1916–21.

Hutchinson M, Fazzini E, Cholinesterase inhibition in Parkinson's disease [Letter]. J Neurol Neurosurg Psychiatry (1996) 61:324–5.

Jagust WJ, Reed BR, Martin EM et al, Cognitive function and regional cerebral blood flow in Parkinson's disease. Brain (1992) 115:521–37.

Janvin C, Aarsland D, Larsen JP, In: Proceedings of 3rd International Workshop on Dementia with Lewy Bodies and Parkinson's Disease Dementia (DLB/PDD), Newcastle upon Tyne, UK (2003a).

Janvin C, Aarsland D, Larsen JP, Hugdahl K, Neuropsychological profile of patients with Parkinson's disease without dementia. Dement Geriatr Cogn Disord (2003b) 15:126–31.

Janvin C, Aarsland D, Larsen JP, Hugdahl K, In: Proceedings of 8th International Congress of Parkinson's Disease and Movement Disorders, Rome, Italy (2004).

Jellinger K, The pedunculopontine nucleus in Parkinson's disease, progressive supranuclear palsy and Alzheimer's disease. J Neurol Neurosurg Psychiatry (1988) 51:540–3.

Jellinger KA, Alpha-synuclein pathology in Parkinson's and Alzheimer's disease brain: incidence and topographic distribution – a pilot study. Acta Neuropathol (Berl) (2003) 106:191–201.

Jellinger KA, Seppi K, Wenning GK, Poewe W, Impact of coexistent Alzheimer pathology on the natural history of Parkinson's disease. J Neural Transm (2002) 109:329–39.

Kieburtz K, McDermott M, Como P et al, The effect of deprenyl and tocopherol on cognitive performance in early untreated Parkinson's disease. Parkinson Study Group. Neurology (1994) 44:1756–9.

Kuhl DE, Minoshima S, Fessler JA et al, In vivo imaging of cholinergic terminals in normal aging, Alzheimer's disease, and Parkinson's disease. Ann Neurol (1996) 40:399–410.

Laakso MP, Partanen K, Riekkinen P et al, Hippocampal volumes in Alzheimer's disease, Parkinson's disease with and without dementia, and in vascular dementia: An MRI study. Neurology (1996) 46:678–81.

Lange KW, Paul GM, Naumann M, Gsell W, Dopaminergic effects on cognitive performance in patients with Parkinson's disease. J Neural Transm Suppl (1995) 46:423–32.

Larsen JP, Dupont E, Tandberg E, Clinical diagnosis of Parkinson's disease: Proposal of diagnostic subgroups classified at different levels of confidence. Acta Neurol Scand (1994) 84:242–51.

Lees AJ, Drugs for Parkinson's disease. J Neurol Neurosurg Psychiatry (2002) 73:607–10.

Leroi I, Brandt J, Reich SG et al, Randomized placebo-controlled trial of donepezil in cognitive impairment in Parkinson's disease. Int J Geriatr Psychiatry (2004) 19:1–8.

Levy G, Marder K, Prevalence, incidence and risk factors for dementia in Parkinson's disease. In: Bedard MA, Agid Y, Chouinard S et al, eds, Mental and Behavioral Dysfunction in Movement Disorders (Humana Press: Totowa, NJ, (2003) 259–70.

Levy G, Tang MX, Cote LJ et al, Motor impairment in PD: Relationship to incident dementia and age. Neurology (2000) 55:539–44.

Levy G, Jacobs DM, Tang MX et al, Memory and executive function impairment predict dementia in Parkinson's disease. Mov Disord (2002a) 17:1221–6.

Levy G, Schupf N, Tang MX et al, Combined effect of age and severity on the risk of dementia in Parkinson's disease. Ann Neurol (2002b) 51:722–9.

Levy G, Tang MX, Cote LJ et al, Do risk factors for Alzheimer's disease predict dementia in Parkinson's disease? An exploratory study. Mov Disord (2002c) 17:250–7.

Levy G, Tang MX, Louis ED et al, The association of incident dementia with mortality in PD. Neurology (2002d) 59:1708–13.

Lewis SJ, Dove A, Robbins TW et al, Cognitive impairments in early Parkinson's disease are accompanied by reductions in activity in frontostriatal neural circuitry. J Neurosci (2003) 23:6351–6.

Lopez OL, Kuller LH, Fitzpatrick A et al, Evaluation of dementia in the Cardiovascular Health Cognition Study. Neuroepidemiology (2003) 22:1–12.

McKeith I, Del Ser T, Spano P et al, Efficacy of rivastigmine in dementia with Lewy bodies: a randomised, double-blind, placebo-controlled international study. Lancet (2000) 356:2031–6.

Marder K, Tang MX, Cote L et al, The frequency and associated risk factors for dementia in patients with Parkinson's disease. Arch Neurol (1995) 52:695–701.

Marder K, Tang MX, Alfaro B et al, Postmenopausal estrogen use and Parkinson's disease with and without dementia. Neurology (1998) 50:1141–3.

Marttila RJ, Rinne UK, Dementia in Parkinson's disease. Acta Neurol Scand (1976) 54:431–41.

Mattay VS, Tessitore A, Callicott JH et al, Dopaminergic modulation of cortical function in patients with Parkinson's disease. Ann Neurol (2002) 51:156–64.

Mattila PM, Rinne JO, Helenius H, Roytta M, Neuritic degeneration in the hippocampus and amygdala in Parkinson's disease in relation to Alzheimer pathology. Acta Neuropathol (Berl) (1999) 98:157–64.

Mattila KM, Rinne JO, Roytta M et al, Dipeptidyl carboxypeptidase 1 (DCP1) and butyrylcholinesterase (BCHE) gene interactions with the apolipoprotein E epsilon4 allele as risk factors in Alzheimer's disease and in Parkinson's disease with coexisting Alzheimer pathology. J Med Genet (2000) 37:766–70.

Mattis S, Dementia Rating Scale. In: Bellak L, Karasu TB, eds, Geriatric Psychiatry. A Handbook for Psychiatrists and Primary Care Physicians (Grune & Stratton: New York, 1976) 108–121.

Mayeux R, Denaro J, Hemenegildo N et al, A population-based investigation of Parkinson's disease with and without dementia. Relationship to age and gender. Arch Neurol (1992) 49:492–7.

Minett TS, Thomas A, Wilkinson LM et al, What happens when donepezil is suddenly withdrawn? An open label trial in dementia with Lewy bodies and Parkinson's disease with dementia. Int J Geriatr Psychiatry (2003) 18:988–93.

Muenter MD, Forno LS, Hornykiewicz O et al, Hereditary form of parkinsonism-dementia. Ann Neurol (1998) 43:768–81.

Ott A, Breteler MM, van Harskamp F et al, Prevalence of Alzheimer's disease and vascular dementia: association with education. The Rotterdam study. BMJ (1995) 310:970–3.

Peppard RF, Martin WR, Carr GD et al, Cerebral glucose metabolism in Parkinson's disease with and without dementia. Arch Neurol (1992) 49:1262–8.

Perry EK, Irving D, Kerwin JM et al, Cholinergic trasmitter and neurotropic activities in Lewy body dementia: Similarity to Parkinson's and distinction from Alzheimer disease. Alzheimer Dis Assoc Disord (1993) 7:69–79.

Perry E, McKeith I, Ballard C, Butyrylcholinesterase and progression of cognitive deficits in dementia with Lewy bodies. Neurology (2003) 60:1852–3.

Petersen RC, Doody R, Kurz A et al, Current concepts in mild cognitive impairment. Arch Neurol (2001) 58:1985–92.

Pimlott SL, Piggott M, Owens J et al, Nicotinic acetylcholine receptor distribution in Alzheimer's disease, dementia with Lewy bodies, Parkinson's disease, and vascular dementia: in vitro binding study using 5-[(125)i]-a-85380. Neuropsychopharmacology (2004) 29:108–16.

Reading PJ, Luce AK, McKeith IG, Rivastigmine in the treatment of parkinsonian psychosis and cognitive impairment: preliminary findings from an open trial. Mov Disord (2001) 16:1171–4.

Reid RT, Sabbagh MN, Corey-Bloom J et al, Nicotinic receptor losses in dementia with Lewy bodies: comparisons with Alzheimer's disease. Neurobiol Aging (2000) 21:741–6.

Reid WG, Hely MA, Morris JG et al, A longitudinal study of Parkinson's disease: clinical and neuropsychological correlates of dementia. J Clin Neurosci (1996) 3:327–33.

Rinne JO, Portin R, Ruottinen H et al, Cognitive impairment and the brain dopaminergic system in Parkinson's disease: [^{18}F]-fluorodopa positron emission tomography study. Arch Neurol (2000) 57:470–5.

Robbins TW, Crofts HS, Cools R, Roberts AC, Catecholamines and cognition: Bridging the gap between the animal studies and the human syndromes. In: Bedard MA, Agid Y, Chouinard S et al, eds, Mental and Behavioral Dysfunction in Movement Disorders (Humana Press: Totowa, NJ, 2003) 194–7.

Roth M, Tym E, Mountjoy CQ et al, CAMDEX. A standardized instrument for the diagnosis of mental disorder in the elderly with special reference to the early detection of dementia. Br J Psychiatry (1986) 149:698–709.

Rusted JM, Newhouse PA, Levin ED, Nicotinic treatment for degenerative neuropsychiatric disorders such as Alzheimer's disease and Parkinson's disease. Behav Brain Res (2000) 113:121–9.

Stevens T, Livingston G, Kitchen G et al, The Islington Study of dementia subtypes in the community. Br J Psychiatry (2002) 180:270–6.

Tiraboschi R, Hansen LA, Alford M et al, Cholinergic dysfunction in diseases with Lewy bodies. Neurology (2000) 54:407–11.

Tison F, Dartigues JF, Auriacombe S et al, Dementia in Parkinson's disease: a population-based study in ambulatory and institutionalized individuals. Neurology (1995) 45:705–8.

Weintraub D, Moberg PJ, Culbertson WC et al, Evidence for impaired encoding and retrieval profiles in Parkinson disease. Cogn Behav Neurol (2004) 17:195–200.

White L, Petrovitch H, Ross GW et al, Prevalence of dementia in older Japanese-American men in Hawaii: The Honolulu-Asia Aging Study. JAMA (1996) 276:955–60.

Whitehouse PJ, Hedreen JC, White CL 3rd, Price DL, Basal forebrain neurons in the dementia of Parkinson's disease. Ann Neurol (1983) 13:243–8.

Ziabreva I, Ballard CG, Aarsland D et al, In: Proceedings of 8th International Congress of Parkinson's Disease and Movement Disorders, Rome, Italy (2004).

Ziabreva I, Ballard CG, Aarsland D et al, Lewy body disease: Thalamic cholinergic activity related to dementia and parkinsonism. Neurobiol Aging (2005) in press.

chapter 18

Other atypical parkinsonian disorders and their differentiation from dementia with Lewy bodies

Niall Quinn

Introduction

Besides the spectrum of primary Lewy body (LB) disease, patients with a range of other diseases may present with, or develop during their course, a combination of parkinsonism, often atypical, and dementia. The commonest of these scenarios are Alzheimer's disease (AD – in which true parkinsonism is late and exceptional), Parkinson's disease (PD) plus AD, cerebrovascular disease, and PD plus cerebrovascular disease. Rarer diseases include progressive supranuclear palsy (PSP), corticobasal degeneration (CBD), multiple system atrophy (MSA – in which dementia is rare), frontotemporal dementia with parkinsonism related to chromosome 17 (FTDP-17), and prion disease (Creutzfeldt–Jakob disease, CJD).

Alzheimer's disease

It has long been accepted that 'extrapyramidal' signs may be seen in patients with AD (Molsa et al, 1984; Ellis et al,1996). There are two important caveats to this view. First, the early literature antedated the realization that many patients clinically labeled as having AD in fact have dementia with Lewy bodies (DLB), with or without additional Alzheimer pathology. Second, the extrapyramidal signs most frequently cited are rigidity (it can be very difficult in a demented patient to confidently distinguish between extrapyramidal rigidity, spasticity and Gegenhalten), slowness of movement or bradykinesia (which is not the same as the progressive decrement and fatiguing of alternating movements that characterizes true extrapyramidal akinesia), and 'parkinsonian' gait (e.g. short steps and en bloc turns). However, tremor is infrequent, rest tremor even less common, and a classical pill-rolling rest tremor, as seen in the vast majority of patients with PD, even rarer. Moreover, patients with AD are commonly treated with dopamine receptor-blocking drugs, which can cause parkinsonism in such individuals, albeit less severely and less commonly than in patients with DLB, who are particularly susceptible to neuroleptics.

Scarmeas et al (2004) have addressed 'motor signs' during the course of AD. They conducted a longitudinal study in 475 patients with clinically diagnosed NINDS/ADRDA-probable AD. Among these cases, 99 came to autopsy, 22% of whom had DLB. The examiners used 11 items from the Unified Parkinson's Disease Rating Scale (UPDRS): five items on rigidity, two on speech and facial expression, two on posture and gait, and one each on body bradykinesia/hypokinesia and tremor at rest (in any limb). At first examination, a score of at least 1 was obtained on at least 1 of the 11 items in 13% of subjects, and at last visit in 36%. Tremor was observed in 4% and 7% respectively. A diagnosis of DLB was present in 24% of patients with 'resting tremor' (not necessarily synonymous with classical pill-rolling rest tremor) and in 19% of those who never had resting tremor. Patients without true parkinsonism can, of course, score on the UPDRS, so the results almost certainly overestimate the incidence of true parkinsonism. However, there is an appreciable rate of at least some parkinsonian features even among the population without LBs, in some cases probably at least partly due to nigral pathology in terms of the presence of neurofibrillary tangles (NFTs) (Liu et al, 1997), and α-synuclein-labeled pathology, without actual LBs (Burns et al, 2005).

Nevertheless, at the Third International Workshop Meeting in Newcastle upon Tyne, none of the participants was able to put their hand on their heart and say that they had definitely encountered convincing true parkinsonism in patients with pathologically proven pure AD.

Other features differentiating 'pure' AD from PD, PD with dementia (PDD) and DLB are the usual absence in the first of hallucinations and fluctuations in cognition and alertness, of REM sleep behavior disorder (RBD – a putative marker for many patients with α-synucleinopathies – Boeve et al, 2003), and of postural hypotension (Horimoto et al, 2003; Thaisetthawatkul et al, 2004), which is seen frequently in patients with LB pathology, although controlled comparative studies with AD are currently lacking.

Parkinson's disease plus Alzheimer's disease

Some of the distinctions outlined above are largely lost when one considers PD plus AD, or DLB with Alzheimer pathology. Basically, the higher the Alzheimer pathology load in such patients, the more the nonmotor features resemble those of AD.

Cerebrovascular disease

Cerebrovascular disease is common in the elderly population. In the case of multiple infarcts, vascular dementia may occur if the infarct load is sufficiently great. In the case of Binswanger change and basal ganglia lacunes, a 'parkinsonian' picture may be seen, with a very variable degree of cognitive impairment. Again, the motor disturbance usually bears only partial or superficial resemblance to true parkinsonism. Thus, rest tremor is exceptional, and there is usually good facial expression and spontaneous upper limb activity, without the fatiguing and decrement of repetitive alternating movements that characterizes true akinesia in the arms. However, the legs are disproportionately involved ('lower-body parkinsonism' – Thompson and Marsden, 1987), sometimes with slow alternating movements and sometimes with true fatiguing, and may also show start hesitation or freezing. The gait may be wide-based, with very short, but not shuffling, steps ('marche à petits pas'), and the posture is typically erect. In some cases, the degree of striatal or nigrostriatal vascular involvement may be sufficient to cause true parkinsonism. Some of these patients, particularly those with lesions in or close to the nigrostriatal pathway (Zijlmans et al, 2004), respond to levodopa. Thus, if the dementia is not too severe, and the parkinsonism is causing functional disability, a trial of a levodopa preparation is worthwhile.

Parkinson's disease plus cerebrovascular disease

Many elderly people with PD develop additional cerebrovascular disease, which may modify their clinical picture. Thus, it may increase the probability of dementia, or may modify the motor disorder or its response to levodopa. Such patients may have typical levodopa-responsive parkinsonism in their upper body, yet (often subacutely) develop, or display, refractory gait abnormality or postural instability, producing a 'mismatch' between their upper body and their gait and balance.

Progressive supranuclear palsy

The population prevalence of clinically diagnosed PSP is about 6 in 100 000 (Schrag et al, 1999). The pathological characteristics comprise tau-associated NFTs, neuroglial pathology (mainly tufted astrocytes), and neuropil threads associated with fibrillary astrogliosis and neuronal loss in selected areas (Hauw and Agid, 2003). These include the striatum, pallidum, subthalamic nucleus, nucleus basalis of Meynert, brainstem (including colliculi, tegmentum, periaqueductal gray, red nucleus and basis pontis) and dentate nucleus. There is also a variable degree of cerebral cortical involvement.

Patients with 'classical' PSP experience early postural instability with falls, often in the first year, a frontal cognitive profile with a dysexecutive syndrome incorporating perseveration, and a memory deficit for recall rather than registration. They also develop the characteristic supranuclear (upper motor neuron) gaze 'palsy' (paresis) that gives the disease its name, and without which one cannot diagnose the condition in life (Litvan et al, 1996). The examination of eye movements is therefore critical in this condition and also in CBD (see below). More caveats are needed. In a patient with severe dementia, an adequate examination of eye movements may be impossible, because of poor comprehension and cooperation. An elderly subject may display a limitation of upward voluntary gaze that, considered alone, is entirely nonspecific, unless associated with falls in the first year. However, a limitation of downward gaze is always pathological. Nevertheless, even in the absence of downgaze limitation, a careful eye movement examination may suggest PSP (or, with different features, CBD).

With normal voluntary saccades, whether hypometric or not, an observer cannot track the movement of the patient's globes – they occur too fast for the trajectory itself to be witnessed (Leigh and Riley, 2000). When the movement of the globe can be followed, a saccade is definitely slow. Even if a PSP patient has nonspecific restriction only of upward gaze, if the residual vertical saccades are slow then this is significant, and usually suggests PSP, although spinocerebellar ataxia type 2 (SCA2) also causes slow saccades

(Wadia et al, 1998), but not dementia. The latency to initiate saccades, by contrast, is normal in PSP.

In PSP, the parkinsonism is usually symmetrical. Sometimes, it is almost exclusively axial, with minimal or no distal parkinsonism, particularly in the arms. Despite this, patients may display 'fast micrographia'. A gruff dysarthria, terminating in repetitive groaning noises in the late stages, is characteristic. Dysphagia and coughing at mealtimes are frequent. Levator inhibition and, less often, blepharospasm are frequent. The patient displays 'motor recklessness', rising from a chair like a rocket and then falling back again, or sitting down 'en bloc'. A minority of patients display tremor, sometimes even pill-rolling. Levodopa preparations are often of little help, but some patients respond, at least initially. Dyskinesias are rare, except for tightening of the muscles of the lower face and jaw. The average age at onset is 63–66 years and the average survival from first symptom to death is between 5 and 9 years (Birdi et al, 2002; Josephs and Dickson, 2003; Williams et al, 2005), although one pathologically proven case surviving 24 years has been reported (Birdi et al, 2002)

The clinical spectrum of PSP can vary. Thus, some patients develop the supranuclear gaze palsy late, or even not at all, during life; many do not fall in the first year, so can never achieve more than NINDS/SPSP-possible status during life. Tremor, psychosis, early dementia, asymmetric findings and absent H1 haplotype are unusual (Josephs and Dickson, 2003). Nevertheless, 32% of 107 cases in the Queen Square Brain Bank were characterized by asymmetric onset, tremor and some response to levodopa (Williams et al, 2005). These authors have called such cases 'PSP–parkinsonism', as opposed to the majority of cases with a classical picture, which they have called 'Richardson's syndrome'. For a recent review of PSP, see Burn and Lees (2004).

Corticobasal degeneration

This condition, first described by Rebeiz et al (1968) under the name 'cortico-dentatonigral degeneration with neuronal achromasia', is also, like PSP, a tauopathy, but is considerably rarer. Its relationship to PSP is debated but, interestingly, both share in common overrepresentation of the H1/H1 tau haplotype (Houlden et al, 2001) However, pathologically classical cases clearly differ clinically from the picture in PSP.

The pathological changes, as indicated by the name, predominantly involve the cortex and basal ganglia, with cortical atrophy (usually frontoparietal and asymmetric) and caudate and pallidonigral atrophy. There are swollen/ achromatic/ballooned neurons and superficial spongiosis in the cortex, tau-positive corticobasal bodies (globose NFTs) and other neurofibrillary lesions in the cortex, basal ganglia and thalamus, and widespread neuropil threads; there are also astrocytic plaques in the cortex and oligodendroglial coiled bodies (Dickson and Litvan, 2003).

CBD typically presents in the sixth to eighth decades of life (average 63 years), and the average survival is 7–9 years. Its classical motor presentation is with varying combinations of unilateral akinesia, rigidity, fixed dystonia, apraxia, cortical sensory loss, myoclonus and sometimes tremor, in one arm – all of these may be present in the fully developed case, except that the severity of all the other features may mean that apraxia cannot be identified in that arm, but may be only evident in the contralateral, subsequently affected, arm. The 'alien limb' phenomenon of a wandering arm that 'has a mind of its own' is seen in up to 50% of patients at some stage (Rinne et al, 1994).

The motor disorder spreads over time to other limbs, and includes the development of a supranuclear eye movement disorder. Its classical characteristics are the opposite of those seen in PSP. Thus, there is (often asymmetric, or lateralized) difficulty in initiating voluntary saccades, particularly to command, with prolonged latency, but, when the eyes finally move, they do so with normal saccadic velocity (Rivaud-Pechoux et al, 2000).

Atypical motor presentations include leg onset, symmetrical disease, falls or drop attacks, and generalized myoclonus. A CBD-like syndrome can be seen in AD, prion disease, cerebrovascular disease, Sneddon's syndrome (with lupus anticoagulant), progressive multifocal leukoencephalopathy (PML) and sudanophilic leukodystrophy (Bhatia et al, 2000). In the 1980s and 1990s, most reported cases of CBD were described by movement disorder neurologists, with emphasis on the 'classic' motor presentation, and dementia was said to be uncommon, usually mild, and late. However, more recently, it has become clear, mainly from postmortem verification of cases (usually misdiagnosed in life) in dementia brain banks, that CBD often presents with a dementia (Grimes et al, 1999; Graham et al, 2003). It may present with language dysfunction, reduced speech output and memory impairment, and a frontal dysexecutive syndrome before parietal symptoms, including apraxia, become more prominent.

For recent reviews on CBD, see Lang (2003) and Mahapatra et al (2004).

Multiple system atrophy

This progressive neurodegenerative disease, formerly reported under the rubrics of Shy–Drager syndrome, striatonigral degeneration and sporadic olivopontocerebellar atrophy (sOPCA), causes varying combinations of autonomic failure, parkinsonism (usually poorly or nonresponsive to levodopa) and cerebellar signs. The population prevalence of clinically diagnosed cases is about 4 in 100 000 (Schrag et al, 1999).

The pathological hallmark is neuronal loss and gliosis in the striatonigral and olivopontocerebellar systems, with additional spinal cord involvement, accompanied by the presence of α-synuclein-positive oligodendroglial cytoplasmic inclusions (GCIs) (Papp et al, 1989). Cortical involvement is usually mild and dementia is uncommon, and therefore used as a clinical exclusion criterion (Gilman et al, 1998). Nevertheless, more severe cortical involvement can sometimes be seen (Konagaya et al, 2002), and mild dementia has been reported in about 20% of pathologically proven cases in the literature, although moderate or severe dementia is decidedly rare (Wenning et al, 1997). The average age at onset is 57 years, and the mean survival from first symptom to death was 7 years in a series of 100 cases from the Queen Square Brain Bank (Ozawa et al, 2004). Many older patients initially suspected of having MSA because of the presence of parkinsonism with autonomic failure and who progress to show evidence of cognitive impairment and develop fluctuations in cognition and arousal, and (usually drug-induced) hallucinations turn out instead to have DLB or PDD (Horimoto et al, 2003; Thaisetthawatkul et al, 2004). However, RBD is even more common in MSA than in PD or DLB.

For a recent review of MSA, see Wenning et al (2004).

Frontotemporal dementia with parkinsonism linked to chromosome 17

This condition, due to mutations in the *tau* gene on chromosome 17, is much rarer than those above. It is dominantly inherited and so far has been identified in about 80 families in total, although a few apparently sporadic cases with mutations have also been reported. The average age at onset is 49 (range 25–76) years, and the average clinical course is 8.5 (range 2–26) years. The pathological changes are due to tau protein deposition in neurons and glia in the frontal and temporal cortex, cerebellum, caudate and pigmented brainstem nuclei (Ghetti et al, 2003). This gives rise to a clinical picture comprising at least two of behavioral and personality disturbances, cognitive deficits, and a motor disorder, usually levodopa-unresponsive parkinsonism. There is considerable clinical variability even within one family, and additional features that may be present include supranuclear gaze palsy, eyelid 'apraxia', upper and lower motor neuron signs, myoclonus, and seizures. Cases may be misdiagnosed as PSP (Morris et al, 2003) or CBD (Kertesz et al, 2000).

Creutzfeldt–Jakob disease

Typical CJD looks and behaves very differently to most other causes of dementia – moreover, significant parkinsonism is uncommon, so that misdiagnosis is relatively rare. Nevertheless, in atypical cases, difficulty can arise. Thus, there are reported instances where cases of DLB and AD have been suspected in life to have been CBD (Haik et al, 2000; Tschampa et al, 2001), and others where cases of CJD have been suspected in life to have instead been FTDP-17 (Nitrini et al, 2001) or CBD (Anschel et al, 2002).

Imaging and differential diagnosis

Conventional magnetic resonance imaging (MRI) is normal in PD. It may show stroke, lacunes or deep white matter changes in cerebrovascular disease, cortical and hippocampal atrophy in AD, and cortical atrophy, sometimes with hipocampal atrophy (if there is superimposed Alzheimer pathology), in PDD and DLB.

In MSA, one may find supra and/or infratentorial changes (Schrag et al, 2000). The former include a hyperintense slitlike appearance at the lateral border of the putamen, which correlates with the highest ferric iron levels, and microgliosis and astrogliosis. However, this has also been described in some cases with PSP, CBD and Huntington's disease. There may be putaminal atrophy or posterior putaminal hypointensity. Infratentorially, one may see a hyperintense 'cross' appearance in the pons, secondary to pontine atrophy. Degeneration of the pontine nuclei and transverse pontine fibers leads to conspicuous retention of the superior cerebellar peduncles and pyramidal tracts. This appearance may also be found in spinocerebellar ataxias 2 and 3 (SCA2 and SCA3), and has been reported in some patients with PSP, CBD and vasculitis. Hyperintensity of the middle cerebellar peduncles is also common in MSA, but is often also seen in the fragile X-associated tremor/ataxia syndrome (Brunberg et al, 2002). Cerebellar atrophy is common in MSA, but very nonspecific.

In PSP, one may see high signal in midbrain or midbrain atrophy, with splaying of the cerebral peduncles to give the so-called 'Mickey mouse ears' appearance in axial, and the so-called 'hummingbird sign' in sagittal, images, with a slender head and tapering beak in the midbrain region (Kato et al, 2003). A recent volumetric study has also shown reduced volume of the superior cerebellar peduncles in PSP (Paviour et al, 2005). One may sometimes see generalized cerebral atrophy in both PSP and (more rarely) in MSA.

In CBD, it is characteristic to see asymmetric posterior frontal and parietal atrophy (Savoiardo, 2003), but this is not always the case. FTDP-17 cases show variable degrees of frontotemporal atrophy. Most sporadic CJD cases show high signal changes in the putamen and the head of the caudate, whereas new variant cases usually show hyperintensity of the pulvinar (posterior nuclei) of the thalamus (Collie et al, 2001).

Other MRI techniques, including thin-section MRI, diffusion-weighted MRI, voxel-based morphometry and MR spectroscopy, are being investigated in the differential diagnosis of parkinsonian syndromes. At present imaging does not feature in the diagnostic criteria for, for example, MSA, PSP or CBD, other than to exclude other causes.

A variety of functional imaging techniques have also been applied, mainly on a research basis. The most widely available of these, dopamine transporter single-photon emission computed tomography (SPECT) scanning, may help to distinguish AD from DLB, but will not separate DLB from PD, PDD, MSA, PSP or CBD (Marshall and Grosset, 2003).

Other causes of dementia and an akinetic–rigid syndrome

The conditions considered above cover the commonest causes of parkinsonism combined with cognitive impairment, together with selected rarer causes. However, the differential diagnosis in individual patients may be much wider. A (nonexhaustive) list of causes is given in Table 18.1.

Table 18.1 Causes of dementia plus an akinetic–rigid syndrome

Lewy body disease (dementia with Lewy bodies, DLB/Parkinson's disease with dementia, PDD)
  ± cerebrovascular disease
  ± Alzheimer pathology
Progressive supranuclear palsy (PSP)
Multiple system atrophy (MSA)
Corticobasal degeneration (CBD)
Frontotemporal dementia with parkinsonism linked to chromosome 17 (FTDP-17) (D)
Huntington's disease (HD) (D)
Wilson's disease (r)
Neuroacanthocytosis (r)
Ceroid lipofuscinosis (r)
Neurodegeneration with brain ion accumulation (NBIA) (r)
Frontotemporal lobar degeneration (FTLD) ± motor neuron disease (MND)
Basal ganglia calcification (Fahr's disease)
Creutzfeldt–Jakob disease (CJD)
Toxins (e.g. manganese)
Vasculitis (systemic lupus erythematosus (SLE), polyarteritis nodosa (PAN), etc.)
Cerebral anoxia
Dementia pugilistica
Infections (e.g. syphilis, HIV)
Normal-pressure hydrocephalus (NPH)
Parkinsonian/dementia/amyotrophic lateral sclerosis (ALS) complex of Guam

(D), domiant; (r), recessive.

Conclusions

Many disorders, or combinations thereof, can sometimes be confused with DLB. Many of these are rare or inherited, or display other features that usually prevent such confusion. The most frequent scenarios remain varying combinations of the three common scourges of the elderly: Lewy body pathology (of variable degree), Alzheimer pathology (of variable degree) and cerebrovascular disease (of variable severity).

References

Anschel DJ, Simon DK, Llinas R, Joseph JT, Spongiform encephalopathy mimicking corticobasal degeneration. Mov Disord (2002) 17:606–7.

Bhatia KP, Lee MS, Rinne JO et al, Corticobasal degeneration look-alikes. Adv Neurol (2000) 82:169–82.

Birdi S, Rajput AH, Fenton M et al, Progressive supranuclear palsy diagnosis and confounding features: report on 16 autopsied cases. Mov Disord (2002) 6:1255–64.

Boeve BF, Silber MH, Parisi JE et al, Synucleinopathy pathology and REM sleep behaviour disorder plus dementia or parkinsonism. Neurology (2003) 61:40–5.

Brunberg JA, Jacquemont S, Hagerman RJ et al, Fragile X premutation carriers: characteristic MR imaging findings of adult male patients with progressive cerebellar and cognitive dysfunction. Am J Neuroradiol (2002) 23:1757–66.

Burn DJ, Lees AJ, Progressive supranuclear palsy: Where are we now? Lancet Neurol (2002) 1:359–69.

Burns JM, Galvin JE, Roe CM et al, The pathology of the substantia nigra in Alzheimer disease with extrapyramidal signs. Neurology (2005) 64:1397–1403.

Collie DA, Sellar RJ, Zeidler M et al, MRI of Creutzfeldt–Jakob disease: imaging features and recommended MRI protocol. Clin Radiol (2001)56:726–39.

Dickson D, Litvan I, Corticobasal degeneration. In: Dickson DW, ed, Neurodegeneration: The Molecular Pathology of Dementia and Movement Disorders (ISN Neuropath Press: Basel, 2003) 115–23.

Ellis RJ, Galigiuri M, Galasko D et al, Extrapyramidal motor signs in clinically diagnosed Alzheimer disease. Alzheimer Dis Assoc Disord (1996) 10:103–14.

Ghetti B, Hutton M, Wszolek ZK, Frontotemporal dementia and parkinsonism linked to chromosome 17 associated with tau gene mutations (FTDP-17T). In: Dickson DW, ed, Neurodegeneration: The Molecular Pathology of Dementia and Movement Disorders (ISN Neuropath Press: Basel, 2003) 86–102.

Gilman S, Low PA, Quinn N et al, Consensus statement on the diagnosis of multiple system atrophy. J Auton Nerv Syst (1998) 74: 189–92.

Graham NL, Bak TH, Hodges JR, Corticobasal degeneration as a cognitive disorder. Mov Disord (2003) 18:1224–32.

Grimes DA, Lang AE, Bergeron CB, Dementia as the most common presentation of cortico-basal ganglionic degeneration. Neurology (1999) 53:1969–74.

Haik S, Brandel JP, Sazdovitch V et al, Dementia with Lewy bodies in a neuropathologic series of suspected Creutzfeldt–Jakob disease. Neurology (2000) 55:1401–4.

Hauw J-J, Agid Y, Progressive supranuclear palsy (PSP) or Steele–Richardson–Olszewski disease. In: Dickson DW, ed, Neurodegeneration: The Molecular Pathology of Dementia and Movement Disorders (ISN Neuropath Press: Basel, 2003) 103–114.

Horimoto Y, Matsumoto M, Akatsu H et al, Autonomic dysfunction in dementia with Lewy bodies. J Neurol (2003) 250:530–533.

Houlden H, Baker M, Morris HR et al, Corticobasal degeneration and progressive supranuclear palsy share a common tau haplotype. Neurology (2001) 56:1702–6.

Josephs KA, Dickson DW, Diagnostic accuracy of progressive supranuclear palsy in the Society for Progressive Supranuclear Palsy brain bank. Mov Disord (2003) 18:1018–26.

Kato N, Arai K, Hattori T, Study of the rostral midbrain atrophy in progressive supranuclear palsy. J Neurol Sci 2003, 210, 57–60.

Kertesz A, Martinez-Lage P, Davidson W et al, The corticobasal degeneration syndrome overlaps progressive aphasia and frontotemporal dementia. Neurology (2000) 55:1368–75.

Konagaya M, Konagaya Y, Sakai M et al, Progressive cerebral atrophy in multiple system atrophy. J Neurol Sci (2002) 195:123–127.

Lang AE, Corticobasal degeneration: selected developments. Mov Disord (2003) Suppl 6:S51–6.

Leigh RJ, Riley DE Eye movements in parkinsonism: it's saccadic speed that counts. Neurology (2000) 54:1018–19.

Litvan I, Agid Y, Calne D et al, Clinical research criteria for the diagnosis of progressive supranuclear palsy (Steele–Richardson–Olszewski syndrome): Report of the NINDS-SPSP International Workshop. Neurology (1996) 47:1–9.

Liu Y, Stern Y, Chun MR et al, Pathological correlates of extrapyramidal signs in Alzheimer's disease. Ann Neurol (1997) 41:368–74.

Mahapatra RK, Edwards MJ, Schott JM et al, Corticobasal degeneration. Lancet Neurol (2004) 3: 736–43.

Marshall V, Grosset D, Role of dopamine transporter imaging in clinical practice. Mov Disord (2003) 18:1415–23.

Molsa PK, Marttila RJ, Rinne UK, Extrapyramidal signs in Alzheimer's disease. Neurology (1984) 34: 1114–6.

Morris HR, Osaki Y, Holton J et al, Tau exon 10+16 mutation FTDP-17 presenting clinically as sporadic young-onset PSP. Neurology (2003) 61:102–4.

Nitrini R, Teixeira da Silva LS, Rosemberg S et al, Prion disease resembling fronto-temporal dementia and parkinsonism linked to chromosome 17. Arq Neuropsiquiatr (2001) 59:161–4.

Ozawa T, Paviour D, Quinn NP et al, The spectrum of pathological involvement of the striatonigral and olivopontocerebellar systems in multiple system atrophy: clinicopathological correlations. Brain (2004) 12:2657–71.

Papp MI, Kahn JE, Lantos PL, Glial cytoplasmic inclusions in the CNS of patients with multiple system atrophy (striatonigral degeneration, olivopontocerebellar atrophy and Shy–Drager syndrome). J Neurol Sci (1989) 94:79–100.

Paviour DC, Price SL, Stevens JM et al, Quantitative MRI measurement of superior cerebellar peduncle in progressive supranuclear palsy. Neurology (2005) 64:675–9.

Rebeiz JJ, Kolodny EH, Richardson EP Jr, Corticodentatonigral degeneration with neuronal achromasia. Arch Neurol (1968) 18:20–33.

Rinne JO, Lee MS, Thompson PD et al, Corticobasal degeneration. A clinical study of 36 cases. Brain (1994) 117:1183–96.

Rivaud-Pechoux S, Vidailhet M, Gallouedec G et al, Longitudinal ocular motor study in corticobasal degeneration and progressive supranuclear palsy. Neurology (2000) 54:1029–32.

Savoiardo M, Differential diagnosis of Parkinson's disease and atypical parkinsonian disorders by magnetic resonance imaging. Neurol Sci (2003) 24 (Suppl 1): S35–7.

Scarmeas N, Hadjigeorgiou GM, Papadimitriou A et al, Motor signs during the course of Alzheimer disease. Neurology (2004) 63:975–982.

Schrag A, Ben-Shlomo Y, Quinn NP, Prevalence of progressive supranuclear palsy and multiple system atrophy: a cross-sectional study. Lancet (1999) 354:1771–75.

Schrag A, Good CD, Miszkiel K et al, Differentiation of atypical parkinsonian syndromes by routine MRI. Neurology (2000) 55:697–702.

Thaisetthawatkul P, Boeve BF, Benarroch EE et al, Autonomic dysfunction in dementia with Lewy bodies. Neurology (2004) 62:1804–9.

Thompson PD, Marsden CD, Gait disorder of subcortical arteriosclerotic encephalo-pathy: Binswanger's disease. Mov Disord (1987) 2:1–8.

Tschampa HJ, Neumann M, Zerr I et al, Patients with Alzheimer's disease and dementia with Lewy bodies mistaken for Creutzfeldt–Jakob disease. J Neurol Neurosurg Psychiatry (2001) 71:33–9.

Wadia N, Pang J, Desai J et al, A clinicogenetic analysis of six Indian spinocerebellar ataxia (SCA2). The significance of slow saccades in diagnosis. Brain (1998) 121:2341–55.

Wenning GK, Tison F, Ben Shlomo Y et al, Multiple system atrophy: a review of 203 pathologically proven cases. Mov Disord (1997) 12:133–47.

Wenning GK, Colosimo C, Geser F et al, Multiple system atrophy. Lancet Neurol (2004) 3: 93–103.

Williams DR, de Silva R, Paviour DC et al, Clinical, genetic and biochemical characteristics of two distinct clinical phenotypes in pathologically proven progressive supranuclear palsy: Richardson's syndrome and PSP–parkinsonism. Brain (2005) 128: 1247–58.

Zijlmans JC, Katzenschlager R, Daniel SE et al, The L-dopa response in vascular parkinsonism. J Neurol Neurosurg Psychiatry (2004) 75:545–7.

Index